# Lecture Notes
# Clinical Pharmacology & Therapeutics

## John L. Reid

DM FRCP FRSE
Regius Professor of Medicine and Therapeutics
University of Glasgow

## Peter C. Rubin

DM FRCP
Professor of Therapeutics
University of Nottingham

## Matthew R. Walters

MD FRCP
Senior Lecturer in Clinical Pharmacology
University of Glasgow

Seventh Edition

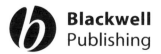

Blackwell
Publishing

© 2006 John Reid, Peter Rubin and Matthew Walters
Published by Blackwell Publishing Ltd
Blackwell Publishing, Inc., 350 Main Street, Malden, Massachusetts 02148-5020, USA
Blackwell Publishing Ltd, 9600 Garsington Road, Oxford OX4 2DQ, UK
Blackwell Publishing Asia Pty Ltd, 550 Swanston Street, Carlton, Victoria 3053, Australia

First published 1982
Second edition 1985
Third edition 1989
Fourth edition 1992
Fifth edition 1996
Sixth edition 2001
Seventh edition 2006

1 2006

Library of Congress Cataloging-in-Publication Data

Reid, John L.
    Lecture notes. Clinical pharmacology and therapeutics / John L. Reid,
Peter C. Rubin, Matthew R. Walters.—7th ed.
        p. ; cm.
    Rev. ed. of: Lecture notes on clinical pharmacology / John L. Reid,
Peter C. Rubin, Brian Whiting. 6th ed. 2001.
    Includes bibliographical references and index.
    ISBN-13: 978-1-4051-3519-1
    ISBN-10: 1-4051-3519-0
    1. Clinical pharmacology.
[DNLM: 1. Pharmacology, Clinical.   2. Drug Therapy. QV 38 R356La
2006] I. Rubin, Peter C.   II. Walters, Matthew R.   III. Reid, John L.
Lecture notes on clinical pharmacology.   IV. Title.

RM301.28.R45 2006
615'.1—dc22
                                        2006004770

ISBN-13: 978-1-4051-3519-1
ISBN-10: 1-4051-3519-0

A catalogue record for this title is available from the British Library

Set in 8/12 Stone Serif by TechBooks, India
Printed and bound in Singapore by C.O.S. Printers Pte Ltd

Commissioning Editor: Vicki Noyes
Development Editor: Fiona Pattison
Production Controller: Kate Charman

For further information on Blackwell Publishing, visit our website: http://www.blackwellpublishing.com

# Lecture Notes: Clinical Pharmacology & Therapeutics

# Contents

# Contributors

The following have contributed substantially to the writing, revision and rewriting of the chapters in the seventh edition of Lecture Notes in Clinical Pharmacology & Therapeutics.

**NICHOLAS BATEMAN** Scottish Poisons Information Bureau, Royal Infirmary of Edinburgh
*Chapter 20, Poisoning and drug overdose*

**SUSAN BRECHIN** Obstetrics and Gynaecology, University of Aberdeen
*Chapter 12, Drugs and the reproductive system*

**JENNIFER CLAYTON** Division of Therapeutics and Molecular Medicine, University of Nottingham
*Chapter 18, Drugs and endocrine disease*

**TOM EVANS** Division of Immunology, Infection and Inflammation, University of Glasgow
*Chapter 7, Antimicrobial therapy*

**IAN HALL** Division of Therapeutics and Molecular Medicine, University of Nottingham
*Chapter 8, Respiratory disease*

**ANDREW SEATON** Brownlee Centre, Gartnavel General Hospital, Glasgow
*Chapter 19, Travel medicine and tropical disease*

# Preface

Clinical pharmacology bridges the gap between laboratory science and the practice of medicine. Its primary aim is the promotion of safe and effective drug use: to optimize benefits and minimize risks. In the third millennium, there are increased responsibilities on the medical profession to base therapeutic decisions on clinical evidence and justify choices and actions, both to colleagues and patients.

Developments in medicine, pharmacology and physiology have led to a better understanding of disease processes and a more rational use of drugs. Many drugs are designed to interact with specific receptors or enzyme systems. In addition, the application of genetic, biochemical and immunological techniques has led to a clearer appreciation of the mechanisms involved in drug action.

For many years we have taught clinical pharmacology to medical practitioners and undergraduate students. We were persuaded by our students that there was a need for a brief, clearly written and up-to-date review of clinical pharmacology. Lecture Notes on Clinical Pharmacology & Therapeutics was prepared to meet this need in 1982 and now enters its seventh edition. The new edition has been extensively revised and updated: several chapters have been rewritten. We have not attempted to be comprehensive, but have tried to emphasize the principles of clinical pharmacology, areas which are developing rapidly and topics which are of particular clinical importance. The book was based on a course of lectures and seminars in clinical pharmacology and therapeutics for medical students at the University of Glasgow. In addition, we have drawn on our experience of organizing courses for postgraduate students, general practitioners and medical specialists. Thus, while intended primarily for medical students, we believe this book will also be of use to those preparing for higher examinations and doctors in established practice who wish to remain well-informed of current concepts and new developments in clinical pharmacology.

It is nearly 30 years since Lecture Notes in Clinical Pharmacology was first conceived and nearly 25 years since the first edition appeared. In the seventh edition Brian Whiting who has retired from medical practice has stepped down from his role as an author and editor of Lecture Notes. Brian has been replaced by Matthew Walters a Senior Lecturer in the University of Glasgow. In the preparation of the seventh edition we have rigorously reviewed—with the considerable help of a range of specialist colleagues—all the topics included, and made several changes to the structure and organisation of chapters reflecting some of the changes in clinical practice and prescribing since the last edition. We have however aimed to adhere to the original ethos of the book: to describe with brevity and clarity the scientific background of rational prescribing while giving an insight into practical aspects of therapeutics.

Recent developments in medical education have emphasized self-learning using a problem-based approach. There has been a tendency to reduce the influence of didactic teaching and the perception of the need to require and retain factual information. Whether learning is problem-based or more traditional, it must be underpinned by clear understanding of the principles of the pathophysiology of disease, the molecular mechanisms of drug action in humans, and an appreciation of drug therapy in the context of overall health care.

For those who use it, we hope this book will provide a clear understanding not only of how but also when to use drugs.

**John L. Reid**
**Peter C. Rubin**
**Matthew R. Walters**

# Acknowledgements

We acknowledge the help and assistance freely given by many colleagues, commenting, reviewing and updating chapters related to their specialist interest and expertise. We particularly acknowledge the input and contribution of Jonathan Cavanagh, Jonathan Hicks, Gordon Lowe, Yash Mahida, Brian McCreath, Gordon McInnes, Iain McInnes, John McMurray, James Overell, Naashika Quarcoo and Roger Sturrock.

We are grateful to Laura Brown and Louise Sabir for their role in collecting, collating and coordinating the text and revisions.

# Part 1

# Principles of clinical pharmacology

# Chapter 1

# Pharmacodynamics and pharmacokinetics

Prior to the twentieth century, medical practice depended largely on the administration of mixtures of natural plant or animal substances. These preparations contained a number of pharmacologically active agents in variable amounts. Their actions and indications were empirical and based on historical or traditional experience. Their use was rarely based on an understanding of the mechanism of disease or careful measurement of effect.

During the last 100 years an increased understanding has developed of biochemical and pathophysiological factors that influence disease. The chemical synthesis of agents with well-characterised, specific actions on cellular mechanisms has led to the introduction of many powerful and effective drugs. Additionally, advances in the detection of these compounds in body fluids have facilitated investigation into the relationships between the dosage regimen, the profile of drug concentration against time in body fluids, notably the plasma, and corresponding profiles of clinical effect. Knowledge of this concentration–effect relationship and the factors that influence drug concentrations are used to determine how much drug an individual patient will require, and how often it should be given.

More recently the elucidation of the human genome with the development of genomics and proteomics has provided new insights and opportunities for drug development, understanding adverse reactions and potentially individualising drug therapy.

## Principles of drug action (pharmacodynamics)

Pharmacological agents are used in therapeutics to:
1 Cure disease:
 • Chemotherapy in cancer or leukaemia
 • Antibiotics in specific bacterial infections
2 Alleviate symptoms:
 • Antacids in dyspepsia
 • Non-steroidal anti-inflammatory drugs in rheumatoid arthritis
3 Replace deficiencies:
 • Thyroxine in hypothyroidism
 • Insulin in diabetes mellitus
4 Prevent or delay end-stage consequences of degenerative diseases, ageing, etc.

A drug is a single chemical entity that may be one of the constituents of a medicine.

A medicine may contain one or more active constituents (drugs) together with additives to facilitate administration.

## Mechanism of drug action

### Action on a receptor

A receptor is a specific macromolecule, usually a protein, to which a specific group of drugs or naturally occurring substances (such as neuro-transmitters or hormones) can bind.

An agonist is a substance that stimulates or activates the receptor to produce an effect.

e.g. salbutamol at the $\beta_2$-receptor

An antagonist prevents the action of an agonist but does not have any effect itself.

e.g. losartan at the angiotensin II receptor

A partial agonist stimulates the receptor to a limited extent, while preventing any further stimulation by naturally occurring agonists.

e.g. pindolol at the $\beta_1$-receptor

The biochemical events that result from an agonist–receptor interaction and which produce an effect, are complex. There are many types of receptors and in several cases subtypes have been identified which are also of therapeutic importance (Table 1.1).

## Action on an enzyme

Enzymes, like receptors, are protein macro-molecules with which substrates interact to produce activation or inhibition. Drugs in common clinical use which exert their effect through enzyme action generally do so by inhibition.

**Table 1.1** Some receptors involved in the action of commonly used drugs.

| Receptor | Subtype | Main actions of natural agonist | Drug agonist | Drug antagonist |
|---|---|---|---|---|
| Adrenoceptor | $\alpha_1$ | Vasoconstriction | | Prazosin |
| | $\alpha_2$ | Hypotension, sedation | | Moxonidine |
| | $\beta_1$ | Heart rate | Dopamine | Atenolol |
| | | | Dobutamine | Metoprolol |
| | $\beta_2$ | Bronchodilation | Salbutamol | |
| | | Vasodilation | Terbutaline | |
| | | Uterine relaxation | Ritodrine | |
| Cholinergic | Muscarinic | Heart rate | | Atropine |
| | | Secretion | | Benzatropine (benztropine) |
| | | Gut motility | | Orphenadrine |
| | | Bronchoconstriction | | Ipratropium |
| | Nicotinic | Contraction of striated muscle | Suxamethonium | |
| | | | Tubocurarine | |
| Histamine | $H_1$ | Bronchoconstriction | | Chlorphenamine (chlorpheniramine) |
| | | Capillary dilation | | Terfenadine |
| | $H_2$ | ↑Gastric acid | | Cimetidine |
| | | | | Ranitidine |
| | | | | Famotidine |
| 5-Hydroxy-tryptamine | | | Fluoxetine | Ondansetron |
| | | | Fluvoxamine | Granisetron |
| | Dopamine | CNS neurotransmitter | Bromocriptine | Chlorpromazine |
| | | | | Haloperidol |
| | | | | Thioridazine |
| Opioid | | CNS neurotransmitter | Morphine, pethidine, etc. | Naloxone |

1 Digoxin inhibits the membrane bound $Na^+/K^+$ ATPase.

2 Aspirin inhibits platelet cyclo-oxygenase.

3 Enalapril inhibits angiotensin-converting enzyme.

4 Selegiline inhibits monoamine oxidase B.

5 Carbidopa inhibits dopa decarboxylase.

6 Allopurinol inhibits xanthine oxidase.

Drug receptor antagonists and enzyme inhibitors can act as competitive, reversible antagonists or as non-competitive, irreversible antagonists. The duration of the effect of drugs of the latter type is much longer than that of the former. Effects of competitive antagonists can be overcome by increasing the dose of endogenous or exogenous agonists, while effects of irreversible antagonists cannot usually be overcome.

*Atenolol* is a competitive β-adrenoceptor antagonist used in hypertension and angina. Its effects last for hours and can be overcome by administering an appropriate dose of a β-receptor agonist like isoprenaline.

*Vigabatrin* is an irreversible inhibitor of gamma aminobutyric acid (GABA) aminotransferase and is used in epilepsy. Its action and adverse effects may persist for days as a result of irreversible binding to the target enzyme.

## Action on membrane ionic channels

The conduction of impulses in nerve tissues and electromechanical coupling in muscle depend on the movement of ions, particularly sodium, calcium and potassium, through membrane channels. Several groups of drugs interfere with these processes:

1 Anti-arrhythmic drugs

2 Calcium slow channel antagonists

3 General and local anaesthetics

4 Anticonvulsants.

## Cytotoxic actions

Drugs used in cancer or in the treatment of infections may kill malignant cells or micro-organisms.

Often the mechanisms have been defined in terms of effects on specific receptors or enzymes. In other cases chemical action (alkylation) damages DNA or other macromolecules and results in cell death or failure of cell division.

## Dose–response relationship

In clinical practice dose–response relationships rarely follow the classical sigmoid pattern of experimental studies. It is uncommon for the upper plateau or maximum effect to be reached in humans or to be relevant therapeutically. Additionally, variability in the relationship between dose and concentration means that it is often difficult to detect a dose–response relationship. Consequently, concentration–response relationships are often more clinically relevant.

Dose– (or concentration–) response relationships may be steep or flat. A steep relationship implies that small changes in dose will produce large changes in clinical response or adverse effects, while flat relationships imply that increasing the dose will offer little clinical advantage (Fig. 1.1).

The potency of a drug is relatively unimportant; what matters is its efficacy or the maximum effect that can be obtained. In clinical practice the maximum therapeutic effect may often be unobtainable because of the appearance of adverse or unwanted effects: few, if any, drugs cause a single pharmacological response. The concentration–adverse response relationship is often different in shape and position to that of the concentration–therapeutic response relationship. The difference between the concentration that produces the desired effect and the concentration that causes adverse effects is called the therapeutic index and is a measure of the selectivity of a drug (Fig. 1.2).

The shape and position of dose–response curves for a group of patients is variable because of genetic, environmental and disease factors. However, this variability is not solely an expression of differences in response to drugs. It has two important

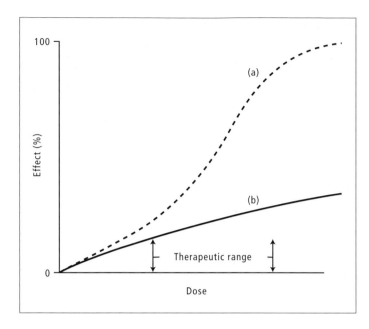

Figure 1.1 Schematic examples of a drug (a) with a steep dose– (or concentration–) response relationship in the therapeutic range, e.g. warfarin as an oral anticoagulant; and (b) a flat dose– (or concentration–) response relationship within the therapeutic range, e.g. thiazide diuretics in hypertension.

components: the dose–plasma concentration relationship and the plasma concentration–effect relationship.

$$Dose \rightarrow Concentration \rightarrow Effect$$

With the development of specific and sensitive chemical assays for drugs in body fluids, it has been possible to characterise dose–plasma concentration relationships so that this component of the variability in response can be taken into account when drugs are prescribed for patients with various disease states. For drugs with a narrow therapeutic index it may be necessary to measure plasma concentrations to assess the relationship between dose and concentration in individual patients.

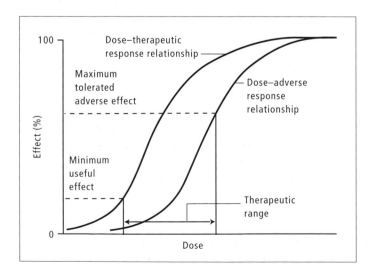

Figure 1.2 Schematic diagram of the dose–response relationship for the desired effect (dose–therapeutic response) and for an undesired adverse effect. The therapeutic index is the extent of displacement of the two curves within the normal dose range.

---

**Clinical pharmacology: What are kinetics and dynamics?**

The description of a drug concentration profile against time is known as pharmacokinetics and its application in clinical practice is clinical pharmacokinetics (Chapter 2). The residual variability in the relationship between dose and response is the concentration–effect component—a true expression of drug response, and a measure of the sensitivity of a patient to a drug. This is known as pharmacodynamics. Clinical pharmacology seeks to explore the factors that underlie variability in pharmacokinetics and pharmacodynamics and to use this information to optimise drug therapy for individual patients.

---

**Table 1.2** Several drugs that undergo extensive first-pass metabolism.

| Analgesics | Drugs acting on CNS |
|---|---|
| Aspirin | Clomethiazole (chlormethiazole) |
| Morphine | Chlorpromazine |
| Paracetamol | Imipramine |
| Pethidine | Levodopa |
| | Nortriptyline |
| *Cardiovascular drugs* | |
| Glyceryl trinitrate | *Respiratory drugs* |
| Isoprenaline | Salbutamol |
| Isosorbide dinitrate | Terbutaline |
| Labetalol | |
| Lidocaine (lignocaine) | *Oral contraceptives* |
| Metoprolol | |
| Nifedipine | |
| Prazosin | |
| Propranolol | |
| Verapamil | |

## Principles of pharmacokinetics

### Absorption

Drug absorption after oral administration has two major components: absorption rate and bioavailability. Absorption rate is controlled partially by the physicochemical characteristics of the drug but in many cases is modified by the formulation. A reduction in absorption rate can lead to a smoother concentration–time profile with a lower potential for concentration-dependent adverse effects and may allow less frequent dosing.

*Bioavailability* is the term used to describe the fraction of the dose that is absorbed into the systemic circulation and is usually designated $F$. It can range from 0 to 1 (0–100%) and depends on a number of physicochemical and clinical factors. Low bioavailability may occur if the drug has low solubility or is destroyed by the acid in the stomach. Changing the formulation can affect the bioavailability of a drug and it can also be altered by food or the co-administration of other drugs. For example, antacids can reduce the absorption of quinolone antibiotics by binding them in the gut. Other factors influencing bioavailability include metabolism by gut flora, the intestinal wall or the liver.

*First-pass metabolism* refers to metabolism of a drug that occurs en route from the gut lumen to the systemic circulation. For the majority of drugs given orally, absorption occurs across the portion of gastrointestinal epithelium that is drained by veins forming part of the hepatoportal system. Consequently, even if they are well absorbed, drugs must pass through the liver before reaching the systemic circulation. For drugs that are susceptible to extensive hepatic metabolism, a substantial proportion of an orally administered dose can be metabolised before it ever reaches its site of pharmacological action. Drugs with a high first-pass metabolism are listed in Table 1.2.

The importance of first-pass metabolism is twofold:

1 It is one of the reasons for apparent differences in drug absorption between individuals. Even healthy people show considerable variation in liver metabolising capacity.

2 In patients with severe liver disease first-pass metabolism may be dramatically reduced, leading to the appearance of greater amounts of parent drug in the systemic circulation.

### Distribution

Once a drug has gained access to the bloodstream it begins to distribute to the tissues. The extent of this distribution depends on a number of factors including plasma protein binding, the $pK_a$ of the drug, its partition coefficient in fatty tissue and regional blood flow. The volume of distribution $V_D$ is the *apparent volume* of fluid into which a drug distributes based on the *amount* of drug in the body and the *measured concentration* in the plasma or serum. If a drug was wholly confined to the plasma, $V_D$ would equal the plasma volume—approximately 3 l in an adult. If, on the other hand, the drug was distributed throughout the body water, $V_D$ would be approximately 42 l. In reality, drugs are rarely distributed into physiologically relevant volumes. If most of the drug is bound to tissues, the plasma concentration will be low and the apparent $V_D$ will be high, while high plasma protein binding will tend to maintain high concentrations in the blood and a low $V_D$ will result. For the majority of drugs, $V_D$ depends on the balance between plasma binding and sequestration or binding by various body tissues, for example, muscle and fat. Volume of distribution can vary therefore from relatively small values (e.g. an average of 0.14 l/kg body weight for aspirin) to large values (e.g. an average of 200 l/kg body weight for chloroquine) (Table 1.3).

**Table 1.3** Average volumes of distribution of some commonly used drugs.

| Drug | Volume of distribution (l/kg) |
| --- | --- |
| Chloroquine | 200 |
| Nortriptyline | 20 |
| Digoxin | 7 |
| Propranolol | 4 |
| Phenytoin | 0.65 |
| Theophylline | 0.50 |
| Gentamicin | 0.25 |
| Aspirin | 0.14 |
| Warfarin | 0.10 |

In general, a small $V_D$ occurs when:
**1** Lipid solubility is low.
**2** There is a high degree of plasma protein binding.
**3** There is a low level of tissue binding.
A high $V_D$ occurs when:
**1** Lipid solubility is high.
**2** There is a low degree of plasma protein binding.
**3** There is a high level of tissue binding.

## Plasma protein binding

In the blood, a proportion of a drug is bound to plasma proteins—mainly albumin (acidic drugs) and $\alpha_1$-acid glycoprotein (basic drugs). Only the unbound, or free, fraction distributes because the protein-bound complex is too large to pass through membranes. Movement of the drug between the blood and other tissues proceeds until equilibrium is established between the unbound drug in plasma and the drug in tissues. It is the unbound portion that is generally responsible for clinical effects—both the target response and the unwanted adverse effects. Changes in protein binding (e.g. resulting from displacement interactions) generally lead to a transient increase in free concentration and are rarely clinically relevant because the equilibrium becomes re-established with the same unbound concentration. However, a lower total concentration will be present and the measurement might be misinterpreted if the higher free fraction is not taken into account. This is a common problem with the interpretation of phenytoin concentrations, where free fraction can range from 10% in a normal patient to 40% in a patient with hypoalbuminaemia and renal impairment.

## Clinical relevance of volume of distribution

Knowledge of volume of distribution ($V_D$) can be used to determine the size of a *loading dose* if an immediate response to treatment is required. This assumes that therapeutic success is closely related to the plasma concentration and that there are no adverse effects if a relatively large dose is suddenly administered. It is sometimes employed when drug response would take many hours or days to develop if the regular maintenance dose was given from the outset, e.g. digoxin.

A loading dose can be calculated as follows:

$$\text{Loading dose} = V \times \text{Desired concentration}$$
(Eqn. 1.1)

In practice, because most values for $V_D$ are related to weight, this calculation is often simplified to a mg/kg dose.

## Clearance

Clearance is the sum of all drug-eliminating processes, principally determined by hepatic metabolism and renal excretion. It can be defined as the theoretical volume of fluid from which a drug is completely removed in a given period of time.

When a drug is administered continuously by intravenous infusion or repetitively by mouth, a balance is eventually achieved between its input (dosing rate) and its output (the amount eliminated over a given period of time). This balance gives rise to a constant amount of drug in the body which depends on the dosing rate and clearance. This amount is reflected in the plasma or serum as a steady-state concentration (Css). A constant rate intravenous infusion will clearly yield a constant Css, while a drug administered orally at regular intervals will result in fluctuation between peak and trough concentrations (Fig. 1.3).

The average Css in any dosage interval may be *approximated* by the concentration one-third of the way between the trough and the peak.

The relationship between the average Css, drug input and drug output for a constant rate infusion can be written as

$$Css_{average} = \frac{Input\ rate}{Output\ rate} = \frac{Infusion\ rate}{Clearance}$$

(Eqn. 1.2)

or for oral therapy,

$$Css_{average} = \frac{F \times Dose}{Clearance \times Dosage\ interval}$$

(Eqn. 1.3)

Equations 1.2 and 1.3 highlight the important fact that if an estimate of clearance is available, it can be used to determine the *maintenance dose* for any desired Css, thus

$$Infusion\ rate = Clearance \times Desired\ Css_{average}$$

(Eqn. 1.4a)

or for oral therapy,

$$maintenance\ dose = Clearance$$
$$\times Desired\ Css_{average}$$
$$\times Dosage\ interval/F$$

(Eqn. 1.4b)

Clearance depends critically on the efficiency with which the liver and/or kidneys can eliminate a drug; it will vary in disease states that affect these organs *per se*, or that affect the blood flow to these organs. In stable clinical conditions, clearance remains constant and Eqns. 1.2 and 1.3 show that the $Css_{average}$ is directly proportional to dose rate. The important implication is that if the dose rate is doubled, the $Css_{average}$ doubles: if the dose rate is halved, the $Css_{average}$ is halved. This is illustrated in Fig. 1.4. If each $Css_{average}$ is plotted against its corresponding dose rate, the direct proportionality becomes obvious (Fig. 1.5). In pharmacokinetic terms this is referred to as a first-order or linear process, and results from the fact that the rate of elimination is proportional to the amount of drug present in the body.

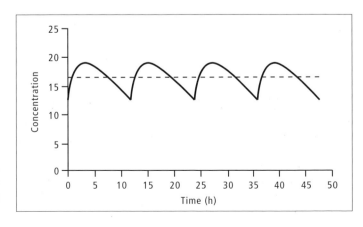

**Figure 1.3** Steady-state concentration–time profile for an oral dose (——) and a constant rate intravenous infusion (- - - - -).

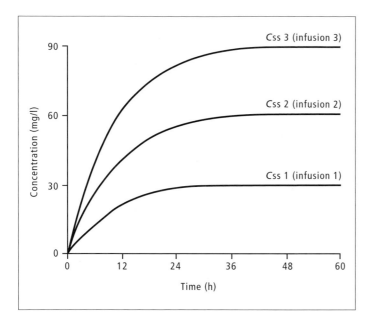

**Figure 1.4** Plots of concentration vs. time for three infusions allowed to reach steady state. Infusion 2 is at a rate twice that of infusion 1; infusion 3 is at a rate three times that of infusion 1. The three steady-state concentrations ($C$ss 1, 2 and 3) are directly proportional to the corresponding infusion rates.

## Single intravenous bolus dose

A number of other important pharmacokinetic principles can be appreciated by considering the concentrations that result following a single intravenous bolus dose (see Fig. 1.6a). If we assume that the drug distributes instantaneously into its volume of distribution $V_D$, then its initial concentration $C_0$ depends only on the dose ($D$) and $V_D$; thus

$$C_0 = \frac{D}{V_D} \qquad \text{(Eqn. 1.5)}$$

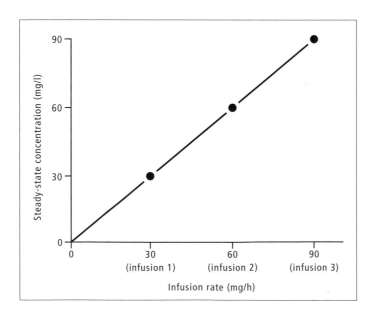

**Figure 1.5** Three steady-state concentrations plotted against corresponding infusion rates showing the linear relationship between dose and $C$ss$_{\text{average}}$.

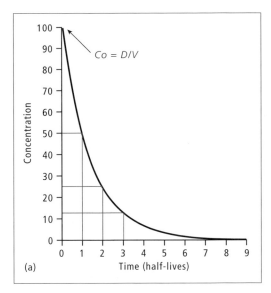

(a)

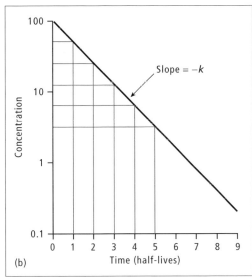

(b)

**Figure 1.6** (a) Plot of concentration vs. time after a bolus intravenous injection. The intercept on the y-(concentration) axis, $C_0$, is the concentration resulting from the instantaneous injection of the bolus dose. (b) Semi-logarithmic plot of concentration vs. time after a bolus intravenous injection. The slope of this line is $-k$; the elimination rate constant (Eqns. 1.6 and 1.7) and the elimination half-life of the drug can be easily determined from such a plot by noting the time at which the concentration has fallen to half its original value.

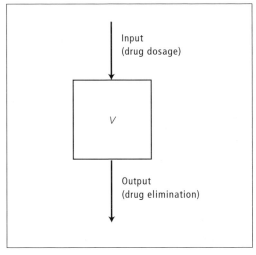

**Figure 1.7** The body depicted as a single compartment of volume $V$.

This is based on the concept that the body can be depicted as a single homogeneous compartment of volume $V$, as shown in Fig. 1.7. The concentration will then decline by a constant proportion per unit time, giving rise to an exponential decline. The concentration at any time $t$ after the dose can therefore be determined from the exponential expression

$$C(t) = \frac{D}{V}e^{-kt} \qquad \text{(Eqn. 1.6)}$$

where $k$ is the elimination rate constant of the drug, $t$ is any time after drug administration and $e^{-kt}$ is the fraction of drug remaining at time $t$. If the concentrations are plotted on a logarithmic scale, a linear decline will be obtained with slope-$k$ and intercept $\ln D/V$; thus

$$\ln C(t) = \ln\frac{D}{V} - kt \qquad \text{(Eqn. 1.7)}$$

Semi-logarithmic graph paper allows $C_0(D/V)$ to be determined directly (Fig. 1.6b). $k$ represents the constant fraction of the volume of distribution from which a drug is eliminated in a given period of time and therefore depends on both clearance and volume of distribution; thus

$$k = \frac{\text{Clearance}}{\text{Volume of distribution}} \qquad \text{(Eqn. 1.8)}$$

$k$ can also be expressed in terms of the half-life of a

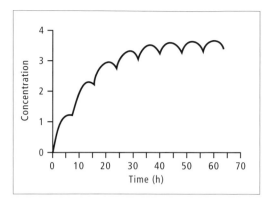

**Figure 1.8** Plot of concentration vs. time illustrating the accumulation to steady state when a drug is administered by regular oral doses.

drug. The half-life $t_{1/2}$ is the time required for the plasma concentration to fall to half of its original value and can be derived either graphically (Fig. 1.6) or from the expression

$$t_{1/2} = \frac{\ln 2}{k} \qquad \text{(Eqn. 1.9)}$$

where ln 2 is the natural logarithm of 2, or 0.693. It can be used to predict the time at which steady state will be achieved after starting a regular treatment schedule or after any change in dose. As a rule, in the absence of a loading dose, steady state is attained after four to five half-lives (Fig. 1.8). Furthermore, when toxic drug levels have been inadvertently produced, it is very useful to estimate how long it will take for such levels to reach the therapeutic range, or how long it will take for all the drug to be eliminated once the drug has been stopped. Usually, elimination is effectively complete after four to five half-lives (Fig. 1.6).

The elimination half-life can also be used to determine dosage intervals to achieve a target concentration–time profile. For example, in order to obtain a gentamicin peak of 8 mg/l and a trough of 0.5 mg/l in a patient with an elimination half-life of 3 h, the dosage interval should be 12 h. (The concentration will fall from 8 mg/l to 4 mg/l in 3 h, to 2 mg/l in 6 h, to 1 mg/l in 9 h and to 0.5 mg/l in 12 h.) However, for many drugs, dosage regimens should be designed to maintain concentrations within a range that avoids high (potentially toxic) peaks or low, ineffective troughs. Excessive fluctuations in the concentration–time profile can be prevented by giving the drug at intervals of less than one half-life or by using a slow-release formulation.

## Linear vs. non-linear kinetics

In the discussion on clearance, it was pointed out that the hallmark of linear pharmacokinetics is the proportionality between dose rate and steady-state concentration. This arises because the rate of elimination is proportional to the amount of drug in the body, while the clearance remains constant. This is not, however, always the case as is exemplified by the anticonvulsant drug phenytoin. When the enzymes responsible for metabolism reach a point of saturation, the rate of elimination, in terms of amount of drug eliminated in a given period of time, does not increase in response to an increase in concentration (or an increase in the amount of drug in the body) but becomes constant. This gives rise to non-linear or zero-order kinetics.

The general relationship between drug concentration ($C$) and rate of metabolism is shown in Fig. 1.9. The maximum rate at which the enzymes can function, $V_{max}$, corresponds to the plateau attained by the curve.

The equation relating the rate of metabolism to $C$ is the Michaelis–Menten equation

$$\text{Rate of metabolism} = \frac{V_{max} \times C}{K_m \times C} \qquad \text{(Eqn. 1.10)}$$

and the fundamental difference between linear and non-linear kinetics can be appreciated by considering two extreme cases.

1 The serum concentration is considerably less than $K_m$. In this case, the Michaelis–Menten equation can be approximated to

$$\text{Rate of metabolism} = \frac{V_{max} \times C}{K_m} \qquad \text{(Eqn. 1.11)}$$

where $V_{max}/K_m$ is a constant. This means that the rate of change of concentration is then proportional to the concentration (linear kinetics).

2 The serum concentration is considerably greater than $K_m$.

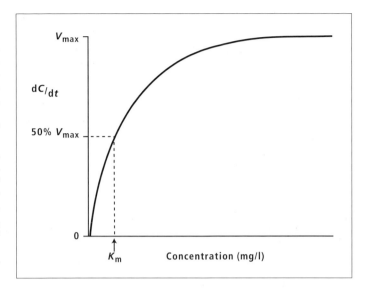

**Figure 1.9** Diagrammatic representation of the general relationship between drug concentration $C$ and the rate of metabolism. $V_{max}$ is the maximum velocity at which the drug-metabolising enzyme can function and is a constant (with units of mass/time). $K_m$ is the concentration at which $V_{max}$ is 50%. The $K_m$ is usually much higher than therapeutic concentrations and the rate of metabolism vs. $C$ is essentially linear (Eqn. 1.11). With a few drugs, notably phenytoin, therapeutic plasma concentrations are in the region of $K_m$ so that rate of metabolism vs. $C$ is non-linear and governed by the relationship shown in Eqn. 1.10.

In this case, the Michaelis–Menten equation can be approximated to

$$\text{Rate of metabolism} = V_{max} \qquad \text{(Eqn. 1.12)}$$

which indicates that the rate of elimination is a constant.

At steady state, dose rate can be substituted for rate of metabolism, i.e.

$$\text{Steady-state dose rate} = \frac{V_{max} \times C_{ss}}{K_m + C_{ss}}$$
$$\text{(Eqn. 1.13)}$$

For phenytoin, $V_{max}$ has a typical value of 7.2 mg/kg per day and $K_m$ has a typical value of 4.4 mg/l (17.6 μmol/l). In the case of phenytoin, the range of concentrations used clinically encompasses and exceeds $K_m$. Consequently, the relationship between the steady-state concentration and dose rate will alter as the concentration changes. At low concentrations, the increase in concentration will be proportional to the dose rate (linear pharmacokinetics). At higher concentrations, the increase will be much greater than would have been anticipated (non-linear pharmacokinetics). Steady state will not be achieved if the dose rate exceeds $V_{max}$. This can be seen in Fig. 1.10.

*Comment.* The clinical relevance of non-linear kinetics is that a small increase in dose can lead to a large increase in concentration. This is particularly important when toxic side effects are closely related to concentration, as with phenytoin.

## Principles of drug elimination

### Drug metabolism

Drugs are eliminated from the body by two principal mechanisms: (i) liver metabolism and (ii) renal excretion. Drugs that are already water-soluble are generally excreted unchanged by the kidney. Lipid-soluble drugs are not easily excreted by the kidney because, following glomerular filtration, they are largely reabsorbed from the proximal tubule. The first step in the elimination of such lipid-soluble drugs is metabolism to more polar (water-soluble) compounds. This is achieved mainly in the liver, but can also occur in the gut and may contribute to first-pass elimination. Metabolism generally occurs in two phases:

*Phase 1* Mainly oxidation (sometimes reduction or hydrolysis) to a more polar compound.

*Phase 2* Conjugation, usually with glucuronic acid or sulphate, to make the compound substantially more polar.

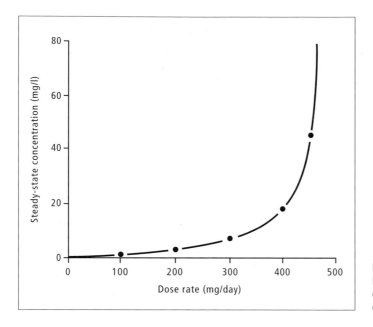

**Figure 1.10** The $C_{ss}$ vs. dose rate relationship for phenytoin. This is governed by Michaelis–Menten kinetics (Eqn. 1.13).

## Phase 1 metabolism

Oxidation can occur in various ways, including aromatic or aliphatic hydroxylation, oxygenation at carbon, nitrogen or sulphur atoms and N- and O-dealkylation. These reactions are catalysed by the cytochrome P-450-dependent system of the endoplasmic reticulum. Knowledge of P-450, which exists as a superfamily of similar enzymes (isoforms), has increased greatly recently. The P-450 superfamily is divided into a number of families and subfamilies, where genes encoding for proteins within a family have at least 40% nucleotide sequence homology and subfamilies have over 65% homology. Although numerous P-450 isoforms are present in human tissue, only a few of these have a major role in the metabolism of drugs. These enzymes, which display a distinct but overlapping substrate specificity, are listed in Table 1.4.

Phase 1 metabolites usually have only minor structural differences from the parent drug, but may exhibit totally different pharmacological actions. For example, the metabolism of azathioprine produces the powerful antimetabolite 6-mercaptopurine.

## Phase 2 reactions

These involve the addition of small endogenous molecules to the parent drug, or to its phase 1 metabolite, and almost always lead to abolition of pharmacological activity. Multiple forms of conjugating enzymes are also known to exist, although these have not been investigated to the same extent as the P-450 system.

## Metabolic drug interactions

The wide range of drugs metabolised by the P-450 system provides the opportunity for interactions of two types, namely enzyme induction and inhibition.

### Induction

Enzyme induction, which may be defined as the increase in amount and activity of drug-metabolising enzymes, is a consequence of new protein synthesis resulting from prolonged exposure to the inducing drug. While a drug may induce its own metabolism, it can also accelerate the metabolism and clearance of unrelated compounds. Many

**Table 1.4** Major human P-450 enzymes involved in drug metabolism.

| Major human P-450s | Typical substrates |
|---|---|
| CYP1A2 | Theophylline, caffeine, tacrine, fluvoxamine, oestradiol, phenacetin ($R$)-warfarin |
| CYP2C9 | ($S$)-Warfarin, tolbutamide, glipizide, losartan, ibuprofen, diclofenac, phenytoin |
| CYP2C19 | ($S$)-Mephenytoin, omeprazole, diazepam, citalopram, proguanil, moclobemide |
| CYP2D6 | ($S$)-Metoprolol, bufuralol, dextromethorphan, fluoxetine, desipramine, nortryptiline |
| CYP2E1 | Enflurane, halothane, chlorzoxazone, ethanol |
| CYP3A4 | Astemizole, terfenadine, cisapride, pimozide, nisoldipine, midazolam, indinavir, lovastatin, St. John's wort |

compounds are known to act as enzyme inducers in animals at toxicological dose levels, but relatively few drugs produce clinically significant induction in humans when used at therapeutic dose levels.

The compounds shown in Table 1.5 are the most potent enzyme inducers in clinical use and have produced numerous clinically significant drug interactions, related primarily to increases in the metabolism of CYP2C9, CYP2C19 and CYP3A4 substrates. For example, the anticonvulsants phenytoin and carbamazepine, as well as the herbal remedy St. John's wort, induce the enzymes that metabolise the constituents of oral contraceptives. If a woman receiving an oral contraceptive starts taking one of these drugs, the metabolism of the oestrogen and progestogen in the oral contraceptive increases, with the risk of contraceptive failure. Enzyme induction is not, however, limited to drug administration. Cigarette smoking, for example, results in enzyme induction with increased metabolism of CYP1A2 substrates, such as theophylline, and ethanol is an inducer of CYP2E1.

**Table 1.5** Some of the most potent enzyme inducers in humans.

| |
|---|
| Carbamazepine |
| Phenytoin |
| Rifampicin |

### Inhibition

Concurrently administered drugs can also lead to inhibition of enzyme activity, with many P-450 inhibitors showing considerable isoform selectivity. Some of the most clinically relevant inhibitors are listed in Table 1.6, together with the isoform inhibited. For example, ketoconazole decreases the metabolism of the CYP3A4 substrate, terfenadine, leading to potentially dangerous adverse effects, e.g. QT interval prolongation and torsades de pointes.

**Table 1.6** P-450 inhibitors involved in drug interactions.

| Major human P-450s | Typical inhibitors |
|---|---|
| CYP1A2 | Furafylline, fluvoxamine, ciprofloxacin |
| CYP2C9 | Fluconazole, ketoconazole, sulfaphenazole |
| CYP2C19 | Omeprazole, ketoconazole, cimetidine |
| CYP2D6 | Quinidine, fluoxetine, ritonavir |
| CYP2E1 | Disulfiram |
| CYP3A4 | Ketoconazole, itraconazole, ritonavir, erythromycin, diltiazem |

**Table 1.7** Major enzymes displaying genetic polymorphism.

| Enzyme | Typical substrates | Characteristics |
|---|---|---|
| CYP2C19 | (S)-Mephenytoin, diazepam, omeprazole | About 2–5% of white people are poor metabolisers, but 18–23% of Japanese people have this phenotype |
| CYP2D6 | Propafenone, flecainamide, desipramine | About 7% of white people are poor metabolisers, but this frequency is only about 2% in black Americans and <1% in Japanese/Chinese |
| N-Acetyl- transferase | Hydralazine, sulphonamides, isoniazid, procainamide | About 50% of white people are slow acetylators |

As with induction, P-450 inhibition is not limited to drug administration. Grapefruit juice is a fairly potent inhibitor of CYP3A4 activity and produces clinically significant interactions with a number of drugs, including midazolam, simvastatin and terfenadine. This type of information, together with some knowledge of the enzymes involved in a particular drug's clearance, makes it much easier to understand and predict drug interactions.

*Comment.* Enzyme induction produces clinical changes over days or weeks, but the effects of enzyme inhibition are usually observed immediately. In most circumstances, these changes are manifest as decreases in efficacy resulting from induction, or as increases in adverse effects resulting from inhibition. Clinical relevance occurs when drug therapy needs to be altered to avoid the consequences of the drug interaction and this is most common and most serious in compounds that have a narrow therapeutic index. Clearly, pronounced enzyme inhibition, which may result in plasma concentrations of the inhibited drug being many times higher than intended, can be a major safety issue. For example, co-administration of ketoconazole or ritonavir with the hypnotic drug midazolam increases the midazolam plasma AUC by 15–20 times, a situation which should be avoided.

## Genetic factors in metabolism

The rate at which healthy people metabolise drugs is variable. Although part of this variability is a consequence of environmental factors, including the influence of inducers and inhibitors, the main factor contributing to interindividual variability in metabolism is the underlying genetic basis of the drug-metabolising enzymes. Although there is probably a genetic component in the control of most P-450 enzymes, some enzymes (e.g. CYP2C19 and CYP2D6) actually show genetic polymorphism. This results in distinct subpopulations of poor and extensive metabolisers, where the poor metabolisers are deficient in that particular enzyme. There are a number of enzymes under polymorphic control and some clinically important examples are shown in Table 1.7. As with enzyme inhibition, genetic polymorphism is primarily a concern for drugs that have a narrow therapeutic index and that are metabolised largely by a single polymorphic enzyme. In such cases, the phenotype of the patient should be determined and lower doses of the drug used, or alternative therapy should be considered.

## Renal excretion

Three processes are implicated in renal excretion of drugs:

1 *Glomerular filtration*. This is the most common route of renal elimination. The free drug is cleared by filtration and the protein-bound drug remains in the circulation where some of it dissociates to restore equilibrium.

2 *Active secretion in the proximal tubule*. Both weak acids and weak bases have specific secretory sites in proximal tubular cells. Penicillins are

eliminated by this route, as is about 60% of procainamide.

**3** *Passive reabsorption in the distal tubule.* This occurs only with un-ionised, i.e. lipid-soluble, drugs. Urine pH determines whether or not weak acids and bases are reabsorbed, which in turn determines the degree of ionisation.

If renal function is impaired, for example by disease or old age, then the clearance of drugs that normally undergo renal excretion is decreased.

# Chapter 2

# Clinical pharmacokinetics: dosage individualisation

## Dosage individualisation

If a dose of a drug is prescribed for a number of patients, the blood concentrations achieved can be quite variable. There are several reasons for this.

---

**Reasons for variability in drug concentration**

1 Individual differences in absorption, first-pass metabolism, volume of distribution and clearance
2 Altered pharmacokinetics because of gastrointestinal, hepaatic, renal or cardiac disease
3 Drug interactions
4 Poor compliance with drug therapy

---

For most drugs there is an accepted 'target' range, i.e. a range of concentrations below which the drug is usually ineffective and above which it is usually toxic. In order to maintain drug concentrations within this range, knowledge about factors that influence the relationships between drug dose and blood concentration is used to design dosage regimens. Dosage adjustments based on age, renal function, hepatic function or other drug therapies are often recommended, especially for drugs with a narrow therapeutic index. For example, the initial dose of gentamicin, a renally cleared antibiotic, is based on the patient's renal function. As a consequence of an interaction that increases digoxin concentrations, the dose of digoxin is usually halved when amiodarone is added to a patient's therapy.

## Therapeutic drug monitoring

In many cases it is relatively easy to evaluate the pharmacological effects of a drug by clinical observation, and initial dosage regimens can be modified to increase the therapeutic effect or to eliminate unwanted effects. Measurement of drug concentrations in blood can be performed to help with diagnosis or to optimise therapy for those drugs where response (therapeutic or toxic effects) cannot be readily evaluated from clinical observation alone. Examples of drugs where monitoring can usefully aid clinical judgement, together with target ranges, are shown in Table 2.1.

Because of pharmacokinetic and pharmacodynamic variability, the following factors should be considered when interpreting drug concentration measurements:

1 Is the patient responding to therapy or showing symptoms of toxicity?
2 Was the sample taken at steady state?
3 Was the sampling time appropriate for the drug?
4 Where is the concentration relative to the 'target' range (Table 2.2)?
5 If the patient is not responding or has toxicity, how should the dose be modified? Unexpectedly low concentrations may indicate poor compliance or an absorption problem (e.g. vomiting).

**Table 2.1** Examples of target ranges.

| Drug | Target range Mass units | Molar units |
|---|---|---|
| Digoxin | 0.8–2 µg/l | 1–2.6 nmol/l |
| Carbamazepine | 4–12 mg/l | 20–50 µmol/l |
| Phenobarbital | 10–30 mg/l | 50–150 µmol/l |
| Phenytoin | 10–20 mg/l | 40–80 µmol/l |
| Amikacin[1] | 15–25 mg/l (1 h post-dose) <5 mg/l (trough) | |
| Gentamicin, netilmicin, tobramycin[1] | 5–12 mg/l (1 h post-dose) <2 mg/l (trough) | |
| Vancomycin | 5–10 mg/l (trough) | |
| Lithium | | 0.4–1.0 mmol/l |
| Theophylline | 5–20 mg/l | 28–110 µmol/l |

1 In some hospitals, high aminoglycoside doses (e.g. gentamicin doses of 5–7 mg/kg) are given at intervals of 24–48 h and the normal target peak and trough ranges do not apply. Samples are usually taken 6–14 h after the dose and the dose is adjusted (if necessary) according to a nomogram.

**Table 2.2** Factors influencing theophylline clearance and therefore dose requirements.

| Factor | Adjustments required |
|---|---|
| Smoking | ×1.6 |
| Congestive cardiac failure | ×0.4 |
| Hepatic cirrhosis | ×0.5 |
| Acute pulmonary oedema | ×0.5 |
| Severe chronic obstructive airways disease | ×0.8 |

## Clearance estimates

The clinical significance of clearance is that it determines an individual patient's maintenance dose requirements. It is important to note that clearance varies between individuals and within an individual in response to changes in his or her clinical condition.

The physiological and pathological factors that affect the clearance of a drug depend mainly on which organ is primarily responsible for its elimination. For example, clearance of the bronchodilator theophylline, a drug that is eliminated by hepatic metabolism, is influenced by age, weight, alcohol consumption, cigarette smoking, other drugs, congestive cardiac failure, hepatic cirrhosis, acute pulmonary oedema and severe chronic obstructive airways disease.

Clearance in any individual is most accurately determined from concentration measurements. However, in many cases, relationships between clearance and clinical factors have previously been established. For example, the average value for theophylline clearance is 0.04 l/h per kg and this is modified according to the patient's clinical characteristics by multiplying by the factors shown in Table 2.3. This means that on average, smokers require 1.6 times the theophylline dose of non-smokers and patients with cirrhosis require half the dose of patients without cirrhosis. For drugs primarily excreted by the kidney, e.g. digoxin and

**Table 2.3** Predicted steady-state digoxin concentrations for Mr AR.

| Dose (µg) | Css$_{average}$ (µg/l) | Css$_{trough}$ (mg/l) |
|---|---|---|
| 250 | 3.0 | 2.4 |
| 187.5 | 2.2 | 1.8 |
| 125 | 1.5 | 1.2 |
| 62.5 | 0.75 | 0.6 |

gentamicin, creatinine clearance closely reflects drug clearance. Thus, digoxin clearance can be estimated from the equation:

$$\text{Digoxin clearance} = \text{Creatinine clearance} + 0.33$$
$$\text{(ml/min/kg)} \qquad \text{(ml/min/kg)}$$

$$\text{(Eqn. 2.1)}$$

The 0.33 in this equation represents the elimination by routes other than the kidney, such as metabolism and clearance by the hepatobiliary system.

An estimate of clearance can then be used to calculate the required dose to achieve a target concentration, as shown in Chapter 1, i.e.

$$\text{Maintenance dose rate} = \text{Clearance}$$
$$\times \text{Target } Css_{average}$$

$$\text{(Eqn. 2.2)}$$

$$\text{Maintenance dose} = \text{Clearance}$$
$$\times \text{Target } Css_{average}$$
$$\times \text{Dosage interval}/F$$

$$\text{(Eqn. 2.3)}$$

where $F$ represents oral bioavailability. Factors that influence clearance are now routinely investigated for all new drugs so that dosage adjustments can be made for patients with a low clearance, who might be at risk from toxicity.

## Interpretation of serum concentrations

Serum concentrations can be measured for a number of reasons and it is important to interpret the measured concentration in the light of the clinical situation. If the aim is to assess the patient's maintenance dose requirements, samples should ideally be taken at steady state. However, confirmation of steady state is not necessary if the aim is to confirm toxicity and compliance or to assess the need for a loading dose in a patient who is acutely unwell.

Steady state normally requires that 4–5 half-lives elapse since treatment started or since any change in dose. Doses should be given at regular intervals

and it is important to confirm that no doses have been omitted. If these conditions can be satisfied and the pharmacokinetics of the drug are linear, clearance depends on the ratio of the dosing rate to the average steady-state concentration as can be seen by rearranging Eqn. 2.2:

$$\text{Clearance} = \frac{\text{Maintenance dose rate}}{Css_{average}}$$

$$\text{(Eqn. 2.4)}$$

This means that doses can be adjusted by simple proportion (see Chapter 1), i.e.

$$\text{Maintenance dose}$$
$$= \frac{\text{Desired } Css_{average}}{\text{Measured } Css_{average} \times \text{Current dose}}$$

$$\text{(Eqn. 2.5)}$$

Concentrations that are not at steady state cannot be used in this way; although if accurate details of dosage history and sampling time are available, clearance may be estimated with the help of a pharmacokinetic computer package.

It is important to remember that drugs with non-linear kinetics (such as phenytoin) require special consideration, and different techniques are applied to the interpretation of their concentrations.

Successful interpretation of a concentration measurement depends on accurate information. The minimum usually required is:

1 Time of sample collection with respect to the previous dose. Samples taken at inappropriate times may be misinterpreted. Usually, the simplest approach is to measure a trough concentration (i.e. at the end of the dosage interval). However, for some drugs (e.g. the aminoglycoside antibiotics), peaks may also be measured.

2 An accurate and detailed dosage history—drug dose, times of administration and route(s) of administration. This information can be used to assess whether the sample represents steady state. Samples taken without knowledge of dosage history can result in an inappropriate clinical action or dosage adjustment.

3 Patient details such as age, sex, weight, serum creatinine (or creatinine clearance) and assessments of cardiac and hepatic function. This information helps to determine expected dose requirements and is necessary for all computerised

interpretation methods. Knowledge about the stability of the patient can help to determine the frequency of monitoring, especially if the drug is renally cleared and renal function is changing.

4 Changes in other drug therapy that might influence the pharmacokinetics of the drug being measured.

5 The reason for requesting a drug analysis should be considered carefully. 'On admission' or 'routine' requests are usually of little value and are a waste of valuable resources.

**Table 2.4** Predicted steady-state phenytoin concentrations for Mrs DL.

| Dose (mg/day) | Steady-state concentration | |
| --- | --- | --- |
| | (mg/l) | ($\mu$mol/l) |
| 225 | 6 | 24 |
| 250 | 7 | 28 |
| 275 | 9 | 36 |
| 300 | 13 | 52 |
| 325 | 18 | 72 |
| 350 | 28 | 112 |
| 375 | 55 | 220 |

## Examples of therapeutic drug monitoring

### Digoxin

Mr AR, a 78-year-old man weighing 72 kg and with a creatinine clearance of 24 ml/min, has been taking 250 $\mu$g digoxin daily to control atrial fibrillation. He presents to his general practitioner with anorexia and nausea a month after starting therapy. A digoxin concentration of 3.6 $\mu$g/l (4.6 nmol/l) is measured.

#### (i) Is this concentration expected?

His expected digoxin clearance can be calculated from Eqn. 2.1, i.e.

$$\text{Digoxin clearance} = \frac{24}{72} + 0.33 (\text{ml/min/kg})$$
$$= 0.663 \text{ ml/min/kg}$$
$$= 2.9 \text{ l/h}$$

His average steady-state concentration can be estimated from Eqn. 1.3, i.e.

$$\text{Predicted } Css_{\text{average}} = \frac{0.6 \times 250\,\mu g}{2.9 \times 24\,h}$$
$$= 2.2\,\mu g/l\ (2.8\,nmol/l)$$

where 0.6 represents the bioavailability of digoxin tablets.

The reason for which the measured concentration is higher than expected should be investigated. In this case, it was found that the sample had been withdrawn 2.5 h after the dose. Digoxin is absorbed quickly but distributes slowly to the tissues. Samples taken before distribution is complete (i.e. less than 6 h after the dose) cannot be interpreted. As concentrations fall only by about 20% from 6 to 24 h after the dose, samples can be taken at any time during this period.

A further (trough) sample withdrawn 24 h after the last dose measured 2.4 $\mu$g/l (3.1 nmol/l). This result is more consistent with the expected concentration but suggests that the dose is too high and may be contributing to his symptoms.

#### (ii) What dose adjustment should be made?

Because digoxin has linear pharmacokinetics, the new dose can be determined by simple proportion. Table 2.3 shows that there are three dosage options for Mr AR. A reduction to 125 $\mu$g daily is the most obvious first choice, but further adjustment (up or down) could be made if necessary on clinical grounds (e.g. poor control of atrial fibrillation or persistence of adverse effects).

*Comment.* This case illustrates the importance of sampling time for the correct interpretation of digoxin concentrations. Although digoxin is traditionally prescribed to be taken in the morning, changing to a night-time dose can reduce the chances of samples being withdrawn during the distribution phase. Digoxin has a long elimination half-life (50–100 h) and elimination is slow beyond 6 h after the dose. If samples are taken at steady state, dosage adjustment can be performed by simple proportion.

## Gentamicin

Mr JL, a 64-year-old man who weighs 80 kg and has an estimated creatinine clearance of 35 ml/min, requires gentamicin therapy for a suspected gram-negative infection. The aim is to achieve a peak concentration around 8 mg/l and a trough around 1 mg/l.

### (i) What dosage regimen should be prescribed?

Gentamicin is cleared by excretion through the kidneys and its clearance can be approximated by creatinine clearance. The volume of distribution of gentamicin is around 0.25 l/kg (Table 1.3). A dosage interval of about 3 half-lives will allow the concentration to fall from 8 mg/l to 1 mg/l (8 → 4 → 2 → 1). The elimination half-life can be calculated from Eqn. 1.9, i.e.

$$t_{1/2} = \frac{\ln 2}{k}$$

$$t_{1/2} = \frac{0.693 \times V}{Cl}$$

$$t_{1/2} = \frac{0.693 \times 0.25 \, l/kg \times 80 \, kg}{35 \, ml/min \times (60/1000)}$$

$$= \frac{0.693 \times 20 \, l}{2.1 \, l/h}$$

$$= 6.6 \, h$$

It will therefore take $3 \times 6.6 = 20$ h for the concentration to fall from 8 mg/l to 1 mg/l. Because the 'peak' is measured 1 h after the dose, the dosage interval should be 21 h. A 'practical' dosage interval is therefore 24 h. The dose administered should increase the concentration by 7 mg/l (i.e. from 1 to 8 mg/l). It can be calculated from the volume of distribution, i.e.

$$\text{Dose (mg)} = 7mg/l \times 0.25l/kg \times 80 \, kg$$

$$= 140 \, mg$$

Mr JL was started on a daily dose of 140 mg and after two days of therapy his peak concentration (1 h post-dose) was 6 mg/l and his trough (24 h post-dose) was 0.5 mg/l.

### (ii) Has steady state been reached?

Mr JL's estimated elimination half-life is 6.6 h; therefore, steady state should be reached in $5 \times 6.6 = 33$ h. He will be at steady state after 2 days of therapy.

### (iii) How should the dose be adjusted?

The peak is slightly lower than the target and the trough is satisfactory. As these represent steady-state concentrations and gentamicin has linear pharmacokinetics, the dose can be adjusted by proportion. Increasing the dose to 200 mg daily should achieve a peak of $(200/140) \times 6 = 8.6$ mg/l and a trough of $(200/140) \times 0.5 = 0.7$ mg/l.

*Comment.* Elimination half-life is a useful guide to dosage interval and is particularly important when the target concentration–time profile includes both peak and trough concentrations. In this case, because the peaks and troughs were both low, the dose can be adjusted by direct proportion. If the trough had been high, an increase in the dosage interval would also have been necessary.

## Phenytoin

Mrs DL, a 38-year-old woman who weighs 55 kg, was prescribed phenytoin at a dose of 300 mg daily (5.5 mg/kg per day) after carbamazepine failed to control her epilepsy. She attended the outpatient clinic 3 weeks later and her 24-h post-dose trough phenytoin concentration was 6 mg/l (24 μmol/l). As her seizures were not well controlled, her dose was increased to 350 mg daily (6.4 mg/kg per day). She presented to her general practitioner 2 weeks later complaining of fatigue and difficulty in walking properly. Her trough phenytoin concentration was 28 mg/l (112 mol/l).

### (i) Why was the first concentration so low?

There are two possibilities: the dose was too low, or she was not complying with her prescribed dose. As patients generally require phenytoin maintenance doses in the range 4.5–5 mg/kg per day, both doses were higher than average. Phenytoin has non-linear pharmacokinetics at concentrations normally seen clinically, and standard pharmacokinetic equations cannot be used. The relationship between dose rate and average steady-state concentration is controlled by $V_{max}$ (the maximum amount of drug that can be metabolised by the enzymes per day) and $K_m$ (the concentration at half $V_{max}$). Using average values of $V_{max}$ (7.2 mg/kg per day) and $K_m$ (4.4 mg/l), Mrs DL's expected concentration can be calculated from the Michaelis–Menten equation (Eqn. 1.13), i.e.

$$\text{Dose rate} = \frac{V_{max} \times Css}{K_m + Css}$$

$$Css = \frac{\text{Dose rate} \times K_m}{V_{max} - \text{Dose rate}}$$

$$Css = \frac{300\,\text{mg/day} \times 4.4\,\text{mg/l}}{(7.2 \times 55)\,\text{mg/day} - 300\,\text{mg day}}$$

$$= \frac{1320}{96}$$

$$= 14\,\text{mg/l}\,(55\,\mu\text{mol/l})$$

The measured concentration of 6 mg/l is much lower than expected and suggests poor compliance with therapy.

## (ii) Why was the second concentration so high?

The predicted concentration on her increased dose can be calculated as before, i.e.

$$Css = \frac{350\,\text{mg/day} \times 4.4\,\text{mg/l}}{(7.2 \times 55)\,\text{mg/day} - 350\,\text{mg/day}}$$

$$= \frac{1540}{46}$$

$$= 33\,\text{mg/l}\,(147\,\mu\text{mol/l})$$

In this case, the measured concentration was reasonably consistent with the predicted value and her actual $V_{max}$ can therefore be estimated from the measured concentration, i.e.

$$V_{max}\,(\text{mg/day}) = \frac{\text{Dose rate} \times (K_m + Css)}{Css}$$

$$V_{max}\,(\text{mg/day}) = \frac{350\,\text{mg/day} \times (4.4 + 28)\,\text{mg/l}}{28\,\text{mg/l}}$$

$$= 450\,\text{mg/day}$$

Using her actual $V_{max}$ and a $K_m$ of 4.4 mg/l, average steady-state concentrations can be predicted for various doses (Table 2.4). Note that a small change in the dose produces a disproportionately large increase in concentration, especially at higher concentrations.

(*N.B.: A number of nomograms and graphical approaches are available to estimate $V_{max}$ and $K_m$ but they are beyond the scope of this text.*)

It is known that a concentration of 6 mg/l does not control her seizures and she experiences toxicity with 28 mg/l. Her ideal dose is therefore likely to lie in the range 275–325 mg daily. It would be sensible to start with 300 mg daily and adjust the dose (if necessary) according to her response. It would also be useful to emphasise to the patient that she must comply with her prescribed dose in order to obtain the maximum benefit from her therapy.

*Comment.* This case illustrates the non-linearity of phenytoin dose–concentration relationships and the difficulty of interpreting phenytoin concentrations when dosage history is uncertain (as frequently occurs with outpatients). It also demonstrates the value of using serial measurements (the two results were clearly inconsistent with each other) and average dose requirements to assess compliance.

# Chapter 3

# Influence of disease and age on pharmacokinetics and pharmacodynamics

Drugs are usually considered in terms of their effect on disease processes. However, several diseases can influence the pharmacokinetics of a drug or its pharmacological effect on target organs. This is of considerable clinical importance when diseases of the liver or kidney modify drug elimination, or drug distribution and elimination are altered in congestive cardiac failure.

## Influence of gastrointestinal disease

### Oesophageal dysmotility

In our increasingly aged population non-specific disorders of oesophageal motility are more common. Although relatively rare, oesophageal spasm in presenting elderly patients may be associated with neurodegenerative diseases such as Parkinson's disease. In such patients there is an increased risk of drug-induced oesophageal injury. Tablet or pill size makes a considerable difference to the ease of swallowing; large round objects are more difficult to swallow and show significantly higher incidence of impaction in the oesophagus (when wetted) when muco-adhesive coats rather than film coats are used. The precise nature of the drug is not always relevant because any tablet that impacts and releases its contents locally will cause irritation, owing to hypertonicity. The chemical nature of the substance may in some cases be relevant, e.g. iron tablets that are directly toxic.

## Achlorhydria

Achlorhydria occurs in around 10% of the elderly population, usually as a result of *Helicobacter*-induced atrophic gastritis. Iatrogenic achlorhydria is becoming increasingly common mainly in patients taking proton pump inhibitors (PPIs) for reflux oesophagitis. This will inhibit the absorption rate of drugs such as doxycycline monohydrate and ketaconazole, whose dissolution and absorption is optimum with an acid gastric pH. Theophylline absorption appears to be increased because of slower small intestinal transit. The absorption rate of solid formulations of aspirin is increased because the higher pH increases its rate of dissolution.

Achlorhydria is induced deliberately by PPIs in order to enhance the bioavailability of acid labile drugs, and in particular macrolides such as clarithromycin. This is important in the treatment of *Helicobacter pylori*; the amount of clarithromycin that remains after 1 h at pH 1 is about 10% but the use of PPIs to raise the pH to 6 can increase this to 90%. PPIs also increase the bioavailability of acid labile penicillins such as benzylpenicillin.

## Coeliac disease

There are several pathophysiological factors that can influence drug absorption. Loss of absorptive surface area decreases absorption along with impairment of fat absorption. However, first-pass metabolism by enterocytes is also decreased and this increases the bioavailability of drugs such as oestrogens, which are usually inactivated by enterocyte sulphatases. Other changes are an increased surface mucosal pH related to the loss of villi and increase in crypt/villous ratio. This enhances the absorption of some drugs, e.g. propranolol, but decreases that of folic acid, a weak acid whose ionisation will increase at the higher pH and, hence, reduce the amount of the most readily absorbed, un-ionised form of the drug.

As a result of these varying influences, the outcome is hard to predict with some drugs showing decreased absorption, e.g. amoxicillin (amoxycillin) and pivampicillin, but with others showing increased absorption, e.g. cefalexin (cephalexin). Decreased absorption of dietary folate contributes to the frequent low red cell folate and may increase the risk of bone marrow toxicity from cotrimoxazole.

Dapsone, which may be given to treat coeliac-associated dermatitis herpetiformis, has an impaired absorption in untreated coeliac patients who may need to go on a gluten-free diet to get the full benefit of dapsone.

Drugs that are lipid-soluble or are absorbed after dissolution in micelles such as vitamin D are usually malabsorbed and may best be given by injection.

## Crohn's disease

The characteristic features are focal inflammation with fibrosis and fistulation affecting either the small or large intestine or both. There are subtle defects with villous atrophy reducing the upper small intestinal absorptive area, although this effect is probably small. The biggest effect is diarrhoea, possibly through cytokine-mediated mechanisms and the presence of anaerobic bacteria within the small bowel when colo-intestinal fistulae develop. This bacterial contamination induces fat malabsorption and will impair the absorption of fat-soluble drugs. Rapid transits through the colon and lower small intestine will induce a degree of impairment of the enterohepatic recirculation. This may make certain

drugs less effective, e.g. enterohepatic recirculation of oestrogen is important in maintaining efficacy of the oral contraceptive pill.

The greatest effect is seen after bowel resection, which, if repeated, may end up with a short bowel syndrome with malabsorption of many substances including drugs and nutrients and water. Terminal ileal resections may impair vitamin $B_{12}$ absorption. *Comment.* Many factors can influence drug absorption when the gastrointestinal tract is abnormal. The presence of a malabsorption syndrome does not imply that drugs are necessarily malabsorbed; the absorption of some can actually increase. Currently there is insufficient information to comment on the clinical importance of these changes, but, theoretically, treatment failure may occur because of malabsorption and drug toxicity may be a consequence of increased absorption. Clinically relevant changes in drug absorption are most likely to result from fat malabsorption and diarrhoea.

## Influence of impaired renal function

---

**Impaired renal function can influence drug therapy for the following reasons**

1 Pharmacokinetics may be altered as result of:
  • Decreased elimination of drugs that are normally excreted entirely or mainly by the kidneys.
  • Decreased protein binding.
  • Decreased hepatic metabolism.
2 Drug effect may be the altered.
3 Existing clinical condition may be worsened.
4 Adverse effects may be enhanced.

---

## Altered pharmacokinetics

### Elimination

Because the kidney represents one of the major routes of drug elimination, a decline in renal function can influence the clearance of many drugs. If a drug normally cleared by the kidney is given to someone with decreased renal function without altering the dose, the steady-state blood concentrations of that drug will be increased. This is of considerable importance in the case of drugs showing concentration-related effects, particularly those that have a narrow therapeutic range.

When such drugs are given to patients with renal dysfunction, the general aim is to achieve similar concentrations to those seen in patients with normal kidneys.

Therapeutic concentrations can be maintained by:

1 Determining renal function, usually by estimating creatinine clearance.

2 Modifying the dose using a nomogram, either by increasing the dosage interval, or by giving a lower dose at the same interval or by altering both the dose and the interval. The extent and precision of dose modification depend very much on the toxicity of the drug concerned. In the case of the aminoglycosides, even minor impairment of renal function requires some dosage alteration, while the dose of penicillins need only be reduced in severe renal failure (creatinine clearance <10 ml/min). Guidance on dosage modification is readily available for most commonly used drugs. It should be noted that the loading dose is usually not changed by renal impairment because this depends more on the volume of distribution of the drug than its rate of elimination.

3 Monitoring drug concentrations. This is useful for drugs with concentration-related adverse effects, such as the aminoglycosides, digoxin, aminophylline, phenytoin and carbamazepine, and mandatory for lithium, ciclosporin (cyclosporin) and methotrexate. Nomograms are useful guides to the doses likely to be appropriate, but every patient is different. Concentrations of drugs in the blood can be used to assess clearance and to determine the most appropriate dose for individual patients.

## Decreased protein binding

The following changes occur in patients with impaired renal function:

1 Acidic drugs are less bound to serum albumin and the decrease in binding correlates with the severity of renal impairment. The binding of basic drugs (to $\alpha_1$-acid glycoprotein) undergoes little or no change.

2 The structure of albumin is changed in renal failure and endogenous compounds may compete with drugs for binding.

3 Haemodialysis does not return binding to normal, but renal transplantation does.

In most cases changes in protein binding have limited clinical relevance and do not require alterations in dose. However, protein binding is important for the interpretation of serum phenytoin concentrations.

## Hepatic metabolism

The hepatic metabolism of some drugs (e.g. nicardipine, propranolol) may be decreased in patients with renal failure. The reasons for this are not clear, but may indicate the presence of a metabolic inhibitor in uraemic plasma because regular haemodialysis appears to normalise the clearance of these compounds.

## Altered drug effect

There are several examples of increased drug sensitivity in patients with renal failure. Opiates, barbiturates, phenothiazines and benzodiazepines all show greater effects on the nervous system in patients with renal failure than in those with normal renal function. The reasons are not known, but increased meningeal permeability is one possible explanation.

Various antihypertensive drugs have a greater postural effect in renal failure. Again the reasons are not clear, but changes in fluid balance and autonomic dysfunction may be partly responsible.

## Worsening of the existing clinical condition

Drug therapy can result in deterioration of the clinical condition in the following ways:

1 By further impairing renal function. In patients with renal failure it is clearly advisable to avoid drugs that are known to be nephrotoxic and for which alternatives are available. Examples include aminoglycosides, amphotericin,

cisplatin, gold, mesalazine, non-steroidal anti-inflammatories, penicillamine and vancomycin.

2 By causing fluid retention. Fluid balance is a major problem in the more severe forms of renal failure. Drugs that cause fluid retention should therefore be avoided, e.g. carbenoxolone and non-steroidal anti-inflammatory drugs (NSAIDs) such as indometacin (indomethacin).

3 By increasing the degree of uraemia. Tetracyclines, except doxycycline, have an anti-anabolic effect and should be avoided.

## Enhancement of adverse drug effects

In addition to decreased elimination, digoxin is more likely to cause adverse effects in patients with severe renal failure if there are substantial electrolyte abnormalities, particularly hypercalcaemia and/or hypokalaemia.

Because potassium elimination is impaired in renal failure, diuretics that also conserve potassium (amiloride, spironolactone) are more likely to cause hyperkalaemia.

## Influence of liver disease

> **Impaired liver function can influence the response to treatment**
>
> 1 Altered pharmacokinetics:
> • Increased bioavailability resulting from reduced first-pass metabolism or, potentially, decreased first-pass activation of pro-drugs.
> • Decreased protein binding.
> • Worsening of metabolic state.
> 2 Altered drug effect.
> 3 Worsening of metabolic state.

## Altered pharmacokinetics

The liver is the largest organ in the body, has a substantial blood supply (around 1.5 l/min) and is interposed between the gastrointestinal tract and the systemic circulation. For these reasons it is uniquely suited for the purpose of influencing drug pharmacokinetics.

## Decreased first-pass metabolism

A decrease in hepatocellular function decreases the capacity of the liver to perform metabolic processes, while portosystemic shunting directs drugs away from sites of metabolism. Both factors are usually present in patients with severe cirrhosis.

Knowledge of the drugs that undergo first-pass metabolism is important in situations where it is decreased as a result of disease. Considerably greater quantities of active drug then reach the site of action and any given dose of drug has unexpectedly intense effects.

Examples of changes in bioavailability found in some patients with severe cirrhosis are:
• Clomethiazole (chlormethiazole) (100% increase)
• Labetalol (91% increase)
• Metoprolol (65% increase)
• Nicardipine (500% increase)
• Paracetamol (50% increase)
• Propranolol (42% increase)
• Verapamil (140% increase)

Conversely, first-pass activation of pro-drugs such as many ACE inhibitors (e.g. enalapril, perindopril, quinapril) may potentially be slowed or reduced.

## Decreased elimination by liver metabolism and decreased protein binding

### High extraction drugs

These are drugs which the liver metabolises at a very high rate. Their bioavailability is low and their clearance is dependent mainly upon the rate of drug delivery to the enzyme systems. The clearance of these drugs is therefore relatively sensitive to factors that can influence hepatic blood flow, such as congestive cardiac failure, and relatively insensitive to small changes in enzyme activity or protein binding. Examples include labetalol, lidocaine, metoprolol, morphine, propranolol, pethidine, nortriptyline and verapamil.

### Low extraction drugs

In low extraction drugs the rate of metabolism is so sufficiently low that hepatic clearance is relatively insensitive to changes in hepatic blood flow, and dependent mainly on the capacity of the liver enzymes. Examples include chloramphenicol, paracetamol and theophylline. The hepatic clearance of drugs in this group that are also highly protein-bound, such as diazepam, tolbutamide, phenytoin and valproic acid, depends on both the capacity of the enzymes and the free fraction. It is thus difficult to predict the consequences of hepatic disease on total drug concentration. However, as with renal disease, care must be taken in the interpretation of concentrations of highly protein bound drugs such as phenytoin.

The influence of liver disease on drug elimination is complex; the type of liver disease is critical. In acute viral hepatitis the major change is in hepatocellular function, but drug-metabolising ability usually remains intact and hepatic blood flow can increase. Mild to moderate cirrhosis tends to result in decreased hepatic blood flow and portosystemic shunting, while severe cirrhosis usually shows reduction in both cellular function and blood flow. Cholestasis leads to impaired fat absorption with deficiencies of fat-soluble vitamins and impairment of absorption of lipophillic drugs. Alcoholic liver disease is common and chronic ethanol abuse is associated with increased activity of the microsomal ethanol-oxidising system. This effect is a result primarily of induction by ethanol of a specific cytochrome P-450 (CYP2E1) responsible for enhanced oxidation of ethanol and other P-450 substrates and, consequently, for metabolic tolerance to these substances. This may lead to enhanced clearance and, hence, decreased response to certain drugs such as benzodiazepine sedatives, anticonvulsants (phenytoin) and warfarin. By contrast, simultaneous alcohol ingestion may decrease clearance of drugs metabolised via the P-450 (CYP2E1) enzyme system.

*Comment.* Unlike the measurement of creatinine clearance in renal disease, there is no simple test that can predict the extent to which drug metabolism is decreased in liver disease. A low serum albumin, raised bilirubin and prolonged prothrombin time give a rough guide.

The fact that a drug is metabolised by the liver does not necessarily mean that its pharmacokinetics is altered by liver disease. It is not easy, therefore, to extrapolate the findings from one drug to another. This is because superficially similar metabolic pathways are mediated by different forms of cytochrome P-450.

The documentation of modestly altered pharmacokinetics does not necessarily imply clinical importance. Even normal subjects show quite wide variations in pharmacokinetic indices and therefore pharmacokinetics should not be viewed in isolation from alterations in drug effect, which are much more difficult to assess. However, if a drug is known to be subject to substantial pharmacokinetic changes, clinical significance is much more likely.

If it is clinically desirable to give a drug that is eliminated by liver metabolism to a patient with cirrhosis, it should be started at a low dose and the drug levels or effect monitored very closely.

## Altered drug effect

### Deranged brain function

The more severe forms of liver disease are accompanied by poorly understood derangements of brain function that ultimately result in the syndrome of hepatic encephalopathy. However, even before encephalopathy develops, the brain is extremely sensitive to the effects of centrally acting drugs and a state of coma can result from administering normal doses of opiates or benzodiazepines to such patients.

### Decreased clotting factors

Patients with liver disease show increased sensitivity to oral anticoagulants. These drugs exert their effect by decreasing the vitamin K dependent synthesis of clotting factors II, VII, IX and X. When the production of these factors is already reduced by liver disease, a given dose of oral anticoagulant has a greater effect in these patients than in subjects with normal liver function.

## Worsening of metabolic state

### Drug-induced alkalosis

Excessive use of diuretics can precipitate encephalopathy. The mechanism involves hypokalaemic alkalosis, which results in conversion of $NH_4^+$ to $NH_3$, the un-ionised ammonia crossing easily into the central nervous system (CNS) to worsen or precipitate encephalopathy.

### Fluid overload

Patients with advanced liver disease often have oedema and ascites secondary to hypoalbuminaemia and portal hypertension. This problem can be worsened by drugs that cause fluid retention, e.g. NSAIDs, and antacids that contain large amounts of sodium. NSAIDs should be avoided anyway, because of the increased risk of gastrointestinal bleeding.

### Hepatotoxic drugs

Where an acceptable alternative exists, it is wise to avoid drugs that can cause liver damage (Table 3.1), e.g. sulphonamides or rifampicin, and repeated exposure to halothane anaesthesia.

## Influence of congestive heart failure

### Altered pharmacokinetics

### Decreased gastrointestinal absorption

The main factors involved are:
1 Mucosal oedema
2 Reduced epithelial blood supply
3 Splanchnic vasoconstriction
4 Reduced secretion of bile salts leading to fat malabsorption.

The most important effect is impaired absorption of fat-soluble vitamins A, D, E and K, which is common in childhood cholestatic disease. This leads to osteomalacia, prolonged clotting and neurological defects. Oral vitamin supplements may need to be replaced in the more advanced stages

**Table 3.1** Drugs that can cause liver damage.

| |
|---|
| *Hepatitis* |
|     Halothane (repeated exposure) |
|     Isoniazid |
|     Rifampicin |
|     Methyldopa |
|     Phenelzine |
|     Trimipramine |
|     Desipramine |
|     Carbimazepine |
|     Trasidone |
|     Propylthiouracil |
|     Augmentin |
|     Erythromycin |
|     Nitrofurantoin |
|     Chloroguanidee |
|     Tienilic acid |
|     Dihydralazine |
|     Azothiaprine |
|     Sulfasalazine (sulphasalazine) |
|     Naproxen |
|     Amiodarone |
| *Cholestasis with mild hepatic component* |
|     Phenothiazines |
|     Carbamazepine |
|     Tricyclic antidepressants |
|     Non-steroidal anti-inflammatory drugs (especially phenylbutazone) |
|     Rifampicin, ethambutol, pyrazinamide |
|     Sulphonylureas, trimethoprin |
|     Sulphonamides, ampicillin, nitrofurantoin, erythromycin estolate |
|     Oral contraceptives (stasis without hepatitis) |
| *Cirrhosis* |
|     Methotrexate |

by the better absorbed alphacalcidol (vitamin D analogue) and (sc)D(/sc)-α-tocopheryl polyethylene glycol 1000 succinate (vitamin K analogue). This latter preparation is a water-soluble form of vitamin K that forms micelles, and when given with vitamin D it actually enhances its absorption.

### Altered volume of distribution

Decreased volume is thought to result from decreased tissue perfusion and is clearly documented for lidocaine. Therefore, for any given dose, higher blood concentrations are achieved. The practical importance of this is that initial loading doses should be correspondingly reduced. Conversely, increased volumes can be observed for water-soluble drugs (such as the aminoglycosides) in the presence of oedema. In this case, higher doses would be required to achieve target peak concentrations.

## Decreased elimination

The main factors involved for the liver are:
1 Decreased perfusion
2 Decreased oxidising capacity due to hypoxia
3 Decreased metabolising capacity due to congestion

For the kidney they are:
1 Decreased glomerular filtration rate
2 Increased tubular reabsorption

The clearance of lidocaine is dependent upon liver blood flow and in heart failure it can be reduced by up to 50%. For theophylline the metabolic capacity of the liver is important and again clearance is reduced in heart failure (Chapter 2, Table 2.2). As these drugs have concentration-related toxicity, the rate of administration must be reduced in heart failure and therapeutic drug monitoring may be used to adjust therapy.

## Influence of thyroid disease

Thyroid disease alters a patient's response to digoxin. Hyperthyroid patients are relatively resistant to the drug, while hypothyroid patients are extremely sensitive to it. The reasons are in part kinetic and in part dynamic. The volume of distribution of digoxin is lower in hypothyroidism and higher in hyperthyroidism and its clearance is roughly proportional to thyroid function. Consequently, for any given dose, lower concentrations are achieved in hyperthyroid patients and higher concentrations are achieved in hypothyroid patients compared to normal patients. In addition, hypothyroid pa-

tients may experience adverse effects at relatively low concentrations while hyperthyroid patients often require higher concentrations, and possibly additional drugs, to control atrial fibrillation.

Lithium can cause hypothyroidism by inhibiting the release of thyroid hormone from the gland. It is important to recognise this complication in order to avoid mistaking hypothyroidism for a relapse in the depressive illness. Thyroxin can be prescribed concurrently with lithium.

## Influence of ageing

The elderly (65 years and over) constitute approximately 16% of the population, yet they consume 40% of the drug prescriptions in the United Kingdom. Two-thirds of those over the age of 65 receive regular medication. This high consumption of drugs is related to an increasing prevalence of acute and chronic disease, resulting in increasing numbers of prescriptions (see p. 19). Multiple drug prescribing can lead to problems with compliance and carries increased risk of side effects. The overall incidence of drug side effects in the elderly is up to three times that seen in the young. Adverse drug reactions in the elderly tend to be dose related rather than idiosyncratic and are related to changes in pharmacokinetics and pharmacodynamics. The drugs that have the highest incidence of side effects in the elderly are those that are most commonly prescribed (sedatives, diuretics and non-steroidal anti-inflammatory drugs). However, in one study, insulin and nitrofurantoin had the highest incidence of adverse effects when related to the total number of doses administered.

Drug absorption, distribution, metabolism, excretion and activity can all change as a result of ageing. However, the presence of multiple pathology in the old frequently has a greater effect than ageing alone.

## Drug absorption

Ageing is associated with increased gastric pH, delayed gastric emptying, decreased intestinal motility and reduced splanchnic blood flow. Despite these changes, there is little evidence to suggest that intestinal drug absorption changes with age. For example, the rate of absorption of digoxin is slower in the elderly but the overall bioavailability remains the same.

## Drug distribution

Age-related changes in body composition, in protein binding and in organ blood flow can all affect drug disposition.

Ageing is associated with a relative increase in body fat and corresponding reduction in body water. The volume of distribution of water-soluble drugs is smaller and this tends to cause an increase in initial drug concentration (e.g. digoxin and cimetidine). Lipid-soluble drugs tend to have an increased volume of distribution (e.g. nitrazepam and diazepam), which prolongs the elimination half-life and may prolong effect.

The extent of plasma protein–drug binding changes little with age but the plasma albumin may fall considerably with the onset of disease. There is no strong evidence that protein-binding interactions are more common in the elderly than in the young.

## Drug metabolism and age

There is evidence for age-related changes in the rates of metabolism of some drugs. In general, drugs that undergo microsomal oxidation (e.g. chlordiazepoxide) are likely to be metabolised more slowly in the elderly. Despite this, there is no evidence that the concentration or activity of hepatic microsomal oxidising enzymes is reduced in the elderly. The age-related reduction in oxidising capacity may be related to the reduction in hepatic volume and blood flow that occurs in the elderly. Conjugation pathways do not appear to be affected by age. Overall, the changes in metabolism with age alone are not of great clinical significance.

First-pass metabolism may be reduced considerably in the elderly (see below). This is probably the consequence of the age-associated reduction in liver mass and blood flow. As a result, drugs that undergo extensive first-pass metabolism (e.g. labetolol and propranolol) may show considerably increased bioavailability in the elderly.

This effect is amplified by the presence of chronic liver disease.

## Renal excretion

In old age there is a fall in both renal blood flow and renal function. Glomerular filtration falls by approximately 30% by the age of 65 years, as compared to young adults. Digoxin and the aminoglycoside antibiotics are excreted mainly by glomerular filtration and these will tend to accumulate in the elderly if the dose is not reduced. Renal tubular function also declines and drugs such as penicillin and procainamide, which undergo active tubular secretion, have a marked reduction in clearance. In addition, the elderly are more likely to suffer a further reduction in renal function as a result of renal tract disease such as infection. Illness in the elderly is frequently accompanied by dehydration and this reduces renal function even further. The overall effect of physiological ageing and disease considerably diminishes the elderly kidney's capacity to excrete drugs.

## Receptor sensitivity

In practice, it is very difficult to assess accurately drug receptor numbers or sensitivity. In most cases information is derived from drug effect related to drug plasma concentration. Using this approach it can be shown that the elderly are more sensitive to the effect of benzodiazepine drugs such as nitrazepam, temazepam and diazepam. Warfarin is more potent in the elderly because of a greater effect on coagulation factor synthesis and this is a reflection of the increased receptor affinity to warfarin that occurs in the elderly.

Perhaps most is known about the effects of ageing on the autonomic receptors. On the one hand there is a modest decline in the tachycardia produced by stimulation of $\beta_1$-adrenoceptors;

on the other, there appears to be no age-related change in $\beta_2$-adrenoceptor-mediated vascular or bronchial relaxation. The effect of the vasconstrictor $\alpha_1$-adrenoceptor is also unchanged with age.

## Impairment of homeostasis

The effect of drugs in the elderly may be affected by a loss of homeostatic control that is often seen in the elderly patient.

Cardiovascular postural reflexes are commonly less effective in the aged. Elderly patients tend to fall more easily than the young and this is made worse by the use of drugs that cause postural hypotension. There are many such drugs, including diuretics, antihypertensive agents and sedatives.

The elderly have impaired thermoregulation. Many of the major tranquillisers may precipitate hypothermia. This is the result not only of a direct hypothermic effect, but also of a reduction in physical activity.

## Compliance

There is no evidence that an elderly patient whose mental function is normal is more likely to make mistakes with their medication than a younger patient. However, one of the main contributory factors to poor drug compliance at all ages is polypharmacy—the rate of errors when three drugs are prescribed is approximately 20% but it is close to 100% when 10 drugs are prescribed—and the high consumption of drugs in the elderly results in a greater opportunity to make errors. This is often made worse by the prevalence of mental impairment, which is as high as 25% in those over the age of 85 years. Physical handicap can also contribute to poor compliance. Arthritic hands have great difficulty in opening 'child-proof' containers or 'bubble-packed' drugs.

---

**Prescribing for the elderly**

**1** Make an accurate diagnosis. The presentation of disease in the elderly is often non-specific (e.g. confusion, dizziness and incontinence). It is important to make an accurate diagnosis to allow appropriate therapy.
**2** Treat only important disorders. Elderly patients frequently have multiple pathology. This can lead to polypharmacy with a resultant increase in side effects and poor compliance.
**3** Avoid ineffective drugs. Prescriptions for marginally effective or ineffective drugs can only lead to side effects and poor compliance. It should be remembered that there is no drug treatment for dementia and those advertised for the treatment of atherosclerosis or urinary incontinence have little, if any, measurable effect.
**4** Review drugs regularly. It is important to review the need for each prescription. If a drug is considered necessary, make sure the minimum dose required is used.
**5** Understand the changes in pharmacology with age for each drug used, remembering that relative renal insufficiency is very common in the elderly.

---

## Pharmacokinetics/pharmacodynamics in the elderly

*Reduced first-pass metabolism*
- propranolol (in sick elderly)

*Reduced protein binding (in sick elderly)*
- phenytoin
- diazepam

*Increased volume of distribution
(relative increased body fat)*
- diazepam

*Decreased hepatic oxidation*
- chloridiazepoxide

*Decreased renal excretion*
- digoxin
- gentamicin
- cimetidine

*Decreased drug-receptor sensitivity*
- cardiac $\beta_1$-adrenoceptor drugs

*Increased drug receptor sensitivity*
- warfarin
- benzodiazepines

# Chapter 4

# Drugs in pregnant and breast feeding women

Nearly 40% of women in the United Kingdom take at least one drug during pregnancy, excluding iron, vitamins and drugs used during delivery. Once in the maternal circulation, drugs are separated from the fetus by a lipid placental membrane, which any given drug crosses to a greater or lesser extent depending on the physicochemical properties of the molecule.

Drugs in pregnancy can be viewed from two standpoints:
1 Effect of drugs on the fetus
2 Effect of pregnancy on the drug.

## Effect of drugs on the fetus

Drugs can influence fetal development at three separate stages:
1 Fertilisation and implantation period: conception to about 17 days gestation
2 Organogenesis: 18–55 days
3 Growth and development: 56th day onward.

The possible consequences of drug exposure are quite different at each stage. In addition, drugs given at the end of pregnancy can influence structure or function in the neonate.

## Fertilisation and implantation period

Interference by a drug with either of these processes leads to failure of the pregnancy at a very early and probably subclinical stage. Therefore, very little is known about drugs that influence this process in humans.

## Organogenesis

It is during this period that the developing embryo shows great sensitivity to the teratogenic effects of drugs. A teratogen is any substance (virus, environmental toxin or drug) that produces deformity. Before discussing the teratogenic properties of certain drugs, the following points must be appreciated:
1 Teratogenesis in humans is very difficult to predict from animal studies because of considerable species variation. Thalidomide, the most notorious drug teratogen of recent times, showed no teratogenicity in mice and rats.
2 Serious congenital deformities are present in 1–2% of all babies; therefore, a drug is only readily identified as teratogenic if its effects are frequent, unusual and/or serious. A low-grade teratogen that infrequently causes minor deformities is likely to pass unnoticed.

Table 4.1 lists some drugs that are known to be teratogenic. It is important to realise that, even for known teratogens, first trimester use often results in a normal baby, e.g. phenytoin is teratogenic in about 5% of exposures and warfarin in up to 25%. Also, there will be occasions, such as the use of warfarin in women with prosthetic heart valves, where the risks to the mother of not using the drug outweigh the risks of exposure in the fetus.

**Table 4.1** Drugs that are known to be teratogenic.

| Drug | Deformity |
| --- | --- |
| Danazol | Virilisation of female fetus |
| Lithium | Cardiac (Ebstein's complex) |
| Phenytoin | Craniofacial; limb |
| Carbamazepine | Craniofacial; limb |
| Retinoids | Central nervous system |
| Valproate | Neural tube; possible neurodevelopment |
| Diethylstilbestrol (stilboestrol) | Adenocarcinoma of vagina in teenage years |
| Warfarin | Multiple defects; chondrodysplasia punctata |

*Comment.* The greatest risk of teratogenesis occurs at a time when a woman might not even be aware that she is pregnant. Only a few drugs are known definitely to be teratogenic, but many more could be under certain circumstances. When prescribing for a woman of childbearing age, remember that she might be pregnant and ask yourself if the benefits of drug use outweigh the risks, however small, of teratogenesis.

## Growth and development

During this stage major body structures have been formed, and it is their subsequent development and function that can be affected:

1 Antithyroid drugs cross the placenta and can cause fetal and neonatal hypothyroidism.
2 Tetracyclines inhibit bone growth and discolour teeth.
3 Angiotensin-converting enzyme inhibitors can seriously damage fetal kidney function.
4 Warfarin can cause bleeding into the fetal brain.
5 Drugs with dependence potential, e.g. benzodiazepines and opiates, which are taken regularly during pregnancy can result in withdrawal symptoms in the neonate.

## Drugs given at the end of pregnancy

1 Aspirin in analgesic doses can cause haemorrhage in the neonate.

2 Indometacin (and possibly other non-steroidal anti-inflammatory drugs) causes premature closure of the ductus arteriosus with resulting pulmonary hypertension.
3 Central nervous system (CNS) depressant drugs (e.g. opiates, benzodiazepines) can cause hypotension, respiratory depression and hypothermia in the neonate.

## Effect of pregnancy on drug absorption, distribution and elimination

The substantial physiological changes that occur in pregnancy can influence drug disposition, while pathological conditions in pregnancy can accentuate these changes.

## Drug distribution

Maternal plasma volume and extracellular fluid volume increase by about 50% by the last trimester, and this may decrease the steady-state concentration of drugs with a small volume of distribution. Considerable changes in protein concentration occur during the last trimester, with serum albumin falling by about 20% while $\alpha_1$-acid glycoprotein increases in concentration by about 40% in normal pregnancies. These changes are accentuated in pre-eclampsia, with albumin concentration falling by about 35% and glycoprotein rising by as much as 100%. This means that the free fraction of acidic drugs can increase substantially, while that of basic drugs can be decreased greatly, in the last trimester. Diazepam, phenytoin and sodium valproate have been shown to have significantly elevated free fractions in the last trimester.

## Drug elimination

Effective renal plasma flow doubles by the end of pregnancy but this has been shown to be important in only a few cases; for example, the clearance of ampicillin doubles and the dose must also be doubled for systemic (but of course not for renal tract) infections. The hepatic microsomal mixed function oxidase system undergoes induction in pregnancy, probably as the result of high circulating levels of progesterone. This leads to an increased clearance of drugs that undergo metabolism by this pathway, and there is evidence that the steady-state concentrations of the anticonvulsants sodium valproate, phenytoin and carbamazepine may be decreased to a clinically significant extent during the second and third trimesters. Therefore, higher doses may be required as the pregnancy progresses, with careful monitoring of drug concentrations.

## Drug treatment of common medical problems during pregnancy

### Infection

Urinary tract infections are common during pregnancy. Penicillins are the preferred treatment (subject to appropriate sensitivity testing), because these drugs have never been implicated in teratogenesis and are generally well tolerated. Nitrofurantoin is not harmful to the fetus but frequently causes nausea. Tetracyclines are contraindicated. Trimethoprim should be avoided in early pregnancy since it can possibly cause limb reduction and cleft palate.

Fortunately, severe infections in pregnancy are rare. Aminoglycosides cause fetal eighth nerve damage, and the benefits of their use must be seen in this context. At present there is no evidence to suggest fetal damage from cephalosporins, metronidazole or chloramphenicol. However, chloramphenicol can cause cardiovascular collapse in neonates and should not be used at the end of pregnancy unless absolutely necessary.

In the case of tuberculosis, both isoniazid and ethambutol have been used extensively during pregnancy, including the first trimester, with no fetal defects. The incidence of fetal deformity following rifampicin is three times greater than with isoniazid or ethambutol, and this drug should be avoided in the first trimester if possible. Streptomycin definitely causes auditory deficit and should not be used.

### Asthma

Poorly controlled asthma is associated with increased perinatal mortality. Maternal hypoxia and respiratory alkalosis are the major determinants of fetal distress in asthmatic pregnancies. Theophylline, salbutamol by metered aerosol, and steroids have good safety records at all stages of pregnancy. There has been little experience with newer bronchodilators.

Pregnancy should not alter the general approach to asthma as described in Chapter 8. It is important to control bronchospasm and avoid

**Table 4.2** Commonly used drugs that should be avoided in women who are breast feeding.

| Drug | Effect of drug |
| --- | --- |
| Amiodarone | Iodine content may cause neonatal hypothyroidism |
| Aspirin | Theoretical risk of Reye's syndrome |
| Barbiturates | Drowsiness |
| Benzodiazepines | Lethargy |
| Carbimazole | Hypothyroidism at higher doses |
| Contraceptives (combined oral) | May diminish milk supply and reduce nitrogen and protein content |
| Cytotoxic drugs | Potential problems include immune suppression and neutropenia |
| Ephedrine | Irritability |
| Tetracyclines | Theoretical risk of tooth discoloration |

---

**Management of pregnant epileptics**

**1** Management should begin before conception:
- If a woman has been seizure-free for 2–3 years, consider slowly stopping treatment.
- There is no justification for changing from, for example, phenytoin to a drug about which even less is known. However, control should be optimised on monotherapy if possible.

**2** Discuss the possibility of a birth defect in the context of around a 95% likelihood of a normal child compared to 98% in the general population.

**3** A scan around 20 weeks is likely to detect major structural defects.

---

prolonged abnormalities of blood gases or acid–base balance.

## Epilepsy

The main issues are possible teratogenicity associated with anticonvulsants and the need for therapeutic drug level monitoring to control fits.

The incidence of congenital malformations in children of epileptic mothers is about 5% (see Table 4.1, p. 35), which is three times higher than in the general population. In part, this could reflect a genetic predisposition, but anticonvulsants seem largely to be responsible. Most evidence exists for the older drugs: carbamazepine, phenytoin and valproate, with cleft palate, neural tube defects and congenital heart disease being the most common findings, but there is increasing evidence of neurodevelopmental delay with some anticonvulsants. Co-administration of anticonvulsants produces a greater risk than when either drug is used alone.

At the present time the guidelines shown below seem appropriate to the management of pregnant epileptics.

The pharmacokinetic changes associated with pregnancy are clinically important in the treatment of epilepsy. Concentrations of some anticonvulsants tend to fall during pregnancy (see above). Although partially offset by a decrease in protein binding, this change in drug level can be accompanied by increased seizure frequency. Therefore, concentration monitoring is required at regular intervals during pregnancy. In women whose epilepsy has been well controlled, the aim should be to maintain early or pre-pregnancy concentrations with doses being increased as necessary to achieve this. Following delivery, there is a return to normal kinetics over 5–10 days and monitoring is again required to aid dosage adjustment.

## Hypertension

Methyldopa is widely used in the management of essential hypertension during pregnancy. This drug is now rarely used outside of pregnancy because of a wide range of side effects, notably sedation. However, it has an unrivalled safety record in pregnancy.

Beta-blockers successfully lower blood pressure in pregnancy, but have not been shown conclusively to improve fetal outcome. They are not teratogenic. When given throughout pregnancy, beta-blockers can cause growth retardation of the fetus.

## Hyperthyroidism

Propylthiouracil tends to be used more often than carbimazole during pregnancy. Propylthiouracil is less lipid-soluble and more protein-bound and crosses less well into the fetus and breast milk. The dose should be titrated against maternal thyroid function.

## Breast feeding

The factors that determine the transfer of drugs into breast milk are the same as those influencing drug distribution in general (Chapter 1, see Principles of pharmacokinetics, p. 7).

Most drugs enter breast milk to a greater or lesser extent but, because the concentration has been greatly reduced by distribution throughout the mother's body, the amount of drug actually received by the breast-fed baby is usually clinically insignificant.

Drugs that can safely be given to breast feeding mothers are listed below.

Certain drugs achieve sufficient concentration in breast milk, and they are sufficiently potent that their use in breast feeding mothers should be avoided (Table 4.2).

*Comment.* Most commonly used drugs can be safely used in women who are breast feeding. If in doubt, seek further information.

---

**Drugs safe for breast feeding mothers**

- Penicillins, cephalosporins
- Theophylline, salbutamol by inhaler, prednisolone
- Valproate, carbamazepine, phenytoin

- Beta-blockers, methyldopa, hydralazine
- Warfarin, heparin
- Haloperidol, chlorpromazine
- Tricyclic antidepressants

---

# Part 2

# Aspects of therapeutics

# Chapter 5

# Primary and secondary prevention of cardiovascular disease

Cardiovascular diseases, particularly myocardial infarction and stroke, are not only an important cause of death and disability worldwide but are major contributors to health care costs. While genetic factors contribute to the risk of cardiovascular diseases, reversible environmental factors also play a major role. These include cigarette smoking and obesity in addition to other established risk factors such as high blood pressure, raised low-density cholesterol (and other lipids), diabetes and a pro-thrombotic state. Non-pharmacological approaches including exercise, diet and smoking cessation can make important contributions to prevention of cardiovascular disease. These should be actively pursued in all patients. However, in a large number non-pharmacological approaches will need to be augmented and supplemented with specific drug therapy. The target of such treatment is the reduction of blood pressure and/or cholesterol but the aim is long-term prevention of progression of atherosclerosis and avoidance of cardiac and vascular (cerebral and renal) complications (primary prevention). In patients presenting with heart disease or stroke, prevention of further events by reversal of plaque instability or delaying if not halting progression of atheroma (secondary prevention) is the objective. There is now good evidence from prospective randomised controlled trials of the benefits and safety of lowering blood pressure and cholesterol in both primary and secondary prevention. Patients with diabetes and other high-risk groups appear to show proportionately more benefit from the reduction of blood pressure and cholesterol. In recent years national and international guidelines have recommended that those individuals at moderate or high risk of cardiovascular disease be identified and treated actively. High risk of cardiac disease (greater than 15% 10-year risk) is used as a guide for the need for treatment of cholesterol. Hypertension treatment guidelines use total cardiovascular risk, which includes heart disease and stroke. The latter is usually considered to be about a third higher than the cardiac rate alone and thus greater than 20% 10-year risk corresponds to the high-risk category in hypertension management. Increasing age is an important component of the calculation of both cardiac and cardiovascular risk. A substantial proportion of the population over the age of 55 are candidates for reduction of blood pressure, cholesterol or both.

## Hypertension

### Aim

The aim of treatment is to reduce blood pressure in order to reduce the risk of death or disability from cardiovascular disease, especially stroke, coronary artery disease and cardiac failure. However, because hypertension is often an asymptomatic condition, the treatment should control blood pressure without inducing adverse effects or otherwise

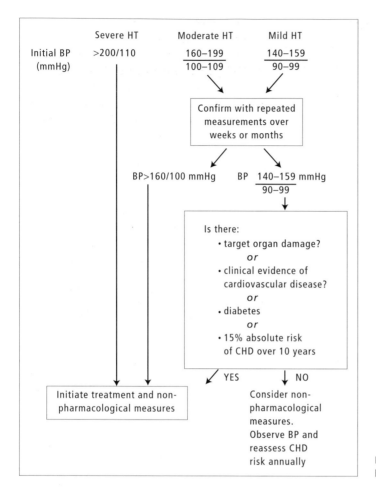

| | Severe HT | Moderate HT | Mild HT |
|---|---|---|---|
| Initial BP (mmHg) | >200/110 | 160–199 / 100–109 | 140–159 / 90–99 |

Confirm with repeated measurements over weeks or months

BP>160/100 mmHg    BP 140–159 mmHg / 90–99

Is there:
- target organ damage?
  *or*
- clinical evidence of cardiovascular disease?
  *or*
- diabetes
  *or*
- 15% absolute risk of CHD over 10 years

YES    NO

Initiate treatment and non-pharmacological measures

Consider non-pharmacological measures. Observe BP and reassess CHD risk annually

**Figure 5.1** Treatment decisions based on observed blood pressure.

interfering with the well-being of the patient. A target blood pressure of ≤140/85 mmHg is generally advocated, although this may be modified for particular patients, e.g. those with co-existent diabetes (target BP <130/80) and patients at the highest risk of cardiovascular disease (Figure 5.1).

## Relevant pathophysiology

Blood pressure is the hydrostatic pressure within the systemic arteries and is determined by total peripheral resistance and cardiac output. Total peripheral resistance is invariably increased in established hypertension, although the causative mechanism is not well understood. Increases in

heart rate or cardiac output are not found consistently.

Blood pressure values are distributed normally (unimodally) in the population and there is no clear cut-off between normotensive and hypertensive values. Long-term prospective epidemiological studies indicate that, for both systolic and diastolic blood pressure, the higher the blood pressure the greater the risk of cardiovascular disease. The definition of hypertension is therefore dependent upon the selection of an arbitrary value for normal blood pressure and the frequency of hypertension varies according to the age, sex and ethnic origin in the population studied.

## Primary and secondary hypertension

Hypertension is either primary or secondary. No underlying cause can be identified in about 95% of cases and the terminology of primary, idiopathic or essential is applied. There is a strong polygenic familial trend and environmental factors such as salt, obesity and alcohol consumption also contribute. Secondary types of hypertension are rare, even in younger age groups, and usually have an endocrine or renal basis.

---

**Causes of secondary hypertension**

1 Renal diseases
Renovascular disease, particularly renal artery stenosis (as a result of fibromuscular hyperplasia in young patients and atheroma in older patients)
  • Glomerulonephritis
2 Endocrine disease
  • Hyperaldosteronism (Conn's syndrome)
  • Phaeochromocytoma
  • Hypercorticism (Cushing's syndrome)
  • Acromegaly
  • Hypothyroidism
3 Coarctation of the aorta
4 Drugs, e.g. oral contraceptives, corticosteroids, NSAIDs, ciclosporin

---

## Benefits of treatment

There is now unequivocal evidence that antihypertensive treatment significantly reduces stroke and the progression of renal and cardiac failure. These benefits have been clearly established in moderate hypertension (systolic 160–199 mmHg and/or diastolic 100–109 mmHg), in severe hypertension (systolic greater than 200 mmHg and/or diastolic greater than 110 mmHg) and in malignant or accelerated phase hypertension. In the treatment of mild hypertension (systolic 140–159 mmHg and/or diastolic blood pressure 90–99 mmHg) there again have been substantial reductions in stroke and also benefits in respect of coronary artery disease. The benefits of treatment in mild hypertension are greatest among those patients who have evidence of target organ damage

(e.g. left ventricular hypertrophy (LVH), retinopathy or proteinuria), diabetes, pre-existing cardiovascular disease (e.g. prior myocardial infarction) or a high risk of cardiovascular disease ($\geq 20\%$ over 10 years) by virtue of other risk factors. Age and systolic hypertension increase risk and benefit. Meta-analysis of randomised trials does not show any convincing benefit of individual drugs or classes but supports the view that in terms of outcome of the treatment, "the lower the achieved blood pressure the better."

---

**Antihypertensive treatment**

1 Hypertension should be confirmed by several measurements of blood pressure over several days, weeks or months.
2 Patients should be counselled about hypertension, and its risk, and the relevance of other risk factors. The reason for long-term treatment should be carefully explained.
3 Hypertension should be treated as part of a management plan for reducing all identifiable cardiovascular risk factors. Mild to moderate hypertension should seldom be treated in isolation and it is important to attempt to modify all of the individual risk factors of the patient including cigarette smoking, hyperlipidaemia and diabetes mellitus and to take account of other factors such as a family history of premature cardiovascular disease.
4 Non-pharmacological approaches should always be considered although long-term compliance is low; For example,
  • For the obese patient, weight reduction of 10 kg may lower blood pressure by about 20/10 mmHg.
  • If salt intake is very high (more than 200 mEq per day), a modest reduction by the simple avoidance of excessively salty foods and the use of table salt may aid blood pressure control.
  • Regular physical exercise.
5 Arrangements should be made for regular and convenient long-term follow-up with blood pressure measurements.
6 As required, a simple and well-tolerated antihypertensive drug regimen should be established.

---

## Principles of antihypertensive treatment

Drugs may be given alone or in rational combinations. With newer treatment targets, patients will often require more than one drug. The simplest regimen is likely to be the most successful. Compliance with treatment is likely to be maintained best if drugs are administered once daily. A wide range of suitable first-line antihypertensive drugs is now available and the classes of drug that are currently in widespread use are thiazide diuretics, beta-blockers, calcium antagonists, angiotensin-converting enzyme (ACE) inhibitors and angiotensin II ($AT_1$) receptor blockers. Whilst a rigid regimen based upon diuretics and beta-blockers either alone or in combination was previously recommended, there is now a tendency to try to select the most appropriate therapy to meet the particular requirements of the individual patient. The response to treatment can then be evaluated over a period of weeks or months and, if the effect is insufficient and if there are no side effects, the dosage can be increased. If side effects occur or if there is clearly no useful blood pressure response to treatment, then it is appropriate to change to another type of therapy. Where blood pressure response is inadequate despite full-dose, well-tolerated monotherapy, combination treatment with more than one drug is advocated. A fixed-dose combination may prove particularly suitable, not only for blood pressure control and compliance but also for satisfying the requirements of the individual patient in terms of other coronary heart disease (CHD) risk factors, or concomitant disease states.

*Clinical comment.* The management of hypertension is a long-term undertaking often in asymptomatic patients. The simplest and most effective treatment should be determined for each individual. Reduction of blood pressure and control of other risk factors is designed to reduce cardiovascular morbidity and mortality without impairing the quality of life. Most patients are started on single-drug therapy but more than half of them will require a second or third drug from different classes to achieve treatment targets of <140/85 mmHg. In patients with diabetes or renal disease the target is <130/80 mmHg.

## Antihypertensive drugs

The following are the most important antihypertensive drug classes (Table 5.1):

1 Thiazide diuretics
2 Calcium antagonists
3 ACE inhibitors
4 $AT_1$ receptor antagonists
5 $\beta$-Adrenoceptor antagonists
6 $\alpha_1$-Antagonists; vasodilators
7 Centrally acting agents.

## Diuretics

### Mechanism of action

These drugs increase sodium excretion and urine volume by interfering with sodium, chloride and water transport across renal tubular cell membranes (Table 5.2). Diuretics are used in states of salt and water overload such as congestive heart failure (Chapter 6, p. 77), nephrotic syndrome and hepatic failure with ascites. The antihypertensive action is not related directly to diuretic efficacy, but upon more subtle alterations to the contractile responses of vascular smooth muscle. Thus, thiazide diuretics are the preferred drugs for the treatment of hypertension. Loop diuretics, such as furosemide, have greater diuretic efficacy but their effects on blood pressure are relatively short-acting and liable to provoke reflex stimulation of the renin–angiotensin system to counter any fall in blood pressure. Potassium-sparing diuretics are the least effective diuretics but use is not associated with potassium loss, which occurs with both thiazide and loop diuretics. Thus, in refractory oedema these agents are very useful in combination with the loop diuretics and in some hypertensive patients potassium-sparing diuretics can usefully be combined with a thiazide diuretic. The antihypertensive effect of thiazide diuretics manifests at relatively low dosages and there is no additional benefit from higher doses in terms of blood pressure reduction. In contrast, it is possible to increase the diuretic response with higher dosages but this also leads to greater potassium loss and other metabolic changes.

### Clinical pharmacology

Thiazides are well absorbed orally, widely distributed and subject to a variable amount of hepatic metabolism. The effects on the kidney depend

**Table 5.1** Indications and contraindications for the major classes of antihypertensive drugs.

| | Indications | | Contraindications | |
|---|---|---|---|---|
| | **Strong** | **Possible** | **Possible** | **Strong** |
| Thiazide diuretics | Old age | — | Dyslipidaemia | Gout |
| Beta-blockers | Myocardial infarction | Heart failure* | Heart failure* | Asthma or COPD heart block |
| Calcium antagonists I (dihydropyridine) | Isolated systolic HT in elderly subjects | Angina in elderly patients | — | — |
| Calcium antagonists II (rate-limiting drugs) | Angina | Myocardial infarction | Combination with beta-blockers | Heart block Heart failure |
| ACE inhibitors | Heart failure LV dysfunction in type I diabetic nephropathy | Chronic renal disease† | Renal impairment Peripheral vascular disease | Pregnancy Reno-vascular HT |
| ANGII antagonists | ACE inhibitor induced cough | Heart failure, intolerance of other antihyper-tensives | Peripheral vascular disease | Pregnancy Reno-vascular HT |

*Note:* ACE, angiotensin-converting enzyme; COPD, chronic obstructive pulmonary disease; HT, hypertension; LV, left ventricular; ANGII, angiotensin II.

* Beta-blockers may worsen heart failure, but in specialist hands may be used to treat heart failure.

† ACE inhibitors may be beneficial in chronic renal failure but should be used with caution under specialist supervision.

**Table 5.2** Classification and site of action of diuretics.

| | Site of action | Comment |
|---|---|---|
| *Thiazides* | | |
| Bendroflumethiazide (bendrofluazide) Hydrochlorothiazide Chlortalidone (chlorthalidone) | Proximal part of the distal tubule | All have an antihypertensive effect. Little evidence that newer agents have any advantages over older established agents |
| *Loop diuretics* | | |
| Furosemide (frusemide) Bumetanide | Ascending limb of loop of Henle | Effective diuretic and saliuretic but less useful for the treatment of hypertension |
| *Potassium sparing diuretics* | | |
| Spironolactone | Distal tubule aldosterone antagonist | May be used in combination with loop diuretics in refractory oedema |
| Triamterene | Sodium potassium exchange | May cause hyperkalaemia in renal failure or in the elderly |

upon excretion of drug into the renal tubule, and thiazide diuretics become less effective with increasing renal impairment, while loop diuretics retain some efficacy. With thiazides, the onset of the diuretic effect is usually observed within 1 h and may last for about 12 h, but with repeated dosing, the acute diuretic effect tends to diminish in the majority of hypertensive patients. The antihypertensive effect, however, is more gradual in onset and more long-lasting so that, at steady state, the antihypertensive effect persists for more than 24 h and once-daily dosing is therefore appropriate for most agents.

## Pharmacologically predictable adverse effects

### Hypokalaemia
Because of the increased urinary loss of potassium there may be a reduction in blood potassium to levels below normal. As severe hypokalaemia may precipitate cardiac arrhythmias (especially in patients also receiving digoxin), it may be necessary to provide potassium supplements or to use a combination diuretic treatment with both a thiazide diuretic and a potassium-sparing diuretic. Persistent hypokalaemia with low-dose thiazide treatment should raise the suspicion of an underlying abnormality of potassium homeostasis such as mineralocorticoid excess (Conn's syndrome).

### Hyperuricaemia
Because thiazide diuretics also interfere with the excretion of uric acid, there may be an increased blood level of uric acid and, rarely, the provocation of acute gout.

### Hyperglycaemia
Long-term diuretic therapy is associated with an impairment of glucose tolerance and an increased incidence of non-insulin-dependent diabetes mellitus. The mechanism appears to be mainly related to interference with the action of insulin in peripheral tissues (so-called 'insulin resistance'). This adverse effect is dose dependent and new onset diabetes is rare with current low doses of thiazides.

### Hypercalcaemia
This is a rare adverse effect of thiazide diuretics resulting from reduced renal excretion of calcium.

## Other adverse effects

### Hyperlipidaemia
By mechanisms that are not entirely clear, long-term use of thiazide diuretics is associated with modest changes in the plasma lipid profile with increases in total and low-density lipoprotein (LDL) cholesterol, increases in triglycerides and a reduction in high-density lipoprotein (HDL) cholesterol.

### Impotence
This is a well-recognised but occasional problem with long-term diuretic treatment especially at higher doses. The mechanism is not known and the problem is usually reversible on treatment withdrawal.

### Others
Thrombocytopenia and skin rash occur rarely.

*Clinical comment.* Thiazide diuretics (for example, bendroflumethiazide (bendrofluazide) 2.5 mg daily; hydrochlorothiazide 12.5 or 25 mg daily; chlortalidone (chlorthalidone) 12.5 or 25 mg daily) are widely used and are effective antihypertensive drugs in mild, moderate and severe hypertension. Where the hypertension is complicated by chronic renal failure (serum creatinine >150 mmol), or is proving refractory to treatment, it may be necessary to try a loop diuretic. Because diuretic-induced hypokalaemia has been associated with poorer outcomes, it may be necessary to add a potassium-sparing drug such as amiloride, triamterene or spironolactone; the combination of a thiazide and a potassium-sparing drug is a popular and effective first-line treatment. Serum potassium tends to rise in renal failure, when a potassium-sparing diuretic should be avoided. As an alternative a combination of low-dose diuretic with an ACE inhibitor or an angiotensin receptor antagonist is a very effective well-tolerated regimen and tends to minimise risks of hypokalaemia. Potassium-sparing diuretics should be avoided in combination with ACE inhibitors or angiotensin receptor antagonists.

## β-Adrenoceptor antagonists (beta-blockers)

### Mechanism of action

Beta-blockers antagonise the effects of sympathetic nerve stimulation or circulating catecholamines. β-Adrenoceptors are widely distributed throughout the body systems and are subclassified as $\beta_1$- and $\beta_2$-receptors according to their location. $\beta_1$-Receptors are predominant in the heart and $\beta_2$-receptors are predominant in other organs such as the lung, peripheral blood vessels and skeletal muscle. This is a clinically useful subclassification but it is not absolutely accurate: for example, there are $\beta_2$-receptors in the heart and there are $\beta_1$-receptors in the kidney.

1 *Heart*: Stimulation of $\beta_1$-receptors in the sino-atrial node causes an increase in heart rate (a positive chronotropic effect) and stimulation of the $\beta_1$-receptors in the myocardium increases the force of cardiac contractility (a positive inotropic effect).

2 *Kidney*: Stimulation of β-receptors in the kidney promotes the release of renin from the juxtaglomerular cells and thereby increases the activity of the renin–angiotensin aldosterone system.

3 *Central and peripheral nervous system*: Stimulation of β-receptors in the brainstem and stimulation of prejunctional β-receptors in the periphery promote the release of neurotransmitters and increased sympathetic nervous system activity.

β-Adrenoceptors are also found in the eye. $\beta_2$-Receptors control the formation of aqueous humour, and beta-blockers applied topically to the eye are used in the treatment of glaucoma. Beta-blockers may block both $\beta_1$-receptors (selective or cardioselective) and blockers.

### Clinical pharmacology

Beta-blockers vary in the extent to which they are eliminated via the kidney or via the liver, usually with extensive first-pass metabolism (Table 5.3). The lipid-soluble beta-blockers, such as propranolol, typically depend upon hepatic metabolism for their clearance, whereas the relatively water-soluble beta-blockers, e.g. atenolol, are eliminated via the kidney. Propranolol is often quoted as a reference example of a drug that undergoes extensive first-pass hepatic metabolism: this is flow-limited because it is directly dependent upon hepatic blood flow (see Chapter 1, p. 7). Thus, particularly for drugs eliminated by the liver, a wide range of doses will be required in clinical practice because of the wide inter-individual variability in bioavailability combined with the inter-individual variability in response. The half-life of most beta-blockers is relatively short: those which depend upon the liver usually require multiple daily dosing, whereas those eliminated via the kidney tend to have longer half-lives and may be suitable for once-daily administration, particularly at high doses.

**Table 5.3** Examples of the pharmacological properties and route of elimination of some beta-blockers in clinical use.

| Clinical class | Approved name | $\beta_1$—Selectivity | Major route of elimination |
|---|---|---|---|
| *Non-selective* | Propranolol | – | Liver |
| *Selective* | Atenolol | ++ | Kidney |
| Bisoprolol | ++ | Liver/kidney | |
| Metoprolol | ++ | Liver | |
| *Additional properties* | | | |
| Intrinsic sympathomimetic activity (also, partial agonist activity) | Pindolol | – | Liver |
| Anti-arrhythmic properties | Sotalol | – | Liver |
| Dual antihypertensive mechanism | Labetalol | – | Liver |

## Pharmacologically predictable adverse effects of $\beta$-receptor blockade

### Bradycardia and impairment of myocardial contractility

An excessive reduction in heart rate and bradycardia is relatively common but seldom symptomatic. Rarely, an excessive reduction in inotropic activity may precipitate or exacerbate cardiac failure in a susceptible individual. Whilst these depressant effects on cardiac function are occasionally deleterious, they also lead to a reduction in cardiac work and a reduction in myocardial oxygen demand which contributes to the anti-anginal efficacy of these agents (see Chapter 7). Although acutely beta-blockers can worsen left ventricular dysfunction, there is now good evidence that, under specialist supervision, $\beta$-adrenoceptor antagonists may improve symptoms and prolong survival in patients with congestive heart failure.

### Peripheral vasoconstriction

The $\beta_2$-receptors in the smooth muscle of peripheral blood vessels subserve a vasodilator role, especially in skeletal muscle beds, and blockade of these receptors leads to a relative vasoconstriction which typically gives rise to impairment of the peripheral circulation with cold hands and feet and, possibly, also the development of Raynaud's phenomenon or the worsening of peripheral vascular disease. This is usually a problem only in critical ischaemia. Because of unnecessary concerns, many patients have been denied the benefits of beta-blockers.

### CNS effects

Blockade of CNS $\beta$-receptors is associated with reduced sympathetic outflow, which is the probable cause of a sense of malaise which may occur insidiously during long-term treatment. Additionally, vivid dreams, nightmares and, rarely, hallucinations may occur with highly lipid-soluble beta-blockers, and propranolol in particular, because of their greater penetration into the CNS.

### Bronchospasm

$\beta_2$-Receptors mediate dilatation of the bronchi, and blockade of these receptors may precipitate bronchospasm in susceptible individuals. Asthma is an absolute contraindication for all beta-blockers which should be used with caution in chronic obstructive pulmonary disease with significant reversibility. In patients with less severe chest disease, beta-blockers can be used without concern.

### Tiredness and fatigue

Stimulation of $\beta_2$-receptors in skeletal muscle is associated with increased muscle activity and blockade of these receptors leads to a sense of tiredness and ready fatigue during exercise.

### Masking of hypoglycaemia

The awareness of hypoglycaemia in the insulin-dependent diabetic depends partly upon sympathetic nervous activation. This response will be blunted by beta-blockers. This effort is marginal with cardioselective beta-blockers.

### Metabolic disturbances

Beta-blockers, especially non-selective agents, increase triglycerides and reduce HDL cholesterol. Beta-blockers in long-term use increase the frequency of diabetes mellitus.

## Additional pharmacological characteristics

1 Partial agonist activity (sometimes known as intrinsic sympathomimetic activity) manifests as a beta-stimulant effect when background adrenergic activity is minimal (e.g. during sleep) but the drug's beta-blocker effect manifests when adrenergic activity is increased (e.g. during exercise).

2 Membrane-stabilising activity: This is a local anaesthetic and anti-arrhythmic effect.

3 Selectivity: The prototype beta-blocker, propranolol, is non-selective as it blocks the responses mediated via both $\beta_1$- and $\beta_2$-receptors. Because many of the potential adverse effects are mediated through $\beta_2$-receptors and many of the desirable effects require blockade of $\beta_1$-receptors in the heart, there has been the development of relatively $\beta_1$-selective (or cardioselective) blockers. It is important to recognise, however, that this selectivity is not absolute. Selectivity is lost at high doses.

4 Additional pharmacological properties: It is possible to augment the beta-blocker molecule

with an ability to also block effects mediated through peripheral $\alpha$-adrenoceptors (e.g. labetalol and carvedilol) or to harness some $\beta_2$-agonist or direct vasodilator activity (e.g. celiprolol).

*Clinical comment.* All beta-blockers, irrespective of their additional characteristics, lower blood pressure to a similar extent. In hypertension those which are $\beta_1$-selective (cardioselective) and which can be administered once daily tend to be preferred, e.g. bisoprolol 10 mg daily, atenolol 25–100 mg daily. Irrespective of their apparent 'cardioselectivity', these drugs are contraindicated in people with asthma and should be introduced with caution in patients at risk of cardiac failure.

In addition to use in hypertension, beta-blockers are also used to treat the following conditions: supraventricular cardiac arrhythmias, angina pectoris, anxiety neurosis, thyrotoxicosis, migraine and glaucoma. There is also some evidence that prophylactic treatment with propranolol reduces the risk of gastrointestinal (GI) bleeding among patients with chronic liver disease and proven oesophageal varices.

## Calcium antagonists

### Mechanism of action

Increased peripheral vascular resistance depends upon increased constrictor 'tone' in peripheral blood vessels, which, in turn, reflects increased contractility of vascular smooth muscle. This process is calcium-dependent, and calcium antagonists (calcium entry blockers) are able to promote vasodilator activity by reducing calcium influx into the cell by interfering with the voltage-operated calcium channels (and to a lesser extent the receptor-operated channels) in the cell membrane of vascular smooth muscle.

Interference with intracellular calcium influx is also important in cardiac muscle, cardiac conducting tissue and the smooth muscle of the GI tract. Thus, the potential cardiac effects of calcium antagonism are negative inotropic, chronotropic and dromotropic activities and the GI effects lead to constipation. These effects vary with different agents according to the ability to penetrate cardiac and other tissues and, in particular, because the

receptor or recognition site close to the calcium channel is slightly different for each drug class.

Thus, although they are often considered as a single class, there are structural and functional distinctions to be made between the three principal types of calcium antagonist drug:

1 Dihydropyridine derivatives: nifedipine, amlodipine

2 Phenylalkalamines: verapamil

3 Benzothiazipine derivatives: diltiazem

The dihydropyridine derivatives have pronounced peripheral vasodilator properties, whereas verapamil and diltiazem also have cardiac effects and reduce heart rate.

### Clinical pharmacology

Most of these agents have low and variable oral bioavailability because all are subject to extensive first-pass metabolism. The exception is amlodipine which, although it is extensively metabolised, has a substantially longer half-life (more than 40 h compared to less than 10 h) (see Table 5.4).

Both diltiazem and verapamil have short half-lives because of extensive first-pass metabolism. During chronic treatment they have a tendency to inhibit hepatic drug metabolism and therefore their own half-lives during steady-state treatment are slightly longer than those following the first dose. This enzyme inhibitory effect is a potential source for drug interactions, e.g. with ciclosporin.

### Pharmacologically predictable adverse effects

1 *Dihydropyridines*: These, particularly with rapid onset and short-acting agents, have a well-recognised pattern of vasodilator side effects with headache and facial flushing and an associated reflex activation of the sympathetic nervous system which provokes cardioacceleration and palpitations. These symptoms usually decline with time. Longer acting agents and the longer acting formulations are less likely to promote these acute vasodilator effects. Swelling of the ankles and occasionally of the hands is a long-term effect of the dihydropyridine derivatives, including the long-acting agents. This does not appear to be attributable to a generalised fluid retention and

**Table 5.4** Clinical classification of calcium antagonist drugs.

| Drugs | | Half-life (h) | Dosing frequency |
|---|---|---|---|
| *Dihydropyridines* | | | |
| Short-acting | Nifedipine | 4–6 | Multiple* |
| | Nicardipine | 4–6 | |
| Intermediate | Isradipine | 8–12 | Once or twice daily |
| Long-acting | Amlodipine | >40 | Once |
| | Nifedipine | (Special formulation) | Once |
| *Verapamil* | | 8–12 | Multiple* |
| *Diltiazem* | | 6–10 | Multiple* |

* Unless special formulation.

instead reflects a drug-related disturbance of the haemodynamics of the microcirculation in the periphery, plus the effect of gravity.

**2** *Verapamil*: The early onset vasodilator effects are less common with verapamil but the cardiac effects may manifest as bradycardia or atrioventricular (AV) conduction delay. Constipation is a well-recognised symptomatic complaint.

**3** *Diltiazem*: The early vasodilator effects are again less apparent but bradycardia and AV conduction effects are recognised. Skin rash occurs occasionally.

*Clinical comment.* All types of calcium-antagonist drugs are effective antihypertensive agents because of their peripheral vasodilator activity. The long-acting dihydropyridine drugs, such as amlodipine or others in long-acting once-daily formulations are generally preferred in the treatment of hypertension. The negative cardiac effects of diltiazem and verapamil lead to reduced myocardial oxygen demand such that these drugs tend to be the preferred types of calcium antagonist as monotherapy in angina (see Chapter 7). Dihydropyridine calcium antagonists may be useful in elderly patients with isolated systolic hypertension.

## ACE inhibitors

### Mechanism of action

ACE inhibitors inhibit competitively the activity of angiotensin-converting enzyme (which is also termed kininase II) to prevent the formation of the active octapeptide angiotensin II from its inactive precursor, angiotensin I. This occurs in blood and in tissues including the kidney, heart, blood vessels, adrenal gland and brain. Angiotensin II has a range of activities but most importantly it is a potent vasoconstrictor, it promotes aldosterone release and it facilitates sympathetic activity both centrally and peripherally. Whilst the reduction in blood pressure following ACE inhibition is greatest in patients with a stimulated renin–angiotensin system (such as in sodium depletion, or diuretic treatment, or renal artery stenosis or malignant phase hypertension), it is now recognised that ACE inhibitors also lower blood pressure in essential hypertensive patients with normal or low activity of the renin–angiotensin system.

The enzyme, kininase II, is also responsible for the breakdown of kinins that have vasodilator and other properties. Inhibition of ACE leads to an accumulation of kinins including bradykinin which promotes vasodilator activity and may make a contribution to the overall effectiveness of ACE inhibitor drugs.

### Clinical pharmacology

All ACE inhibitor drugs are bound to tissues and plasma proteins and this gives rise to a characteristic concentration–time profile whereby free drug is relatively rapidly eliminated by the kidney, predominantly by glomerular filtration, such that there is little evidence of drug accumulation during chronic dosing. However, because of the binding to tissue sites the plasma drug concentration–time profile shows a long-lasting terminal elimination phase of several days.

**Table 5.5** Drugs acting on the renin–angiotensin system.

| ACE inhibitors | Typical dose regimens |
|---|---|
| *First generation* | |
| Captopril | 25 mg two or three times daily |
| Enalapril | 5–20 mg once or twice daily |
| Lisinopril | 5–20 mg once daily |
| *Second generation* | |
| Fosinopril | 10–20 mg once daily |
| Perindopril | 2–4 mg once daily |
| Quinapril | 20–40 mg once or twice daily |
| Ramipril | 2.5–5 mg daily |
| Trandolapril | 1–2 mg daily |

There are significant pharmacological differences between the ACE inhibitors. For example, the prototype drug captopril is absorbed rapidly but has a short duration of action and is usually administered twice or thrice daily. Enalapril, like many of the other later ACE inhibitors, is an inactive pro-drug that requires hydrolysis in vivo of the parent ester to its active acid form enalaprilat. Lisinopril is an analogue of enalapril and is itself active (see Table 5.5).

ACE inhibitors also vary in efficacy and duration of action with some but not others more suitable for once-daily dosing.

The dose–response relationship for blood pressure reduction is linear initially, but a 'plateau' is quickly reached within the therapeutic dose range; further increases in dosage do not increase the intensity of effect, either on blood pressure reduction or on plasma ACE inhibition, but prolong the duration of action. The fall in blood pressure following ACE inhibition is not associated with a change in heart rate; in particular, there is no reflex tachycardia.

## Pharmacologically predictable adverse effects

*Profound hypotension* may complicate the first dose of ACE inhibitor drugs especially in patients with sodium or volume depletion in whom the renin–angiotensin system is activated. Hypotension occurs only rarely in uncomplicated essential hypertension but is more common in patients with cardiac failure.

*Impairment of renal function* is recognised particularly in patients with renovascular disease (bilateral renal artery stenosis). Reversible renal failure may be precipitated. However, ACE inhibitors can protect renal function in patients with chronic renal failure and hypertension.

*Cough* is the most frequent adverse effect and is probably attributable to the effect on the kinin system rather than upon ACE inhibition as it does not occur with angiotensin receptor antagonists (see later). A non-productive, irritant cough is widely reported in the treatment of hypertension in about 15% of patients. The reported incidence is considerably less in patients with cardiac failure, presumably as a reflection of their much higher background incidence of respiratory symptoms.

### Other adverse effects

Angioneurotic oedema is a rare but well-recognised class effect that also has been attributed to the kinin potentiation. Increases in serum potassium and, occasionally, hyperkalaemia occur because ACE inhibitors have potassium-saving effects (mediated via the reduction in aldosterone). Taste disturbance and skin rash occur more frequently with captopril.

*Clinical comment.* Although many of these agents are recommended for once-daily dosing, for some such as enalapril, a more consistent response is produced by twice-daily administration. In elderly patients, or in patients with compromised renal function, or in patients with cardiac failure, it is advisable to initiate treatment with lower than usual dosages. In general these drugs are well tolerated by patients. ACE inhibitor drugs combine well with thiazide diuretics, and with calcium antagonists, to produce overall antihypertensive effects that are additive. However, it is recommended that potassium supplements and potassium-sparing diuretics should not be used in combination because hyperkalaemia may result, especially if there is pre-existing renal impairment. Since the effectiveness of ACE inhibitors in both hypertension and cardiac failure may be compromised by non-steroidal anti-inflammatory drugs (NSAIDs), if possible, NSAIDs should be avoided in these patients.

ACE inhibitors (and angiotensin receptor antagonists) are associated with a lower (25–30%) incidence of new onset diabetes compared to other classes.

## Angiotensin (AT$_1$) receptor antagonists

Angiotensin II receptors are subclassified into two subtypes, AT$_1$ and AT$_2$. The AT$_1$-receptor mediates all of the classical pharmacological effects of angiotensin II, e.g. vasoconstriction and aldosterone release, whereas the functional role of the AT$_2$-receptor remains unclear. Because many tissues contain enzymatic pathways capable of converting angiotensin I to angiotensin II, independently of ACE, there are theoretical advantages in blocking the renin–angiotensin system via AT$_1$-receptor antagonism. Losartan was the first AT$_1$-receptor antagonist; irbesartan, valsartan, candesartan and others have followed (Table 5.6). All are well absorbed after oral administration but differ slightly in their pharmacokinetic and pharmacodynamic properties. Losartan is converted to an active metabolite, EXP 3174; candesartan is the active metabolite of the pro-drug candesartan cilexetil. Irbesartan, valsartan, candesartan and EXP 3174 bind to the AT$_1$-receptor in a manner which is competitive but only slowly surmountable, so the duration of blood pressure lowering effect is longer than the apparent half-life of the drug.

The angiotensin II antagonists produce reductions in blood pressure similar to ACE inhibitors

and other antihypertensive classes, but they seem to be particularly well tolerated with very few side effects. Because AT$_1$-receptor antagonists do not influence kinin metabolism, these drugs are not associated with the dry cough seen with ACE inhibitors. Angiotensin II antagonists may also offer additional benefit to patients with type II diabetes complicated by hypertension and nephropathy and can be useful in congestive heart failure together with ACE inhibitors or in ACE I in tolerant patients. Like ACE inhibitor treatment, regimens based on AT$_1$-receptor antagonists reduce the risk of new onset diabetes. Since diabetes carries a huge risk of long-term cardiovascular complications, this is likely to represent a major advantage for drugs that block the renin–angiotensin system.

## $\alpha_1$-Antagonists

Prazosin and doxazosin act via selective blockade of peripheral $\alpha_1$-adrenoceptors to produce their vasodilator effects but they are not widely used first-line agents. Instead they tend to be used as third-line agents or where other drugs are poorly tolerated.

Alpha-blockers may be associated with a 'first dose' hypotensive effect that constitutes a postural fall in blood pressure after the initial dosage, accompanied by reflex cardioacceleration and palpitations. In susceptible patients who cannot maintain a rapid heart rate there is the risk of a vago–vagal collapse leading to syncope. This first-dose effect was particularly associated with the short-acting prototype agent prazosin and is much less of a problem with longer acting agents such as doxazosin.

**Table 5.6** Angiotensin II (AT$_1$) receptor antagonists used in hypertension.

| Drug | Pro-drug | Route of elimination | Half-life (h) |
|------|----------|---------------------|---------------|
| Losartan | Yes | Hepatic | 6–9 |
| Valsartan | No | Unchanged in urine | 6 |
| Irbesartan | No | Hepatic | 15–17 |
| Candesartan Cilexetil | Yes | Hepatic | 6–12 |

## Centrally acting agents

Agents acting on $\alpha_2$-adrenoceptors, or related imidazoline receptors in the brainstem, reduce sympathetic outflow and lead to a reduction in blood pressure.

Clonidine is an $\alpha_2$-adrenoceptor agonist that can cause sedation and drowsiness, dry mouth and interference with sexual function in men. In addition, this agent may give rise to a rebound hypertensive syndrome on abrupt cessation of treatment at high dose, presumably as a consequence of receptor up-regulation.

$\alpha$-Methyldopa, which acts via its active metabolite $\alpha$-methylnoradrenaline, has a profile similar to that of clonidine but in addition is known to give rise to immunological side effects, including pyrexia, hepatitis and, rarely, haemolytic anaemia.

These centrally acting agents are no longer used widely because of poor side effect profiles (particularly CNS depressant effects) and because of the development of newer, comparably effective but better-tolerated alternative agents. However, $\alpha$-methyldopa is still used to treat hypertension in pregnancy, especially where hypertension precedes pregnancy or is identified in the first or middle trimester. This is justified by the long-term experience of fetal and maternal safety. More recently centrally acting agents have been developed which preferentially bind to imidazoline binding sites in brain. Agents such as moxonidine are reported to have fewer adverse effects although dry mouth remains a problem; moxonidine is used mainly as third-line therapy. These drugs have not been studied in long-term outcome trials.

## Hypertensive emergencies

There are no indications for the rapid (within seconds or minutes) reduction of blood pressure, even where there is severe hypertension and related complications. However, there are some indications for the controlled and progressive reduction of blood pressure (over a period of a few hours) when accelerated or malignant phase hypertension is complicated by hypertensive encephalopathy or acute left ventricular failure, or in other situations such as dissection of the aorta or in eclampsia of pregnancy.

In severe cases, with the above complications, there may be grounds for intravenous treatment that is titrated to produce a gradual and progressive reduction in blood pressure. The preferred agents are glyceryl trinitrate or sodium nitroprusside by infusion where the rate of the infusion can be controlled, minute by minute, according to the blood pressure response. The infusion of glyceryl trinitrate is not associated with significant adverse effects beyond those predicted by the blood pressure reduction, but with sodium nitroprusside there is the additional potential complication of thiocyanate accumulation and cyanide poisoning, especially in patients with impaired renal function. For this reason, and especially with sodium nitroprusside, these manoeuvres should only be undertaken in the setting of an intensive care unit with appropriate monitoring facilities.

## Cholesterol and lipids

### Aim

The overall aim of lipid-modifying treatment is to reduce the circulating levels of atherogenic lipids in order to slow, reverse or ideally prevent the development of atherosclerotic vascular lesions and thereby reduce the long-term risk of cardiovascular disease.

### Relevant pathophysiology

Cholesterol is a major component of lipid-containing atherosclerotic plaques. Raised plasma levels of cholesterol—and related lipid disturbances—have been identified as a major risk factor (along with smoking and hypertension) for atherosclerotic cardiovascular disease and its consequences, particularly myocardial infarction. Cholesterol is derived both from the diet and by endogenous synthesis in the liver and it is a component of all cell membranes, a precursor of steroid hormones and bile salts, and of glycoproteins and quinones.

The biochemistry and metabolism of cholesterol are complex. Cholesterol, and other lipid fractions, are transported in blood via lipoproteins of different densities. Increased total cholesterol and its major component fraction, LDL cholesterol, have been linked to accelerated atherosclerosis and increased coronary artery disease. LDL cholesterol is cleared from the circulation by specific receptors on the cell surface and the function of these receptors plays an important role in determining the plasma levels of LDL cholesterol. In contrast, HDL cholesterol appears to have a protective and anti-atherogenic effect because it is involved in the mobilisation of cholesterol from tissues and its transportation back to the liver.

## Primary and secondary lipid disorders

Disorders of lipid metabolism occur as primary conditions that may be familial or polygenic in origin, or secondary to an underlying disease state or drug treatment.

### Familial hypercholesterolaemia

Very high levels of LDL cholesterol occur in this rare genetic disease which involves the failure to express LDL receptors. It is inherited as an autosomal dominant condition such that homozygotes have no LDL receptors and heterozygotes have only 50% of the normal number of LDL receptors. In this condition LDL cholesterol (and therefore total cholesterol) is very high, and in the homozygotes there will be no response to drug treatments that exert their lipid-lowering effects via the up-regulation of LDL receptors. In such patients it may be necessary to remove cholesterol by physical techniques such as apheresis using LDL affinity columns.

### Polygenic lipid disorders

This is by far the most common type of primary lipid disorder and reflects a variety of factors including a non-specific genetic predisposition, dietary factors such as high calorie and saturated fat intake and lifestyle influences including physical inactivity. In the most common pattern there are moderate increases in LDL and total cholesterol. This is the commonest lipid disorder found in westernised populations. In part, the disturbed

lipid profile reflects down-regulation of LDL receptors.

### Secondary lipid disorders

These manifest as mixed elevations of cholesterol and triglycerides in response to underlying diseases such as hypothyroidism nephritic syndrome and diabetes mellitus, as a manifestation of chronic alcohol abuse, or in response to drug treatments such as thiazide diuretics and beta-blockers.

### Risks of hypercholesterolaemia

The central role of cholesterol in the development of atheroma and atherosclerotic cardiovascular disease is well established. The epidemiological evidence from population studies in different countries and from within the same country identify clear associations between both LDL and total cholesterol and the development of cardiovascular disease, particularly CHD. There are also weaker associations with elevated triglycerides and an inverse relationship with HDL cholesterol.

### Benefits of lipid-lowering treatment

A number of large placebo-controlled randomised clinical trials have been performed to examine the effects of cholesterol-lowering therapy in the primary and secondary prevention of cardiovascular disease. Primary prevention refers to patients who might have one or more cardiovascular risk factors, but in whom overt atherosclerotic disease has not presented clinically. Secondary prevention refers to those patients who have, for example, suffered an acute myocardial infarction or who have angina or intermittent claudication. Clinical trials using statins to lower cholesterol have shown 30–40% reductions in coronary heart disease events in both primary and secondary prevention studies. Cholesterol-lowering therapy also reduces the risk of stroke. The absolute benefits of treatment are proportional to the magnitude of cholesterol reduction and the pre-treatment cardiovascular risk in an individual patient.

## Principles of lipid-lowering treatment

1 Detection: Hypercholesterolaemia can be identified in patients at risk by the measurement of total cholesterol in a non-fasting blood sample. Although a more accurate assessment of the lipid profile can be obtained from a fasting blood sample that can be subfractionated to measure the triglyceride concentration and the HDL and LDL cholesterol fractions, random not fasting lipids are increasingly used to guide treatment in practice.

2 Patients should be counselled about hypercholesterolaemia, and its risk, and the relevance of other concomitant risk factors. The reason for long-term treatment should be carefully explained.

3 Hypercholesterolaemia should be treated as part of a management plan for reducing all identifiable cardiovascular risk factors in the 'at risk' patient and management decision based on overall cardiovascular risk assessment.

4 Secondary types of lipid disorder: These should be identified in order to undertake the specific treatment and management for the underlying condition. Thus, further investigations should be undertaken to exclude significant renal or hepatic disease, hypothyroidism, diabetes mellitus, or alcohol abuse or relevant drug treatments.

5 Non-pharmacological treatment should always be used initially and this centres around dietary modification.

## Lipid-lowering treatment

### Dietary and lifestyle advice

The principles of dietary advice revolve around the reduced intake of saturated animal fats and, in the obese patient, a reduced total calorie intake. In addition, it is desirable to increase the intake of unsaturated fats and, where possible, increase the level of physical activity. Ideally, dietary modification should be planned in discussion with the partner, or other members of the family, and it should take account of some of the social, cultural and economic circumstances of each patient. In a compliant and motivated patient total cholesterol may be reduced by about 10% within a few months of adherence to dietary modification, but in the long term, it is unusual for patients to be able to maintain or exceed this magnitude of change.

## Lipid-lowering drugs

There are several different drugs available for cholesterol reduction and modification of the plasma lipid profile. The major classes in widespread use include 3-hydroxy-3-methoxygluteryl coenzyme A (HMG CoA) reductase inhibitors ('statins'), fibrates, and bile acid sequestrant resins (see Table 5.7).

## HMG CoA reductase inhibitors

### Mechanisms

HMG CoA reductase is the rate-limiting enzyme in the hepatic synthesis of cholesterol and inhibition leads to reduced cholesterol production and, as a consequence, an attempt by the liver to compensate by increasing its extraction of LDL cholesterol from plasma by up-regulating its LDL cholesterol receptors. The principal effect, therefore, is a reduction of LDL cholesterol (and, thereby, total cholesterol) by up to 40%, and there are only modest effects on the other lipid fractions. Some statin drugs also lower triglyceride levels by 15%.

**Table 5.7** Summary of the actions of lipid-lowering drugs.

| Drug | LDL | HDL | Triglycerides |
|---|---|---|---|
| HMG CoA reductase inhibitors | ↓↓ | ↑ | → |
| Fibrates | ↓ | ↑ | ↓ |
| Resins | ↓ | → | → |
| Others | | | |
|   Nicotinic acid | ↓ | ↑ | ↓ |
|   Probucol | ↓ | ↓ | → |

Because cholesterol is synthesised mainly during sleep, these drugs are usually administered at night. HMG CoA reductase inhibitors comprise the family of 'statins'—simvastatin, pravastatin, atorvastatin, fluvastatin and rosuvastatin. While the statins clearly have a major action via lowering LDL cholesterol, there are increasing indications that other mechanisms particularly anti-inflammatory effect may also be important in stabilising atheroma plaques and reducing cardiovascular events.

Side effects reported include headache, GI symptoms and non-cardiac chest pain. Raised liver enzymes can also occur. Rarely rash and hypersensitivity reactions have been reported. The most troublesome side effects are myalgia, muscle cramps and occasionally life-threatening rhabdomyolysis. These symptoms are more common at higher doses and when statin is combined with fibrates, nicotinic acid or immunosuppressants. In severe cases the creatinine kinase in blood is raised.

*Clinical comment.* The impressive clinical evidence from large randomised clinical trials that statin therapy reduces cardiovascular mortality and morbidity in both primary and secondary prevention has led to a dramatic increase in prescribing. From a public health and cost-effectiveness perspective, the challenge has been to target statin therapy at the higher risk patients, i.e. those who will benefit most from cholesterol reduction. Current guidelines in the United Kingdom advocate statin therapy regardless of total cholesterol levels following an acute myocardial infarction and for those patients with angina. For primary prevention the strategy has been to advocate statin therapy for patients who have an absolute risk of a cardiovascular event of 2% or more per year (20% 10-year risk). Various tables have been produced to allow clinicians to quickly risk-stratify an individual patient by entering basic clinical information, e.g. age, smoking status, cholesterol level and blood pressure. Thus, the decision to initiate statin therapy for primary prevention is not based solely on the level of cholesterol, but also on an overall clinical assessment of an individual patient's absolute cardiovascular risk. This approach is supported by the results of prospective studies like the Heart Protection Study which confirmed the benefit of a statin across a wide (including 'normal') range of cholesterol in high-risk patients.

## Fibrates

These drugs lower LDL cholesterol by about 20% and they also cause a significant reduction in total triglycerides and an increase in HDL cholesterol. They have a number of effects on lipid metabolism including the activation of lipoprotein lipase to promote lipolysis of triglyceride-rich particles, which reduces the levels of triglyceride, and they may also inhibit HMG CoA reductase and promote a consequential up-regulation of LDL receptor activity. Bezafibrate and gemfibrozil are examples of fibrates in widespread use and there is evidence (with gemfibrozil) that CHD events can be reduced as part of a primary prevention strategy. As a group, these drugs are absorbed completely from the GI tract and are excreted largely unchanged via the kidney, but are liable to cause GI side effects and there is potential for drug interactions, most notably with oral anticoagulants.

The side effects most commonly associated with fibrates are GI upsets, headaches, fatigue and skin reactions. Less commonly, muscle cramps and loss of libido are reported. The fibrates as a class are thought to increase bile lithogenicity and, although this has not been conclusively demonstrated with the modern agents, these drugs should be regarded as relatively contraindicated in those patients with gall bladder disease or with a strong family history of gallstones.

## Bile acid sequestrant resins

Resins such as colestyramine are not absorbed from the GI tract and as a consequence bind bile salts to prevent their normal enterohepatic recirculation. Hence, hepatic cholesterol synthesis increases and the receptor-mediated uptake of LDL cholesterol from plasma is also increased. The resins primarily lower LDL cholesterol and total cholesterol with associated small increases in HDL cholesterol but no effect on triglycerides. The adverse GI effects of the resins cause major symptomatic problems that few patients are able to tolerate when large doses are administered. For this reason, there is also a significant incidence of poor compliance or non-compliance. The taste and texture of the resins are unpleasant. Symptomatic adverse effects are confined to the GI tract with dyspepsia, flatulence and altered bowel habit.

Use with statins may increase the risk of cramps and myositis.

## Ezetimibe

This agent blocks intestinal absorption of cholesterol and can augment the effects of statin if given in combination. It may also be useful where statin is contraindicated or not tolerated in high doses. This agent appears to be better tolerated than bile acid sequestrants.

## Other lipid-lowering drugs

Nicotinic acid and its derivatives are potent inhibitors of LDL and VLDL formation; probucol lowers LDL cholesterol but also inhibits the production of HDL cholesterol, although the significance of this latter effect remains to be established.

Fish oils, high in unsaturated fatty acids, are particularly useful for reducing excessively high triglyceride concentrations. Both omega-3 acid ethyl esters and marine triglycerides are available.

## Antiplatelet drugs

### Approach to the management of thrombosis

Both antiplatelet drugs and anticoagulants are effective in prevention of arterial, cardiac and venous thromboembolism. Antiplatelet drugs are preferred for routine cardiovascular prevention, because they are less likely to cause excessive bleeding. However, anticoagulants are more effective in treatment of venous thromboembolism and peripheral arterial embolism and are indicated in

specific circumstances such as atrial fibrillation. Thrombolytic agents have a main role in the treatment of acute thrombotic arterial occlusion, especially coronary thrombosis. Anticoagulants, heparin products and thrombolytics are described in Chapter 17.

There are many potential targets for drug action in the biochemical pathways involved in platelet activation. Aspirin is cheap and effective and has been the drug of choice; clopidogrel and dipyridamole are other options.

## Aspirin

### Pharmacology

All of the pharmacological effects of aspirin (acetylsalicylic acid) are based upon inhibition of prostaglandin synthesis. Aspirin is used as an antiplatelet drug in doses lower than those employed for analgesia. Aspirin acetylates and inactivates cyclo-oxygenase, a key enzyme in the platelet biosynthetic pathway for the pro-aggregatory prostaglandin thromboxane $A_2$. The interaction of aspirin with cyclo-oxygenase is irreversible. As platelets are anucleate, recovery of thromboxane synthesis is dependent on the appearance of a new platelet population in the circulation. Recovery from the effects of aspirin therefore takes about 10 days. Aspirin also inhibits endothelial cyclo-oxygenase, in this case leading to a reduction in prostacyclin synthesis, an effect that would be theoretically undesirable. A predominant effect on thromboxane synthesis is achieved because the endothelium can regenerate cyclo-oxygenase activity. Differential sensitivity of the platelet and endothelial enzymes, and pre-systemic hydrolysis of aspirin, limiting endothelial exposure to active drug, may also contribute to the achievement of some selectivity of action (see below). The lower the dose of aspirin, the greater the differential effect; but no dose at which useful inhibition of thromboxane synthesis is achieved is absolutely selective. In practice, aspirin doses of 75–300 mg/day appear as effective as higher doses in thrombosis prevention, and have fewer GI side effects.

## Effects on haemostasis

Administration of aspirin results in prolongation of the skin bleeding time and a characteristic defect on testing platelet aggregation in the laboratory. As would be expected, coagulation tests are unaltered by aspirin. Very large doses of aspirin, e.g. in overdose, can, however, lead to a variable prolongation of the prothrombin time.

## Pharmacokinetics

Aspirin, in standard formulation, is rapidly absorbed from the upper GI tract including both the stomach and duodenum. Slow-release formulations are available which have delayed and incomplete absorption characteristics. Aspirin undergoes extensive pre-systemic hydrolysis to salicylate. Platelet cyclo-oxygenase may therefore be irreversibly inhibited as platelets pass through the portal circulation, whilst the endothelium on the systemic side of the circulation is exposed to smaller concentrations of active aspirin.

## Clinical use of aspirin

Low-dose aspirin has been shown to be clinically beneficial in acute myocardial infarction, unstable angina and acute ischaemic stroke; in the secondary prevention of arterial thrombosis; and in prevention of arterial, venous and cardiac thrombosis in persons at increased risk (see Table 5.8). There are several general points of importance.

**Table 5.8** Clinical conditions in which low-dose aspirin is of proven benefit.

| |
| --- |
| Myocardial infarction (acute and chronic) |
| Unstable angina |
| Ischaemic stroke (acute and chronic) |
| Transient cerebral ischaemia |
| Peripheral vascular arterial disease |
| Post-coronary artery bypass graft |
| Post-peripheral arterial surgery |
| Atrial fibrillation |
| Prophylaxis of venous thromboembolism |
| Primary prevention of cardiovascular disease in high-risk patients (e.g. risk ≥2% per year) |

1 'Low-dose' aspirin refers to a range of doses from 75 to 300 mg daily. Doses less than 100 mg require several days to produce their full effects on thromboxane synthesis. Hence a loading dose of 150–300 mg/day is given in acute myocardial infarction, unstable angina and acute ischaemic stroke.

2 Presentation with one form of arterial disease is often associated with risk of another form of vascular disease on which aspirin may have an impact. For example, treatment of a patient with a transient ischaemic attack reduces not only the risk of ischaemic stroke, but also of myocardial infarction and death from other vascular causes.

3 In acute myocardial infarction, it has been shown that administration of aspirin has additive effects with streptokinase in reduction of mortality.

4 Cerebral haemorrhage should be excluded by brain scanning before administering (or continuing) aspirin to a patient presenting with a stroke.

5 In patients with acute ischaemic stroke who are unable to swallow, aspirin may be given per rectum.

## Adverse effects of aspirin

### Gastric erosions and GI bleeding

1 GI toxicity constitutes the main adverse effect of aspirin. This includes dyspepsia, ulceration and GI bleeding (one excess major bleed per 500 patient-years use). It is related to inhibition of prostaglandin synthesis in the GI tract as well as to the antiplatelet effects of aspirin. The GI effects are dose related, and incidence is reduced but not eliminated by the use of lower doses.

2 Hypersensitivity reactions.

3 Precipitation of asthma.

4 Precipitation of renal failure, especially in patients with renal artery stenosis and in patients taking ACE inhibitor drugs.

5 Intracranial haemorrhage (one per 2500 patient-years).

## Contraindications

1 Peptic ulcer or GI haemorrhage

2 Underlying bleeding disorders, congenital or acquired (including anticoagulant therapy)

3 Severe renal or hepatic impairment
4 Known hypersensitivity to aspirin
5 Intracranial haemorrhage or aneurysm
6 Uncontrolled hypertension (risk of intracranial haemorrhage).

## Clopidogrel

Clopidogrel is a recently introduced antiplatelet drug that has a different mechanism of action on platelets to aspirin. It has an active metabolite that irreversibly modifies the platelet ADP receptor, reducing the aggregability of platelets for the remainder of their lifespan. A dose of 75 mg/day is used clinically, which reduces platelet aggregability and prolongs the skin bleeding time to a similar extent as low-dose aspirin (75–300 mg/day). A recent large study showed that clopidogrel was at least as effective as aspirin in reducing the risk of arterial thrombosis in patients with recent myocardial infarction, recent ischaemic stroke, or chronic peripheral arterial disease. Clopidogrel was also as safe as aspirin, with a lower risk of dyspepsia and GI bleeding, but a higher risk of diarrhoea and skin rash. As it is expensive than aspirin, the main indication is secondary prevention of arterial thrombosis in patients who are intolerant of aspirin or in whom aspirin is contraindicated. The combination of clopidogrel and aspirin appears more effective than aspirin alone (or anticoagulants) in prevention of thrombosis following coronary angioplasty with stenting. Clopidogrel has replaced the related drug, ticlopidine, which has a significant risk of neutropenia requiring monitoring of the white blood cell count.

## Dipyridamole

Dipyridamole is a vasodilator drug that provokes myocardial ischaemia and is used in cardiac stress testing: it is therefore contraindicated in patients with angina. It was observed to reduce platelet aggregation in whole blood but not in plasma: it may act by reducing red blood cell uptake of adenosine, a circulating endogenous platelet inhibitor. Dipyridamole (100 mg thrice daily, or 200 mg sustained release twice daily) appears similarly effective to aspirin in secondary prevention of stroke, but has been less extensively evaluated, is more expensive and has vasodilator side effects including headache. It may be used in secondary prevention of stroke or transient cerebral ischaemia in patients who are intolerant of aspirin or in whom aspirin is contraindicated. Whether or not the combination of dipyridamole and aspirin is more effective than aspirin alone in secondary prevention of cardiovascular events after stroke or transient cerebral ischaemia is controversial.

## Glycoprotein IIb/IIIa receptor antagonists

The final common pathway of platelet aggregation is the exposure in activated platelets of membrane glycoprotein IIb/IIIa receptors, which are linked by fibrinogen in platelet aggregation. Several antagonists of this receptor are currently under investigation as antithrombotic agents. Abciximab is a monoclonal antibody that blocks this receptor: it is used as a single intravenous injection in prevention of thrombosis following high-risk coronary angioplasty.

# Chapter 6

# Management of coronary artery disease and its complications

## Background

Ischaemic heart disease is usually due to coronary atheroma. The previous chapter described the pharmacological approaches that have been proven to modify risk factors of hypertension and hyperlipidaemia and thus prevent or slow the progression of atherosclerosis and cardiac target organ damage. Where these primary prevention approaches are unsuccessful or introduced too late, patients will present with complications and symptoms ranging from angina pectoris to acute myocardial infarction in addition to cardiac arrhythmias and cardiac failure. Heart failure is most commonly a consequence of ischaemic heart disease with myocardial infarction. The prevalence of complications of coronary artery disease, particularly heart failure, increases markedly with advancing age.

The risk of cardiovascular events in an individual patient is greatly increased by pre-existing heart disease whether symptomatic, such as angina or myocardial infarction, or asymptomatic (left ventricular hypertrophy or dysfunction). Therapeutic strategies were previously directed to relieve symptoms including relief of pain, breathlessness or peripheral oedema. These remain an important aspect of management. In recent years randomised clinical trials have confirmed therapeutic approaches that also improve outcome by reducing further cardiovascular events. Aggressive

management of risk factors such as blood pressure and cholesterol is increasingly recognised as an important aspect of secondary prevention of cardiovascular disease (see Chapter 5).

## Angina pectoris, myocardial infarction and acute coronary syndromes

### Aims

Relief of symptoms, prevention of worsening or recurrent angina and myocardial infarction and improved survival; also to prevent non-coronary atherosclerotic problems, e.g. stroke.

### Relevant pathophysiology

Angina is the symptom experienced when myocardial oxygen delivery is insufficient to meet myocardial energy requirements. The major determinants of myocardial oxygen consumption are heart rate and the force of myocardial contraction. Angina occurs in two forms.

### Stable angina

Attacks are predictably provoked by exertion or excitement and recede when the increased energy demand is withdrawn. The underlying pathology is usually chronic coronary artery disease, with moderate to severe fixed stenosis of the coronary arteries with super-added variation in coronary tone. Anaemia and thyrotoxicosis can precipitate or aggravate angina by reducing oxygen delivery and increasing energy requirements, respectively. Treatment can be directed at increasing myocardial oxygen supply (coronary vasodilatation) or reducing myocardial oxygen consumption (reduce heart rate, contractility, preload and afterload). Drugs that reduce heart rate also increase the duration of diastole, the time when most myocardial blood flow occurs.

## Unstable angina

In unstable angina, which is one type of acute coronary syndrome (see below), attacks occur with increasing frequency and severity and on lesser exertion or at rest and are unpredictable. The underlying pathology is usually rupture or dissection of an atheromatous plaque with thrombus formation or extension in the coronary arteries. Spasm may be an additional mechanism. Acute changes in coronary artery pathology are presumed and therapeutic attention directed to halting, reversing or bypassing the coronary arterial occlusive process in the hope of avoiding myocardial infarction. Given the nature of the pathophysiological process, antithrombotic therapy is the key. At the same time, treatment is aimed at reducing myocardial energy requirements. Severe unstable angina can progress to myocardial infarction or death.

In recent years unstable angina and non-ST segment elevation myocardial infarction (non-STEMI), along with ST segment elevation myocardial infarction (STEMI) have, collectively, become known as acute coronary syndromes (ACS). This categorisation reflects how the treatment of ACS is determined by the way in which the patient presents. Unstable angina and non-STEMI may be indistinguishable at presentation (with confirmation of infarction depending on an increase in a cardiac biomarker such as troponin) and are managed similarly with anti-platelet therapy, antithrombotic therapy (e.g. heparin), anti-ischaemic drugs and, increasingly,

early percutaneous coronary intervention (PCI) or coronary artery bypass surgery. There is evidence that early 'revascularisation' for non-STEMI acute coronary syndromes reduces recurrent angina and myocardial infarction. STEMI is managed differently and should be treated by thrombolysis (see Chapter 14) or primary PCI.

## Drugs used in angina

### Glyceryl trinitrate

**Mechanism**

A potent, direct, short-acting, smooth muscle relaxant with widespread vasodilator activity. Whether the predominant effect is a direct action on the coronary arteries to increase flow or a peripheral (systemic) reduction in pre- and afterload is disputed.

**Pharmacokinetics**

Virtually 100% first-pass metabolism and it is therefore given sublingually, bucally, transdermally as a patch or paste, or intravenously. Very rapid clearance by liver metabolism: half-life about 2 min.

**Adverse effects**

These are dose related and result from vasodilatation and hypotension: headache, flushing and postural dizziness. These symptoms can be terminated by swallowing the tablet or spitting it out or by removing the patch.

**Clinical use and dose**

Glyceryl trinitrate (GTN) tablets are generally kept as a 'rescue' treatment for 'breakthrough' angina. Ideally, GTN should be taken to prevent angina. For example, it can be taken sublingually by the patient before carrying out a task known to produce angina. The total daily dose may be determined individually as that required to control symptoms. GTN is also available in patch form. The shelf-life of sublingual GTN is only 6 months. For patients with infrequent angina, GTN by sublingual spray or chewable isosorbide dinitrate have a much longer shelf-life and are more appropriate.

## Isosorbide dinitrate and isosorbide mononitrate

The clinical pharmacology of isosorbide dinitrate is similar to GTN, but it is also effective orally and has a longer half-life of 40 min. Isosorbide mononitrate has an even longer half-life. It is the active metabolite of isosorbide dinitrate and is claimed to have more consistent pharmacokinetics and longer duration of action.

Early trials demonstrated loss of efficacy with long-acting nitrates after several weeks, especially with high doses. This was shown to be a result of tolerance and drug effect could be restored by a short break of treatment. Subsequently it has been shown that a 6- to 8-h nitrate-free interval in every 24 h allows restoration of nitrate efficacy. A long-acting formulation of isosorbide mononitrate can be used once daily, while short-acting formulations of isosorbide dinitrate should be prescribed two to three times per day but with no doses given between 6 p.m. and 8 a.m. (i.e. an eccentric dosing regimen to give a nitrate-free interval). It must be realised that the patient has no anti-anginal cover over this period and, hence, is most vulnerable to a coronary event. If nocturnal angina is troublesome then the nitrate-free interval can be switched to the day time.

### Doses

Isosorbide dinitrate: 30–120 mg daily in two to three doses.
Isosorbide mononitrate: 20–120 mg daily in one dose (or two doses not more than 8 h apart).
Transdermal GTN: 5–15 mg.
*Comment.* Nitrate patches should be removed at night to ensure efficacy during the day.

## Potassium channel activators

Nicorandil, a compound that has several mechanisms of action including activation of potassium channels and nitrate-like activity, is available for the management of angina. Nicorandil's pharmacodynamic profile is very similar to that of nitrates although tolerance may be less of a problem. In an outcome trial nicorandil reduced major coronary events.

## β-Receptor blockers

The detailed clinical pharmacology of these drugs is described in Chapter 5. Their role in angina depends mainly on decreasing myocardial oxygen consumption by:
1 Limiting the increased heart rate associated with exercise and anxiety.
2 Limiting the increased force of contraction associated with the same stimuli.
3 Increasing the length of diastole, the period during which coronary blood flow occurs.

Beta-blockers have been shown to reduce sudden death and reinfarction following a myocardial infarct.

### Adverse effects

Lethargy, fatigue, bradycardia and bronchospasm are common side effects. Rebound worsening of angina, myocardial infarction or tachycardia has been reported when beta-blockers are suddenly withdrawn. Reduce dose over 24–48 h if beta-blockers are being withdrawn in such patients.

### Clinical use

There are no reliable data to say whether $\beta_1$ selective or non-selective beta-blockers should be preferred in stable and unstable angina. The major post-myocardial infarction trials showing beta-blocker benefit used non-selective agents. The only absolute contraindication for a beta-blocker is asthma.

### Doses

Atenolol: 50–200 mg daily in two divided doses.
Metoprolol: 100–400 mg daily in two or three divided doses.
Bisoprolol: 5–20 mg once daily.
Carvedilol 25–50 mg in two divided doses.

These drugs must all be given in an individually titrated dose to control symptoms and attenuate postural and exercise-induced tachycardia.

## Calcium antagonists

There are two major groups:
1 Dihydropyridines including nifedipine, nicardipine, nitrendipine, felodipine and amlodipine.
2 Heart rate limiting ones including verapamil and diltiazem.

Calcium antagonists are further described in Chapter 5. Their principal action is inhibition of the slow calcium-ion channel component of the smooth muscle action potential leading to:
1 Reduction in afterload.
2 Decreased tone in vascular smooth muscle cells including coronary arteries.
3 Decreased contractility in myocardial cells.
4 Depressant effects by verapamil and diltiazem on sinus node and atrioventricular node function and therefore slow heart rate. These drugs have additional anti-arrhythmic activity.

### Pharmacokinetics

All drugs are well absorbed following oral administration. They are cleared by liver metabolism. All undergo extensive first-pass metabolism. Active metabolites may contribute to their effects.

### Adverse effects

Headache, nausea, flushing and ankle swelling with nifedipine and other dihydropyridines. The side effects of nifedipine appear to be diminished markedly by combination with a beta-blocker. Constipation occurs with verapamil.

Short-acting formulations of calcium antagonists, particularly dihydropyridines, should be avoided, especially in patients not treated with a beta-blocker as there is some evidence that rapid onset vasodilatation, leading to a fall in blood pressure and reflex tachycardia, can worsen angina or even precipitate myocardial infarction. Slow-release formulations of nifedipine have a smoother pharmacodynamic profile, as do long-acting calcium antagonists like amlodipine. They have no effect on cardiovascular survival but may reduce the need for intervention.

There is a general perception that beta-blockers may be more effective anti-anginal agents than calcium channel blockers and should be the first choice agent for angina prophylaxis.

### Drug interactions

Verapamil or diltiazem should not be given routinely with beta-blockers since the combined negative inotropic and chronotropic effects can cause bradyarrhythmias and heart block and can rarely precipitate heart failure. Bradycardia may also follow use of these agents with digoxin or amiodarone.

### Clinical use

They may be used in stable or unstable angina. Verapamil and diltiazem are alternative first-line agents to a beta-blocker in intolerant patients in stable or unstable angina. Nifedipine and other dihydropyridines are used to best effect in combination with beta-blockers in severe angina.

### Doses

Verapamil: 40 mg two or three times daily up to 360 mg daily in divided doses or as a single dose of a slow-release preparation.
Nifedipine: up to 120 mg daily as a long-acting preparation.
Amlodipine: 5–10 mg once a day.
Diltiazem: 60 mg two or three times daily up to 480 mg daily in divided doses or as a slow-release formulation once or twice daily.

## General principles of management of angina

There are three major components to the treatment of angina:
1 Management of the risk factors for coronary atherosclerosis (e.g. lipid lowering, aspirin, antihypertensive drugs, cessation of smoking)
2 Treatment of symptoms
3 Preventing or delaying myocardial infarction and death

There is considerable evidence that treating the first two goals will achieve the third goal by default.

There is also evidence that surgical revascularisation of patients with angina and severe coronary artery disease improves prognosis.

Where possible, objective evidence of coronary disease should be sought using electrocardiography and exercise testing. This provides diagnostic confirmation and, importantly, objective evidence of the severity of the underlying ischaemia, providing the indication for coronary angiography.

## Stable angina

1 Modify cardiovascular risk factors such as cigarette smoking, treat hypertension and consider a statin to lower LDL cholesterol.
2 Prescribe prophylactic aspirin; clopidogrel is an alternative in aspirin-intolerant patients.
3 Angiotensin-converting enzyme (ACE) inhibitors such as ramipril, perindopril or trandolapril may prevent cardiovascular events and death in patients with angina or post-infarction.
4 Treat any underlying precipitating cause such as anaemia, thyrotoxicosis or arrhythmias.
5 Prescribe prophylactic therapy with a beta-blocker or a rate-limiting calcium antagonist if a beta-blocker is contraindicated.
6 Prescribe treatment with GTN for breakthrough attacks of angina or to be taken before undertaking the effort or activity that provokes pain.
7 If prophylaxis with a beta-blocker is unsuccessful add a dihydropyridine calcium antagonist, long-acting nitrate or nicorandil.
8 Coronary angiography is indicated under three circumstances:
  • The diagnosis of angina is in doubt.
  • Symptoms are not controlled with medical therapy, i.e. revascularisation by coronary artery bypass graft (CABG) or percutaneous transluminal coronary angioplasty (PTCA) is indicated on symptomatic grounds. Patients who fail to respond to the combination of two anti-anginal drugs should be considered for revascularisation.
  • Stress testing suggests the presence of severe coronary artery disease, i.e. surgical revascularisation might be indicated on prognostic grounds.

## Unstable angina

Once the diagnosis is established (for example by symptoms accompanied by ST segment or T wave changes on the electrocardiogram (ECG)), the patient should be treated with aspirin and low-molecular-weight heparin; clopidogrel should be added in higher risk patients. A beta-blocker (or verapamil if contraindicated) and an intravenous nitrate should be used to relieve symptoms. A high dose of atorvastatin (80 mg daily) has been shown to improve outcome in patients with ACS. If symptoms persist, coronary revascularisation is indicated though addition of a dihydropyridine calcium antagonist may also be considered. Platelet glycoprotein receptor (GPIIb/IIIa) antagonists improve outcome in severe unstable angina and are frequently used in patients requiring emergency revascularisation who should also receive clopidogrel. It is recommended that clopidogrel is continued for 6 to 12 months. Thereafter, patients should be treated as for stable angina.

## Cardiac arrhythmia

Not all electrocardiographically documented arrhythmias require treatment. In each instance, the physician must consider the balance between the symptomatic or prognostic significance of the arrhythmia and the potential side effects of therapy. The indications for active treatment in certain circumstances are clear, such as in the termination or prophylaxis of arrhythmias that are life-threatening, producing major haemodynamic sequelae or troublesome symptoms. Treatment of arrhythmias may involve either pharmacological or non-pharmacological therapy. Where pharmacological therapy is indicated, the choice of the most appropriate anti-arrhythmic drug depends on several factors:
1 Patient-related:
  • Electrocardiographic diagnosis
  • Possible mechanism of the arrhythmia
  • Nature of underlying cardiac disease (if any), especially coronary artery disease and/or left ventricular dysfunction
  • Requirement for acute or long-term therapy

2 Drug-related:
  • Mechanism of drug action—primary and secondary
  • Pharmacokinetics
  • Haemodynamic effects of the drug
  • Electrophysiological effects of the drug, e.g. effects on conduction, QT interval, etc.

Under different circumstances, the aim of the therapy may be termination of a tachycardia with restoration of sinus rhythm (e.g. supraventricular tachycardia), control of ventricular rate without restoration of sinus rhythm (e.g. atrial fibrillation) or prevention of recurrent episodes of tachycardia.

## Relevant pathophysiology

### Normal electrophysiology

Cardiac muscle may be divided into three electrophysiologically distinct types:
1 Tissue with spontaneous pacemaker activity, i.e. the sinoatrial (SA) and atrioventricular (AV) nodes
2 Specialised high-velocity conducting tissue—the His–Purkinje system
3 'Working' atrial and ventricular myocardium

The action potentials of SA and AV nodal cells undergo diastolic depolarisation, which results in the generation of spontaneous action potentials. The upstroke of the cardiac action potential in these cells is dependent on the 'slow' inward calcium current. Conduction velocity in nodal tissue, e.g. AV node, is slow, accounting for the delay between atrial and ventricular systole. The refractoriness of the AV node (i.e. the failure to conduct impulses at short intervals) limits the rate at which atrial impulses are transmitted to the ventricles, of particular importance in atrial fibrillation.

Depolarisation in His–Purkinje tissue and atrial and ventricular myocardium depends on the rapid inward sodium current. The action potential upstroke and conduction velocity are much faster than those in nodal tissue, allowing electrical activation of the atria or ventricles in a short period of time, permitting coordinated contraction. Under normal circumstances, atrial and ventricular myocardium has no intrinsic automaticity,

while that of the His–Purkinje network is slow (30 beats/min).

## Mechanisms of arrhythmias

Arrhythmias may arise either from abnormal automaticity triggered after depolarisation or from disorders of impulse conduction. Most clinically important arrhythmias depend on the latter mechanism, and are examples of the 're-entry' phenomenon. Re-entry can occur when an advancing wave of depolarisation from a premature impulse finds one pathway temporarily inexcitable (refractory) as a result of prematurity, resulting in conduction block. Depolarisation may proceed by another route and reach the distal part of the refractory area after a long enough period to allow partial excitability to have recovered. The impulse can then travel in a retrograde direction through the area of previous conduction block. If the time taken for the impulse to pass around such a circuit exceeds the refractory period of the normal tissue at the site proximal to the area of conduction block, this tissue will be re-excited, and the potential for a continuous 'circus' movement will exist. Atrial flutter and fibrillation, supraventricular tachycardias, ventricular tachycardia secondary to previous myocardial infarction and ventricular fibrillation are all examples of re-entry.

Triggered activity is the likely basis for the arrhythmias of digitalis toxicity as a consequence of intracellular calcium overload.

## Classification of anti-arrhythmic drugs

The most commonly used classification of anti-arrhythmic drug action was proposed by Singh and Vaughan Williams, following observations on the electrophysiological effects of drugs on isolated tissues. Four principal modes of action have been identified (Table 6.1). However, individual drugs may have actions in more than one category, and their effects in abnormal myocardium (e.g. during ischaemia) differ from those under normal physiological conditions. The anti-arrhythmic actions of digitalis and adenosine are not included in the

**Table 6.1** Classification of anti-arrhythmic drug actions.

| Class | Drugs |
| --- | --- |
| I: Fast sodium channel inhibitors | Ia: Quinidine, procainamide, disopyramide |
| | Ib: Lidocaine, phenytoin, mexiletine, tocainide |
| | Ic: Flecainide |
| II: Antisympathetic agents | Beta-blockers |
| III: Prolongation of action potential duration | Amiodarone, bretylium, sotalol |
| IV: Slow calcium channel antagonists | Verapamil, diltiazem |
| Not classified | Digoxin, adenine nucleotides |

Vaughan Williams classification, and are considered separately.

### Class I action

Agents with class I activity block sodium channels and reduce the rapid inward sodium current, resulting in slowing of conduction, an increase in refractory period, or both. This action is sometimes termed 'local anaesthetic' or 'membrane stabilising'. Class I drugs are subdivided according to their subsidiary properties. Class Ia agents lengthen action potential duration moderately and cause minor slowing of intracardiac conduction and widening of the QRS complex in therapeutic concentrations. Class 1b drugs shorten action potential duration and have no effect on intracardiac conduction or the QRS complex in sinus rhythm. Class Ic drugs have no net effect on action potential duration, but slow intracardiac conduction, and widen the QRS complex.

### Class II action

Drugs with class II action decrease the arrhythmogenic effects of catecholamines. This may occur by competitive antagonism at β-adrenoceptors (e.g. beta-blockers), by non-competitive adrenoceptor antagonism (e.g. amiodarone) or by inhibition of noradrenaline release at sympathetic nerve terminals (e.g. bretylium).

### Class III action

Class III activity involves inhibition of outward (repolarising) currents, resulting in lengthening of action potential duration and effective refractory period without interference with the inward sodium current. The basis of this action in clinically available drugs in this category is inhibition of the rapid component of the delayed rectifier current $I_{kr}$. The action of class Ia drugs in lengthening action potential duration is also mediated by $I_{kr}$ inhibition. Currently available drugs in this category possess additional class II (e.g. bretylium, sotalol) or both class I, II and IV activity (e.g. amiodarone), but drugs with 'pure' class III activity are under development and are likely to be licensed shortly.

### Class IV action

Inhibition of the slow inward $Ca^{2+}$ current by this class of drugs results in slowed conduction and increased refractoriness in the AV node. This action is of value in blocking supraventricular tachycardia involving the AV node as one limb of a re-entry circuit, or in slowing the ventricular response to atrial fibrillation.

## Pharmacological vs. non-pharmacological therapy

Anti-arrhythmic drugs exert powerful electrophysiological effects on the heart. While these may be beneficial, it is increasingly recognised that potentially lethal arrhythmias may be provoked by drug action. This phenomenon, termed proarrhythmia, has been identified increasingly in recent years as a result of randomised clinical trials that demonstrated an increased mortality in patients receiving certain anti-arrhythmic drugs compared with placebo. As a result of this problem, and the limited efficacy of drug therapy in many instances, a non-pharmacological approach

**Table 6.2** Non-pharmacological therapy of arrhythmias.

| Arrhythmia | Indication | Technique |
|---|---|---|
| Atrial fibrillation | Termination | DC cardioversion |
| | Rate control | AV nodal ablation/pacemaker |
| | Prophylaxis | Catheter ablation |
| Atrial flutter | Termination | DC cardioversion |
| | Prophylaxis | Catheter ablation |
| Supraventricular tachycardia (AV nodal and AV re-entry) | Termination | Valsalva manoeuvre |
| | Prophylaxis | Catheter ablation |
| Ventricular tachycardia | Termination | DC cardioversion, overdrive pacing Implantable cardioverter- defibrillator. |
| | Prophylaxis | Catheter ablation, surgery |
| Ventricular fibrillation | Termination | DC cardioversion Implantable cardioverter- defibrillator |

is now used for the definitive treatment of arrhythmias, e.g. catheter ablation. In many instances, a non-pharmacological approach is now used for the definitive treatment of arrhythmias. However, drug treatment, by virtue of its ease of administration and widespread availability, is still the commonest initial therapeutic approach. Full discussion of the indications for drug vs. non-pharmacological treatment is beyond the scope of this chapter, but an indication of the arrhythmias in which non-pharmacological approaches are used is given in Table 6.2.

## Class I agents

### General

Although class I drugs have been the mainstay of anti-arrhythmic drug therapy for many years, results from several recent clinical trials have shown them to be inferior to other (class III) agents in terms of efficacy and safety in the prophylaxis of symptomatic arrhythmias. Class I drugs increase the risk of death in patients with asymptomatic ventricular premature beats after myocardial infarction. Overall, the benefit/risk margin for class I agents is narrow, the risks of producing conduction block or exacerbating arrhythmias are considerable and use of these drugs is declining. They should only be used under expert supervision. All class I agents interfere with sodium channel activity, and reduce $Na^+$ influx. This may reduce intracellular $Na^+$ concentrations and, by $Na^+/Ca^{2+}$ exchange, result in a reduced intracellular $Ca^{2+}$ concentration. Thus, all class I agents have a potentially negative inotropic effect and need to be used with great caution in patients with overt or incipient heart failure. In some instances (e.g. quinidine) the negative inotropic effect may be balanced by peripheral vasodilation. Of the subgroups, group Ib agents have the least negative inotropic action, and group Ia the most.

## Class Ia agents

### Quinidine

*Mechanism*
Quinidine reduces the maximal rate of depolarisation, depresses spontaneous phase 4 diastolic depolarisation in automatic cells, slows conduction and also prolongs the effective refractory period of atrial, ventricular and Purkinje fibres.

*Pharmacokinetics*
Seventy per cent of the drug is absorbed from the gut. With conventional preparations measurable levels are obtained within 15 min and the peak effect occurs between 1 and 3 h. However, because the average half-life is of the order of 6 h, slow-release preparations are more commonly

used. It is 80–90% bound to plasma proteins and is metabolised by hydroxylation; the inactive metabolites are excreted in the urine. Antiarrhythmic effects are seen with drug levels of 2.3–5.0 mg/l. In cirrhosis the clearance of quinidine is reduced. There is also less binding to plasma proteins and hence lower plasma levels are effective.

*Adverse effects*
Quinidine has a vagolytic action, which increases AV conduction. This may lead to acceleration in ventricular rate in patients with atrial flutter or fibrillation. Progressive QRS and QT prolongation may occur, the latter leading to atypical ventricular tachycardia (torsades de pointes). Higher concentrations are associated with decreased myocardial contractility, hypotension or electrophysiological effects with possible sinus arrest, SA or AV block. Other adverse effects include gastrointestinal symptoms with nausea, vomiting and diarrhoea; cinchonism; hypersensitivity reactions with fever, purpura, thrombocytopaenia and hepatic dysfunction.

*Drug interactions*
Quinidine increases digoxin plasma levels and may precipitate digoxin toxicity if the dose of digoxin is not reduced to compensate.

*Clinical use and dose*
Quinidine now has limited use. The dose is 200–600 mg orally 6-hourly after an initial test dose.

**Procainamide**
*Mechanism*
Procainamide has similar electrophysiological properties to quinidine.

*Pharmacokinetics*
Procainamide can be administered either intravenously or orally (being 75% bioavailable). However, because it has a relatively short half-life of the order of 3.5 h, it is usually given as a slow-release preparation. The compound is metabolised to N-acetyl procainamide (NAPA), which has class III anti-arrhythmic activity in its own right. Anti-arrhythmic activity of procainamide occurs at

blood levels of 4–10 mg/l and toxic effects are likely with blood levels of 16 mg/l. Relatively high plasma levels of both parent drug and NAPA occur in renal impairment and cardiac failure.

The drug is metabolised by acetylation in the liver by an enzyme that also metabolises isoniazid and hydralazine. The enzyme is bimodally distributed in the population; slow acetylators theoretically require smaller doses for anti-arrhythmic activity than fast acetylators.

*Adverse effects*
Rapid intravenous administration may cause hypotension with vasodilatation and reduced cardiac output. ECG changes include QRS and QT prolongation. In toxic doses PR prolongation may occur, leading ultimately to AV block. On chronic oral therapy at high dosage many patients develop a drug-induced lupus erythematosus syndrome with a positive antinuclear factor.

*Drug interactions*
Procainamide reduces the antimicrobial effect of sulphonamides. The mechanism appears to be formation of *p*-aminobenzoic acid from procaine.

*Clinical use and dose*
Procainamide is used predominantly in the termination or prophylaxis of ventricular tachycardias, including lidocaine-resistant arrhythmias. It is administered intravenously, 50–100 mg every 5 min to a total dose of 1000 mg or until hypotension or QRS widening occurs. It is rarely used in chronic oral form.

**Disopyramide**
*Mechanism*
Disopyramide has electrophysiological properties similar to quinidine.

*Pharmacokinetics*
Disopyramide is 70–80% bioavailable. The half-life in normal subjects is 6–8 h. Fifty per cent is excreted unchanged in the urine; a further 25% is excreted in the form of the main metabolite—the N-dealkylated form of disopyramide. The dose should be reduced in severe renal failure when creatinine

clearance levels are less than 25 ml/min. The therapeutic range is 2–5 mg/l.

*Adverse effects*

Disopyramide has marked negative inotropic actions and should be avoided in patients with left ventricular dysfunction. Other adverse effects are related primarily to anticholinergic activity, with urinary retention, glaucoma and blurred vision. QT prolongation occurs with increasing plasma concentrations, and may predispose to torsades de pointes. Contraindications to therapy include sick sinus syndrome and prostatic hypertrophy.

*Clinical use and dose*

Disopyramide is occasionally used for atrial and ventricular arrhythmias, including those resistant to lidocaine. The dose is 100–200 mg 6-hourly orally or by slow-release preparation. It is also available for slow intravenous injection 2 mg/kg over 20 min.

## Class Ib agents

### Lidocaine (formerly lignocaine)
*Mechanism*

Lidocaine causes only marginal slowing of conduction velocity in Purkinje fibres and in ventricular muscle, but is selectively active in suppressing ventricular premature beats and ventricular tachycardia. Like other class Ib agents, it has no useful action against supraventricular tachycardias.

*Pharmacokinetics*

Lidocaine is not given orally because it is hydrolysed in the gastrointestinal tract and is subjected to extensive first-pass metabolism in the liver so that adequate blood levels are not achieved. Following intravenous administration, the elimination half-life is about 100 min. The clearance of lidocaine is reduced in cardiac failure and lower rates of infusion are required.

*Adverse effects*

Although therapeutic concentrations have little haemodynamic effect, high levels of lidocaine cause bradycardia, hypotension and even asystole.

Nausea and vomiting may also occur. At levels $\geq 5$ mg/l, central nervous system adverse effects may occur with paraesthesiae, twitching and even grand mal seizures.

*Clinical use and dose*

Lidocaine has no action on atrial arrhythmias, but it is used in the termination of haemodynamically stable ventricular tachycardia and the short-term prevention of recurrent ventricular tachycardia or fibrillation after myocardial infarction. Lidocaine is given by the intravenous route, with a loading dose of 1–2 mg/kg body weight by rapid injection followed by an infusion of 1–2 mg/min to maintain arrhythmia suppression. The dose requires reduction in the presence of cardiac failure or liver disease. Therapeutic blood levels are 1.5–5.0 mg/l.

### Mexiletine
*Mechanism*

This primary amine has similar electrophysiological action to lidocaine.

*Pharmacokinetics*

Mexiletine is active after both oral and intravenous administration. It is extensively metabolised to *p*-hydroxy- and hydroxymethylmexiletine and to their corresponding deaminated alcohols by hepatic metabolism. The half-life in normal subjects is 9–12 h. However, this may be increased, particularly following acute myocardial infarction. Oral absorption is reduced when given with morphine or diamorphine.

*Adverse effects*

Toxic effects include nausea, dizziness, drowsiness, tremor and hypotension, common at plasma levels above 2.0 mg/l.

*Clinical use and dose*

Mexiletine is occasionally used in the treatment of ventricular arrhythmias but therapy is commonly limited by patient intolerance. Mexiletine is given initially as a 1–3 mg/kg i.v. bolus injection, then 20–45 µg/kg per min by i.v. infusion, followed by 0.6–1.2 g orally in 24 h. Effective plasma levels are 0.75–2.0 mg/l; the therapeutic range is narrow.

## Phenytoin

Phenytoin has class Ib activity similar to lidocaine. Haemodynamic adverse effects include dose-related impairment of myocardial contractility following intravenous use. Adverse effects are reviewed in the chapter on anticonvulsants. It finds occasional use as an alternative to lidocaine or in digoxin-induced arrhythmias, given in 50–100 mg rapid intravenous doses over 5 min, up to 1000 mg.

## Class Ic agents

### Flecainide

*Mechanism*

Flecainide slows conduction in the atria, His–Purkinje system, accessory pathways and ventricles. In therapeutic concentration it causes lengthening of the PR and QRS intervals. Flecainide is effective against atrial arrhythmias and tachycardias involving accessory pathways (Wolff–Parkinson–White syndrome).

*Pharmacokinetics*

Flecainide is well absorbed orally, and about 27% is excreted unchanged in the urine. The remainder undergoes biotransformation to active metabolites, but the plasma concentrations of the unconjugated, pharmacologically active forms are considerably less than those of the parent drug. Flecainide is not extensively protein-bound. The average elimination half-life in normal subjects is 14 h, permitting twice daily administration. The half-life is increased in cardiac and renal failure.

*Adverse effects*

Flecainide may exacerbate pre-existing conduction disorders and should be used with great care in patients with SA disease, AV nodal disease or bundle branch block. It may cause an acute increase in the ventricular stimulation threshold, with a risk of asystole in pacemaker-dependent patients. Exacerbation of ventricular arrhythmias may occur. These are not normally of the torsades de pointes type, but rather a sustained (often incessant) monomorphic ventricular tachycardia with gross widening of the QRS complex and a

relatively slow rate (120–140/min). Neurological disturbances such as ataxia and taste disturbance may occur at higher doses.

*Clinical use and dose*

Flecainide is effective in the chemical cardioversion of recent-onset atrial fibrillation, and in the maintenance of sinus rhythm after cardioversion or in paroxysmal atrial fibrillation. The drug is also used in the prophylaxis of AV re-entry tachycardia in the Wolff–Parkinson–White syndrome. Flecainide should not be used in patients with prior myocardial infarction or left ventricular dysfunction. It is a potentially hazardous drug, and its use should be restricted to arrhythmia specialists.

Chronic oral doses range from 50 to 150 mg twice daily with target therapeutic plasma concentrations of 0.2–1.0 mg/l. Intravenous flecainide (up to 2 mg/kg) may be given by slow infusion over 30 min.

### Propafenone

This class Ic agent has additional minor beta-blocking and calcium antagonist properties.

*Pharmacokinetics*

Propafenone undergoes variable metabolism. Fast acetylators metabolise the drug rapidly to an active metabolite, in contrast to slow acetylators. There is therefore a marked variability in the plasma half-life of the native drug, but the overall pharmacodynamic properties of the active drug and metabolite are similar. Propafenone exhibits non-linear kinetics as a result of saturation of hepatic metabolism. For this reason, an increase in the daily dose from 300 mg to 600 mg daily results in doubling of the plasma concentration, while a further doubling in plasma concentration occurs when the dose is increased from 600 mg per day to 900 mg per day.

*Adverse effects*

The cardiac and non-cardiac adverse effects of propafenone are similar to those of flecainide. In addition, the weak beta-blocking action may be of significance in patients with asthma in whom the drug is contraindicated. The calcium antagonist properties also render the drug unsuitable for patients with myasthenia gravis.

*Clinical use and dose*
Propafenone is indicated for the prophylaxis of paroxysmal atrial fibrillation or supraventricular tachycardia. As with flecainide, its use should be avoided in patients with prior myocardial infarction or impaired left ventricular function The dosage ranges from 450 to 900 mg daily in two or three divided doses.

## Class II agents

### β-Adrenoceptor antagonists

The pharmacokinetics, adverse effects and mechanisms of action are discussed in Chapter 5.

### Clinical use

These compounds are useful in anti-arrhythmic therapy in view of their freedom from significant pro-arrhythmic effects. They may be used for the control of inappropriate sinus tachycardia, or the prophylaxis of paroxysmal atrial fibrillation or supraventricular tachycardia. Beta-blockers are ineffective in restoring sinus rhythm in atrial fibrillation. However, they are used either singly or in conjunction with digoxin to control the ventricular rate in permanent atrial fibrillation by virtue of their slowing effect on AV nodal conduction. β-adrenoceptor antagonists reduce the risk of sudden death in long-term therapy after myocardial infarction and in congestive heart failure. Other clinical situations in which the beta-blockers have useful anti-arrhythmic action include mitral valve prolapse, and the congenital long QT syndromes.

### Bretylium

This agent has adrenergic neurone blocking activity and suppresses noradrenaline release. It is eliminated by the kidney with a half-life of 7–12 h. Bretylium also has class III action on Purkinje fibres and is effective in ventricular arrhythmias, particularly ventricular fibrillation refractory to lidocaine or procainamide, and repeated electrical defibrillation.

Adverse effects include hypotension.

It is administered by the intravenous route, 5–10 mg/kg, or by the intramuscular route, 5 mg/kg.

## Class III agents

### Amiodarone

#### Mechanism
Amiodarone prolongs the action potential duration and effective refractory period in all cardiac tissues. It is a non-competitive α- and β-adrenoceptor antagonist, and also has class I, II and IV activity.

#### Pharmacokinetics
After oral administration, considerable accumulation occurs in muscle and fat, and the therapeutic action may take several weeks to develop fully. Amiodarone is metabolised in the liver to desethylamiodarone, which is also electrophysiologically active. The steady-state therapeutic plasma concentrations of amiodarone and desethylamiodarone are in the range of 1–2 mg/l. Elimination of amiodarone is complex, with an initial relatively rapid (1–2 days) and extremely slow terminal half-life (more than 30 days).

#### Adverse effects
Amiodarone has little negative inotropic effect, and is the best tolerated of all the anti-arrhythmic agents in heart failure. Amiodarone depresses sinus node automaticity and intra-cardiac conduction; therefore, it should be used with caution in the presence of SA or AV nodal disease. In common with all drugs that prolong ventricular repolarisation, amiodarone may provoke torsades de pointes ventricular tachycardia, but this occurs less frequently than with other class III agents. The use of amiodarone is limited principally by its non-cardiac side effects, of which the most important are pulmonary (alveolitis), hepatic (hepatitis), neurological (tremor, ataxia), thyroid (hyper- or hypothyroidism), testicular (orchitis) and cutaneous (photosensitivity). The last effect occurs in a high percentage of patients, of whom a small minority develop a slate-grey discoloration of light-exposed

areas, especially the nose and cheeks. Corneal micro-deposits occur in almost all patients, but do not interfere with vision.

### Clinical use and dose

Amiodarone is effective in a wide variety of supraventricular and ventricular arrhythmias. In view of its adverse effects, chronic amiodarone therapy should be used only in life-threatening or severely disabling arrhythmias, when other anti-arrhythmic agents have failed or are contraindicated, and non-pharmacological therapy is not appropriate. An oral loading dose of 600–1200 mg daily is given for 2 weeks, and then reduced to 100–400 mg daily. Intravenous amiodarone may be effective in the acute conversion or control of troublesome supraventricular and ventricular arrhythmias, including recent-onset atrial flutter and fibrillation. It has a relatively slow onset of action, which makes its use suitable only for haemodynamically stable arrhythmias. The initial dose is 300 mg i.v. given over 30 min to avoid hypotension, followed by up to 1200 mg/24 h. The intravenous preparation is irritant, and should be given via a central vein.

### Drug interactions

Amiodarone potentiates the effect of warfarin and increases plasma digoxin levels. Dose reduction is required in both cases.

## Sotalol

### Mechanism

Sotalol is a non-selective beta-blocker, which also possesses class III activity and thus prolongs atrial and ventricular action potential duration and refractory period. It has no class I activity at therapeutic concentrations.

### Clinical use

Sotalol appears to be more effective than other beta-blockers, particularly in supraventricular tachycardias involving accessory pathways and in ventricular arrhythmias. It may be used in the prophylaxis of recurrent ventricular tachycardia. The side effects are those of other beta-blockers (see Chapter 5) with the additional predisposition to torsades de pointes. The principal risk factors for this are female gender, bradycardia, left ventricular hypertrophy or dysfunction, high plasma concentrations, co-existing potassium depletion and co-administration of other drugs that lengthen QT interval. The dosage of sotalol in anti-arrhythmic therapy ranges from 80 to 320 mg twice daily.

## Class IV agents

## Verapamil

### Mechanism

Verapamil inhibits the slow inward $Ca^{2+}$ current. Its anti-arrhythmic actions stem from decreasing AV conduction.

### Pharmacokinetics

Bioavailability is only 10–20% owing to extensive first-pass metabolism. It is eliminated by the kidneys.

### Adverse effects

The commonest side effect is constipation. In view of its depressant effects on the SA and AV nodes, verapamil is contraindicated in heart block or SA disease. Verapamil has significant negative inotropic action, and is contraindicated in heart failure. Additional effects include nausea, dizziness and facial flushing.

### Drug interactions

Verapamil potentiates the negative effects of digoxin and beta-blockers on AV nodal conduction. Verapamil and beta-blockers in combination may cause high-grade AV block or asystole, particularly if either is administered intravenously. Beta-blockers also enhance the negative inotropic action of verapamil.

### Clinical use and dose

Verapamil is ineffective in restoring sinus rhythm in atrial flutter and atrial fibrillation, but its effect on increasing AV block allows control of the ventricular rate. Verapamil is useful in terminating re-entry supraventricular arrhythmias by transient block of AV nodal conduction. It should not be used in the termination of undiagnosed wide-complex tachycardias where ventricular tachycardia cannot be excluded. Verapamil can be used by both oral and intravenous routes. Intravenous verapamil is administered by infusion or slow injections over 2–3 min. Oral dosage is 80–120 mg three times daily.

## Diltiazem

This calcium channel blocker has similar anti-arrhythmic properties to verapamil. Dosage is 60–120 mg thrice daily of conventional release diltiazem. Sustained-release preparations may be taken once or twice daily.

*Comment.* Calcium channel blockers of the dihydropyridine class (e.g. nifedipine) do not interfere with AV nodal conduction and have no anti-arrhythmic action.

## Digitalis glycosides

The term digitalis or digitalis glycoside refers to any of the cardioactive steroids that share an aglycone ring structure and have positive inotropic and electrophysiological effects. In the United Kingdom, the vast majority of clinicians use the cardiac glycoside, digoxin.

## Mechanism

A major effect is to decrease sodium transport out of the cardiac cell by inhibiting $Na^+/K^+$ ATPase (the sodium pump). The resulting accumulation of sodium results in an increase of intracellular calcium ions by $Na^+/Ca^{2+}$ exchange, which is responsible for the positive inotropic effects of digitalis glycosides. These drugs exert their anti-arrhythmic effect by virtue of enhancing vagal inhibition of sinus node automaticity and AV nodal conduction. At high concentrations, digitalis glycosides increase myocardial automaticity as a result of intracellular calcium overload.

The three major effects of digitalis glycosides on the heart are:
1 Positive inotropy
2 Decreased ventricular rate in atrial fibrillation or flutter, by decreasing AV conduction. This effect is diminished on exercise as a result of withdrawal of underlying vagal tone
3 Increased myocardial automaticity in high (toxic) concentrations, or at 'therapeutic' concentrations if other factors such as hypokalaemia are present.

## Digoxin

**Pharmacokinetics**

Digoxin can be given orally or intravenously. The average volume of distribution is approximately 7.3 l/kg; this is decreased in patients with renal disease, hypothyroidism and in patients taking quinidine. It is increased in thyrotoxicosis. Clearance varies from individual to individual and is the result of both renal and metabolic elimination mechanisms. In healthy adults, the metabolic component is of the order of 40–60 ml/min per 70 kg, and the renal component approximates creatinine clearance. Metabolic clearance is reduced in congestive cardiac failure. Clearance in any individual can be calculated by the equations discussed in Chapters 1 and 2.

In patients with normal renal function, the elimination half-life is approximately 2 days. This is increased to approximately 4–6 days in severe renal disease.

**Adverse effects**

Adverse effects are determined in part by plasma concentration (>2.5 μg/l for digoxin) and in part by electrolyte balance. Digoxin and potassium compete for cardiac receptor sites and hypokalaemia can precipitate digitalis adverse effects. Hypercalcaemia also potentiates toxicity.

The common extracardiac adverse effects are anorexia, nausea, diarrhoea, vomiting, fatigue or weakness.

Less commonly, neurological symptoms occur, including difficulty in reading, confusion or even psychosis. Abdominal pain is another less common manifestation.

The cardiac adverse effects may include depression of automaticity or conduction resulting in sinus bradycardia, sinus arrest, junctional rhythm or various degrees of AV block, including complete heart block. Additionally, digoxin may produce excitatory effects, resulting in ventricular ectopic beats, atrial or ventricular tachycardia, or ventricular fibrillation. The typical effects of digitalis glycosides on the ECG, i.e. prolonged PR interval and ST segment depression, do not indicate toxicity. Cardiac signs precede extracardiac signs in about 50% of cases of toxicity.

### Drug interactions

Digoxin absorption is decreased by drugs that increase intestinal motility (e.g. metoclopramide), and increased by drugs that decrease motility (e.g. propantheline). Many antacids, particularly magnesium trisilicate, reduce digoxin absorption. Digoxin levels increase if quinidine or amiodarone is co-administered and toxicity can occur. The potential for toxicity is enhanced for all cardiac glycosides when diuretics are co-administered because of hypokalaemia.

### Digitoxin and ouabain

Digitoxin is more lipid-soluble than digoxin and is practically 100% absorbed from the gastrointestinal tract. It is given orally and intravenously. It is extensively metabolised by the liver, and the elimination half-life is 5–7 days. Renal impairment does not appreciably alter digitoxin kinetics, but binding to plasma proteins, normally of the order of 90–97%, may be slightly decreased in uraemia.

It seems likely that digitoxin is excreted in the bile and is then reabsorbed to some extent, i.e. it has an enterohepatic circulation. Colestyramine (cholestyramine), which can bind cardiac glycosides in the gut, can interrupt the enterohepatic circulation; whether it can shorten the duration of digitoxin toxicity is still a matter for speculation.

Ouabain is poorly absorbed from the gut and is administered exclusively by the intravenous route.

Its onset of action is rapid, and it has a somewhat shorter half-life than digoxin, approximately 1 day. Elimination is mainly renal.

### Clinical use and doses

The principal use of cardiac glycosides is in the control of ventricular rate in atrial fibrillation, particularly when a return to sinus rhythm is not expected (e.g. chronic mitral valve disease). Combination therapy with verapamil or beta-blockers provides better control of exercise heart rate with a lower risk of toxicity than high-dose glycosides. The onset of action even after intravenous administration is delayed for several hours. Thus if clinical circumstances require urgent control of ventricular rate, other approaches such as cardioversion or intravenous amiodarone may be more appropriate. Acute digitalisation has been superseded by the use of intravenous adenosine or verapamil in the termination of supraventricular tachycardias. The use of digoxin in patients with heart failure in sinus rhythm is discussed elsewhere.

The dosing schedules used with the cardiac glycosides depend not only on the pharmacokinetic properties of the drug, but also on factors that determine individual susceptibility. The loading dose is determined by the volume of distribution and the desired plasma concentration; the maintenance dose by clearance (Chapters 1 and 2). Nomograms and simple equations are available for dose calculation. However, these must remain approximations and the patient's clinical response must influence long-term management. If a maintenance dose is employed without a loading dose, drug accumulation and activity develop slowly because steady state is not reached for 4–5 half-lives. The major determinant of digoxin clearance is renal function and the maintenance dose for this glycoside must be reduced if renal function is impaired. The average loading dose of digoxin is 1.0–1.5 mg orally, or 0.3–1.0 mg intravenously. The usual oral maintenance dose in the presence of normal renal function is 0.125–0.250 mg daily.

The use of drug monitoring of the glycoside plasma levels has been useful, particularly in renal impairment and toxicity. The normal therapeutic range of digoxin is 1–2 µg/l. Venous sampling should be performed 3–4 h after an i.v. dose or 6–8 h after an oral dose. If blood levels are low then compliance should be checked, and possible causes of malabsorption considered.

### Treatment of digitalis-induced toxicity

Treatment of digitalis-induced arrhythmias is often difficult. The glycoside should be withdrawn, and if hypokalaemia is present, potassium chloride should be administered by infusion at a rate of 20 mmol/h (not exceeding 100 mmol total) with electrocardiographic and biochemical monitoring. Severe digitalis intoxication is treated with specific Fab antidigoxin antibodies, which bind and inactivate digoxin.

Ventricular arrhythmias may require lidocaine or phenytoin administration. Supraventricular arrhythmias may respond to beta blockade or phenytoin. Care must be observed when using verapamil and procainamide, as increased degrees of heart block may occur. Temporary pacing may be required for heart block with haemodynamic effects or in the rare instance of SA node arrest. Intravenous amiodarone infusion has shown promise in digitoxic arrhythmias.

## Adenine nucleotides

### Mechanism

The adenine nucleoside, adenosine, acts via purinergic receptors situated in the SA and AV nodes. Stimulation of these receptors causes hyperpolarisation of the cells resulting in suppression of automaticity and conduction. This results in transient sinus bradycardia and AV block. Adenosine transiently interrupts the re-entrant circuit in AV nodal re-entry tachycardia or in AV re-entry tachycardia involving an accessory pathway, while increasing the degree of AV block in atrial flutter or fibrillation. Adenosine triphosphate (ATP) has similar actions and is used as an anti-arrhythmic in Europe. ATP is rapidly metabolised to adenosine in the plasma and probably exerts its anti-arrhythmic effects as adenosine.

### Pharmacokinetics

Adenosine is metabolised to the inactive inosine. The plasma half-life of adenosine is less than 10 s. Both adenosine and ATP are inactive orally.

### Adverse effects

Adenosine is a vasodilator and produces marked flushing. Bolus injection causes a transient increase followed by a small fall in blood pressure, but the duration of action of a bolus dose is normally insufficient to cause clinically significant hypotension. A feeling of chest tightness or sometimes chest pain is experienced, which may be very unpleasant but is transient. Transient complete heart block lasting a few seconds may occur. Adenosine may precipitate bronchoconstriction in asthmatics.

### Clinical use and dose

Adenosine is the drug of choice for the termination of regular supraventricular tachycardias. Tachycardias involving the AV node as an integral part of the re-entry circuit will be terminated, while atrial tachycardias will demonstrate transient slowing of the ventricular rate, which allows identification of the underlying rhythm, e.g. atrial flutter. Dosing of adenosine is by rapid intravenous bolus injection, using a large or central vein, starting with a bolus of 3 mg, followed by saline. The anti-arrhythmic effect occurs shortly after the onset of flushing, usually 20–30 s after injection. Continuous electrocardiographic recording should be made during the administration and until symptoms have passed, since diagnostic information may be lost otherwise. If the initial dose is ineffective, boluses of 6 mg, followed by 12 mg if necessary, are given at the 2- to 3-min intervals. If a dose of 12 mg is unsuccessful, it may be repeated once. Some patients will respond to 18 mg (although this dose is not licensed in the United Kingdom). The dose may be limited by patient intolerance. Supraventricular tachycardia may recur within minutes, once the action of adenosine has passed. The same previously effective dose can be repeated but if supraventricular tachycardia recurs, verapamil should be considered as an alternative treatment.

## Drug interactions

The effects of adenosine are inhibited by purinoceptor antagonists (methylxanthines, e.g. theophylline and its derivatives) and accentuated by dipyridamole. Adenosine may be given safely to patients already receiving $\beta$-adrenoceptor antagonists or calcium channel blockers.

## Heart failure

### Definition

*Physiological*: An inability of the heart to maintain a cardiac output sufficient to meet the requirements of the metabolising tissues despite a normal filling pressure.

*Clinical*: Symptoms suggestive of heart failure (e.g. exertional breathlessness, ankle swelling, etc.) accompanied by objective evidence (usually by echocardiography) of cardiac dysfunction of sufficient severity to account for these. Most patients with heart failure have left ventricular systolic dysfunction and it is for these patients for which there is evidence-based treatment. The treatment of other causes of heart failure is less evidence-based and empirical. In patients who do not respond to appropriate therapy the diagnosis should be reviewed. The causes of heart failure are summarised in Table 6.3 and the principles of management in Table 6.4.

There is a poor relationship between haemodynamic abnormalities (the physiological definition of heart failure; see above) and symptoms and signs of heart failure (the clinical definition of heart failure).

### Relevant pathophysiology

There is a poor relationship between symptoms and cardiac performance in chronic heart failure. Treatment that improves cardiac function does not necessarily improve symptoms or prognosis and

**Table 6.3** Aetiology/management of heart failure.

*Principal aims*
Improve quality of life by:
- improving symptoms
- avoiding side effects
- preventing major morbid events such as myocardial infarction or stroke
- delaying death

*Secondary aims*
Improve cardiac performance
Improve exercise capacity
Reduce arrhythmias (ventricular and supraventricular)
Maintain renal function
Prevent electrolyte disturbance

*Aetiology*
In westernised countries heart failure is usually caused by one of the following:
- ischaemic heart disease
- hypertension (Chapter 5)
- heart muscle disorders
- valvular heart disease

many treatments that have only modest beneficial effects on cardiac function may have clear beneficial effects on symptoms and prognosis.

In contrast, there may be a relationship between haemodynamics, symptoms and prognosis in patients with acute pulmonary oedema or cardiogenic shock.

Cardiac performance is influenced by:

1 *Preload*: This determines ventricular end-diastolic pressure and volume. In normal hearts an increased preload leads to increased end-diastolic fibre length, which, in turn, causes increased force of contraction. In heart failure this response is reduced or even reversed.

2 *Force of cardiac contraction*: This is determined largely by the intrinsic strength and integrity of the muscle cells. Force of contraction is decreased by:
- Ischaemic heart disease (myocardial infarction or chronic severe ischaemia)
- Specific disorders affecting heart muscle, such as hypertension and myocarditis
- Disorders of heart muscle of unknown cause, e.g. idiopathic dilated cardiomyopathy.

**Table 6.4** Drugs used to treat heart failure.

| |
|---|
| 1. Diuretics: thiazides, loop diuretics<br>  • Decrease peripheral and pulmonary oedema<br>  • Decrease preload by reduction in circulatory volume<br>2. Neuroendocrine antagonists<br>  • ACE inhibitors<br>  • $\beta$-receptor antagonists<br>  • ARBs<br>  • Aldosterone antagonists<br>3. Drugs with a positive inotropic effect<br>  Cardiac glycosides (mainly chronic heart failure)<br>  $\beta$-adrenoceptor agonists (acute heart failure only)<br>4. Vasodilator agents<br>  • Mainly decrease preload: nitrates (glyceryl trinitrate, isosorbide dinitrate and isosorbide mononitrate)<br>  • Mainly decrease afterload: hydralazine<br>  • Decrease preload and afterload: sodium nitroprusside (acute HF only) |

**3** *Myocardial compliance*: This is an important determinant of ventricular filling and therefore of cardiac output. Compliance is decreased by:

- Fibrosis
- Hypertrophy
- Ischaemia.

**4** *Afterload*: This is the ventricular wall tension developed during ejection. Afterload is increased by:

- Systemic arterial vasoconstriction
- Increased arterial pressure
- Obstruction to outflow, e.g. aortic stenosis.

**5** *Neuroendocrine activation*: After an acute cardiac insult plasma concentrations of renin, angiotensin II, aldosterone, noradrenaline, endothelin, antidiuretic hormone (arginine vasopressin) and the natriuretic peptides are increased. If the patient survives and does not require treatment, then activity of the renin–angiotensin–aldosterone system (RAAS) returns to normal, probably a consequence of compensatory salt and water retention, but plasma concentrations of other neuroendocrine systems remain elevated. Once diuretics have been administered, RAAS activity increases, as do the concentrations of other neuro-hormones with the exception of the natriuretic peptides, which may decline. However, as heart failure

progresses, all the above neuroendocrine systems become markedly activated. Increased sympathetic activation via arterial baroreflexes (and possibly a down-regulation of inhibitory activity of baroreceptors) leads to sympathetically mediated increases in renal renin secretion and further increases in angiotensin II and aldosterone. Local haemodynamic factors probably play an important role in activation of other systems.

Neuroendocrine activation may be responsible for many of the characteristic features of heart failure. Examples include:

*Angiotensin II*: vasoconstriction (especially renal), sodium retention, continuing cardiac myocyte damage causing progressive ventricular dilatation (remodelling); stimulates aldosterone secretion.

*Aldosterone*: sodium retention; potassium loss and myocardial fibrosis (both may lead to arrhythmias).

*Sympathetic activation*: vasoconstriction, arrhythmias, hypokalaemia, sodium retention. May initially increase cardiac contractility but has adverse effects on long-term cardiac function as for angiotensin II by progression remodelling following myocardial damage.

## Diuretics

These drugs are first-line treatment for patients with heart failure. In mild failure a thiazide (Chapter 5) may suffice. Moderate or severe failure requires a loop diuretic.

### Loop diuretics

Furosemide (frusemide), bumetanide, torasemide.

*Mechanism*

Inhibition of active chloride reabsorption and also of $Na^+/K^+$ ATPase in the ascending limb of the loop of Henle with increased salt and water loss. The increased delivery of sodium to the distal tubule encourages $Na^+/K^+$ exchange with a tendency to hypokalaemic alkalosis.

*Pharmacokinetics*

Both drugs are well absorbed following oral administration and are also available in intravenous formulations. Elimination is largely by renal excretion with a small contribution by liver metabolism. These drugs have a rapid onset and short duration of action.

*Adverse effects*
Salt and water depletion can occur. May cause prerenal uraemia (increase in blood urea and creatinine concentrations). Regular monitoring of serum potassium is required. Urate retention can occur as with thiazides. Rapid intravenous injection of large doses can cause deafness.

*Drug interactions*
These include potentiation of nephrotoxic effects of gentamicin and cephaloridine. Hypokalaemia enhances the risk of digoxin toxicity. A loop diuretic may be combined usefully with a thiazide diuretic (or thiazide-like diuretic, e.g. metolazone 5–20 mg daily) resulting in an extremely potent diuretic combination. This combination should be used with caution and close monitoring of electrolytes. It is not clear if this combination is superior to the use of large doses of loop diuretic alone. Non-steroidal anti-inflammatory drugs (NSAIDs) may impair diuresis and provoke hyperkalaemia and renal failure. There is an increased risk of ototoxicity when used with an aminoglycoside, decreased excretion of lithium and increased risk of lithium toxicity.

*Doses*
*Furosemide*: Oral—20 mg each morning up to 1 or 2 g each day in very resistant oedema or cardiac failure. Intravenous—20–40 mg slowly. In resistant cases up to 1 g can be infused over 2–4 h.
*Bumetanide*: Oral—0.5–5.0 mg each day. Intravenous—0.5–2.0 mg or infusion up to 5 mg slowly.
*Torasemide*: 5 mg each morning up to 40 mg each day in very resistant oedema or cardiac failure.

*Prevention and treatment of hypokalaemia*
There is no evidence that potassium supplements (other than intravenous) are effective in preventing or treating hypokalaemia in patients with heart failure. Hypokalaemia is much less of a problem in patients with heart failure treated with ACE inhibitors or an angiotensin receptor blocker (ARB) but may still occur in patients taking very large doses of diuretics. There are three occasions where hypokalaemia is likely to be a problem:
1 Administration of high doses of loop diuretics in treating heart failure without an ACE inhibitor
2 Co-administration of digoxin since hypokalaemia potentiates digoxin toxicity
3 Administration of a thiazide diuretic to a patient with a low potassium intake, e.g. the older patient.

In general, persistent serum potassium below 3.5 mmol/l is an indication for potassium correction usually by co-administration of a potassium-sparing diuretic, the most appropriate of which is spironolactone.

## Potassium-sparing diuretics

*Amiloride, triamterene, spironolactone*: These drugs are all diuretics themselves, but their effect is weak and they are rarely used alone. They act mainly on the distal tubule, inhibiting sodium/potassium exchange. Spironolactone acts by inhibiting the effect of aldosterone on the distal tubule and is discussed further under the section Neuroendocrine antagonists (p. 77). Eplerenone is a more selective mineralocorticoid receptor antagonist and causes less gynaecomastia than spironolactone.

The adverse effect common to all of these drugs is hyperkalaemia and is particularly likely in patients with impaired renal function. Potassium supplements should rarely be required with potassium-sparing diuretics. If they are used, close monitoring of serum potassium is necessary. Potassium-sparing drugs (with the exception of spironolactone—see below) should generally be avoided in patients taking ACE inhibitors, as both agents raise potassium and severe hyperkalaemia may occur especially in the presence of renal failure. Note that there are proprietary formulations available which contain the combination of a thiazide or loop diuretic and a potassium-sparing diuretic. Spironolactone should be used only in a low dose and with caution in patients prescribed an ACE inhibitor (see below).

## Doses

*Amiloride*: 5–20 mg/day.
*Triamterene*: 100–200 mg/day.
*Spironolactone*: 12.5–50.0 mg/day for severe heart failure. Higher doses may be used for refractory oedema.
*Eplerenome:* 25–50 mg/day.
*Comment.* Potassium-sparing diuretics are available in proprietary formulations combined with a thiazide or furosemide. Combination tablets are more expensive but may improve compliance by reducing the number of tablets to be taken.

## Neuroendocrine antagonists

### ACE inhibitors

ACE inhibitors not only improve symptoms, but also reduce mortality and morbidity including hospital admissions in all grades of heart failure resulting from left ventricular systolic dysfunction treated with diuretics.

### Mechanism

The precise mechanism of action of ACE inhibitors has yet to be elucidated. The ACE not only converts angiotensin I to angiotensin II, but also degrades bradykinin. Angiotensin II is a powerful vasoconstrictor. It stimulates aldosterone and antidiuretic hormone release, enhances sympathetic activity, causes renal sodium retention and can cause direct damage to cardiac myocytes, increase myocardial fibrosis and stimulate vascular and myocardial hypertrophy. Bradykinin is a powerful vasodilator and also has anti-proliferative effects on smooth muscle and stimulates the production of vasodilator prostaglandins and nitric oxide.

ACE inhibitors produce both arterial and venous dilatation. The latter may be mediated through increased bradykinin or reduced sympathetic activation. ACE inhibitors increase serum and total body potassium by reducing aldosterone and should not, generally, be used with potassium-sparing drugs. (One exception is spironolactone—see below).

### Adverse effects

Profound hypotension may rarely occur after the first dose in patients on diuretics or with hyponatraemia. The magnitude and duration differ between different ACE inhibitors. Other adverse reactions include postural hypotension, renal dysfunction, hyperkalaemia, cough and angioneurotic oedema.

### Drug interactions

These include hyperkalaemia when combined with a potassium-sparing diuretic or an ARB and renal failure when combined with an NSAID or anARB.

### Doses

Captopril was the first orally active ACE inhibitor and has a short duration of action and has to be given two or three times a day. Enalapril, which is a prodrug for the active constituent enalaprilat, is longer acting. Several ACE inhibitors are licensed for heart failure and their long-term benefits are likely to be a class effect.
Agents used include:
Enalapril: 2.5–20.0 mg twice daily.
Lisinopril: 2.5–20.0 mg once daily.
Perindopril: 2–8 mg daily.
Ramipril: 1.25–10.00 mg once daily.

The prospective outcome trials showing benefit used high doses of ACE inhibitors. Dose-ranging studies have not shown a convincing difference between doses on symptoms or prognosis. It would however seem advisable to use in practice the same doses shown to be of benefit in large clinical trials.

### β-Adrenoceptor antagonists

For the last 30 years heart failure has generally been regarded as a contraindication to beta-blockade, although a series of small studies in heart failure consistently suggested benefit. Recent large trials suggest not only that beta-blockers are safe, but also that they reduce symptoms and mortality, as well as progression of heart failure and hospital re-admission. The reduction in morbidity and mortality is substantial and additional to that of ACE inhibitors. About 5–10% of patients will deteriorate within the first few days of receiving a beta-blocker and it may take 2–6 months for benefits to become obvious. The mechanism of action of beta-blockers in heart failure seems to involve retarding or even reversing progressive ventricular dysfunction due to excessive sympathetic activity. Currently, the most promising results have been achieved with bisoprolol, carvedilol and extended release metoprolol; nebivolol may also be beneficial. Beta-blockers must be used very carefully by those experienced in the management of heart failure. In heart failure, beta-blockers are initiated in a very low dose and the dose is up-titrated slowly over 2–3 months.

Bisoprolol: Initially 1.25 mg once daily; target dose 10 mg once daily.

Carvedilol: Initially 3.125 twice daily; target dose 25 mg twice daily orally for heart failure.

### Angiotensin II antagonists

There is evidence that angiotensin II receptor antagonists or blockers (ARBs) have comparable haemodynamic and neurohumoral effects to those of ACE inhibitors in congestive heart failure (CHF). These drugs also improve symptoms. Angiotensin II antagonists have the advantage of not causing troublesome cough and can be used as an alternative to ACE inhibitors if the latter cannot be tolerated. While ARBs do improve outcome in heart failure, there is no good evidence that they are superior to ACE inhibitors.

Recent outcome trials also showed that adding an ARB in patients who remain symptomatic despite treatment with an ACE inhibitor and beta-blocker improved symptoms, lessened the risk of hospital admission for worsening heart failure and, in one trial, reduced cardiovascular mortality.

An ARB should be used like an ACE inhibitor, i.e. initiated at a low dose which should be increased gradually over a week's period with appropriate monitoring of renal function, potassium and for symptoms of hypotension.

Candesartan: Initially 4 mg once daily; target dose 32 mg once daily.

### Aldosterone antagonists

Spironolactone competitively inhibits the effects of aldosterone. It is useful in treating the resistant oedema of conditions associated with excess aldosterone including nephrotic syndrome and cirrhosis. In one trial, spironolactone 25–50 mg daily reduced mortality in patients with New York Heart Association (NYHA) class III and IV heart failure already treated with a diuretic, digoxin and an ACE inhibitor (but not a beta-blocker in most cases).

Spironolactone can cause nausea, gynaecomastia in men and menstrual irregularities in women. It may decrease the renal secretion of digoxin. There is a risk of hyperkalaemia when given with other potassium-sparing diuretics or an ACE inhibitor. Eplerenome is a newer selective mineralocorticoid antagonist which causes less gynaecomastia.

### Hydralazine and isosorbide dinitrate

The combination of hydralazine and isosorbide dinitrate was shown to reduce mortality in patients with heart failure in a relatively small trial conducted before the widespread use of ACE inhibitors and beta-blockers. Recently, the same combination was shown to improve symptoms, reduce admission to hospital for worsening heart failure and increase survival in African-Americans treated with an ACE inhibitor, beta-blocker and, in many cases, spironolactone. The main role of hydralazine and isosorbide dinitrate in non–African-Americans is as an alternative in patients with renal intolerance of an ACE inhibitor or ARB.

## Drugs with a positive inotropic effect

### Digoxin

Digoxin now has a limited role in patients with heart failure in sinus rhythm, usually reserved for those remaining symptomatic despite an ACE inhibitor, beta-blocker and either an ARB or aldosterone antagonist. It remains a more important treatment in patients with heart failure and atrial fibrillation. The pharmacodynamics and pharmacokinetics of digoxin together with clinical uses and doses are discussed in full earlier in this chapter. Digoxin improves cardiac performance in patients with atrial fibrillation by slowing the ventricular rate. In patients with sinus rhythm, digoxin has a positive inotropic effect when given acutely. There has been controversy as to whether this effect is maintained during long-term therapy. Digoxin has autonomic actions that may be useful in heart failure. Double-blind studies have confirmed the long-term beneficial effect of digoxin on symptoms and morbidity (but not mortality) in sinus rhythm, an effect best seen in patients with severe heart failure. If digoxin is used, the dose should be adjusted to take account of renal function.

Monitoring of plasma drug levels is of limited use as there is a poor relationship between therapeutic effect (in terms of symptoms) and plasma level. Toxicity may be best judged by the occurrence of side effects (anorexia, nausea). However, in elderly patients the symptoms of digoxin toxicity are protean and the first evidence may be serious arrhythmia which is increased with hypokalaemia. Monitoring for toxicity may be warranted in this group.

## Adrenoceptor agonists: dopamine and dobutamine

These drugs are currently used only in acute heart failure accompanied by hypotension and poor tissue perfusion. They have established short-term effects when given intravenously.

*Mechanism*
Both drugs produce their inotropic effect by $\beta_1$-adrenoceptor stimulation of the myocardium. The effects of dopamine are dose dependent and result partly from direct action and partly from indirect effects through increased noradrenaline release. Below 5 μg/kg per min the major effect is to increase renal blood flow by stimulation of dopamine receptors. As the dose is increased in the 5–20 μg/kg per min range both

$\beta_1$- and $\alpha$-adrenoceptor stimulant effects are seen with increased cardiac output and a modest rise in blood pressure. Above this dose range, $\alpha$-receptor effects are more marked, with a further rise in blood pressure. This tends to increase afterload and is undesirable. Dobutamine has no renal vasodilator effect, less vasoconstrictor (alpha) effect and a similar inotropic effect to dopamine.

*Pharmacokinetics*
These drugs undergo rapid clearance. Dopamine and dobutamine must be given intravenously.

*Adverse effects*
Mainly tachyarrhythmias from $\beta_1$-receptor stimulation when used in excessive doses. Stimulation of $\beta$-receptors in skeletal muscle can cause hypokalaemia.

*Dose*
Dopamine: 5 μg/kg per min initially, increasing as required by the clinical response.
Dobutamine: 2.5 μg/kg per min initially, increasing as necessary.

## Levosimendan

Levosimendan is believed to act by sensitising the cardiomyocyte contractile proteins to calcium, thus exerting a positive inotropic effect without increasing intracellular calcium or cAMP concentration, undesirable properties of adrenoceptor agonists and phosphodiesterase inhibitors. Levosimendan also causes arterial vasodilatation, possibly by opening ATP-dependent $K^+$ channels in vascular smooth muscle. For this reason, levosimendan has been described as an 'inodilator'. Preliminary clinical studies have confirmed that levosimendan has favourable haemodynamic effects and may improve symptoms and survival in patients with severe heart failure. These early observations require substantiation in larger trials.

## Drugs affecting preload

### Glyceryl trinitrate

Sublingual nitroglycerin leads to direct relaxation of smooth muscle of the systemic venous system, although such treatment is rarely adequate for acute pulmonary oedema. Subsequent venous pooling in cardiac failure leads to a reduction in left ventricular end diastolic pressure and volume, reducing pulmonary congestion. There is usually no associated rise in cardiac output. Intravenous GTN can be used acutely until oral agents can be introduced.

### Isosorbide dinitrate and mononitrate

The combination of intravenous isosorbide dinitrate and intravenous diuretic has been shown to be a better treatment for acute heart failure than high-dose diuretic alone.

## Drugs affecting afterload

### Hydralazine

This has a direct vasodilator effect confined to the arterial bed. Reduction in systemic vascular resistance leads to a considerable rise in cardiac output. Changes in arterial blood pressure, as a consequence of the rise in cardiac output and heart rate resulting from blunting of baroreflexes, are smaller than in patients with hypertension. Its use may be of benefit in chronic heart failure when used in combination with oral nitrates. Doses up to 200 mg daily are used in heart failure. Slow acetylators are at increased risk of a drug-induced lupus syndrome.

### Calcium antagonists

Until recently, heart failure was considered a contraindication to calcium antagonist use with evidence that nifedipine, diltiazem and verapamil could have adverse effects on prognosis after myocardial infarction in patients with heart failure. Recent studies with long-acting dihydropyridine calcium antagonists (amlodipine, felodipine) suggest that these agents may be safe in heart failure.

## Drugs affecting preload and afterload

### Sodium nitroprusside

This is a mixed venous and arteriolar dilator also used for acute reduction of blood pressure (Chapter 5). It must be given intravenously by continuous infusion in a dose range of 25–125 μg/min. Blood pressure falls rapidly and the effects wear off over 1–2 min after stopping the infusion. This agent is particularly useful in acute valvular insufficiency, such as mitral incompetence following an acute infarct or aortic incompetence in bacterial endocarditis. However, randomised controlled trials show a trend to increased mortality in patients with post-infarction heart failure treated routinely with this agent. It should not be used for more than 24–48 h because of accumulation of thiocyanate.

### Nesiritide

Nesiritide is recombinant human b-type natriuretic peptide which acts as an arterial and venous dilator by increasing intracellular cGMP. Intravenous administration of nesiritide reduces pulmonary capillary wedge pressure, increases cardiac output and has been shown to reduce breathlessness in patients with acute decompensated heart failure. Diuresis has not been convincingly demonstrated and there are limited safety data on this agent.

*Comment.* Nitrates (glyceryl trinitrate or isosorbide dinitrate) are the only commonly used intravenous vasodilator used to treat acute heart failure. Oral vasodilators are generally reserved for patients who are intolerant of, or who have contraindications to, ACE inhibitors or ARBs. As discussed above, the combination of hydralazine and isosorbide dinitrate may be an alternative treatment if ACE inhibitor or ARB cannot be used in patients with renal intolerance.

## General principles of management of heart failure

*Acute left ventricular failure or pulmonary oedema* presents with severe breathlessness, orthopnoea or nocturnal dyspnoea.

1 Sit the patient up.

2 100% oxygen.

3 Establish an i.v. line.

4 Give 5 mg diamorphine or 10 mg morphine i.v. (with an antiemetic) because:
- It has a venodilator effect reducing preload.
- It reduces the intense distress of the patient.

5 Give furosemide 40 mg i.v., more if the patient is already receiving a loop diuretic, because:
- It has a rapid off-loading effect resulting from venous dilatation.
- It has a slower off-loading effect resulting from diuresis and natriuresis.

6 If the systolic blood pressure is ≥100 mmHg and obstructive valve disease has been excluded, start on intravenous GTN or isosorbide dinitrate infusion:
- It has a venodilator effect, reducing preload.
- It has an arterial vasodilator effect, reducing afterload.
- It reduces myocardial ischaemia which is often a co-existent problem in patients with acute heart failure.

7 Correct precipitating or aggravating factors, especially arrhythmias, anaemia and ischaemia.

8 Exclude mechanical problems requiring surgery by echocardiography, e.g. valvular lesions, ruptured ventricular septum.

9 In resistant patients, appropriate therapy with an i.v. vasodilator (e.g. sodium nitroprusside) and/or inotropic agent (e.g. dobutamine or levosimendan) should be considered and the choice of drugs may be aided by invasive haemodynamic monitoring. In selected cases, placement of an intra-aortic balloon pump or a left ventricular assist device may also be considered.

*Cardiogenic shock* consists of hypotension and oliguria with clinical signs of poor tissue perfusion. It is usually caused by recent extensive myocardial infarction.

1 Where possible monitor both arterial and pulmonary wedge pressure.

2 Give 100% oxygen.

3 Improve cardiac performance with dobutamine or a similar inotropic drug.

4 Low-dose dopamine intravenously may improve renal function.

5 If this fails, then depending on the haemodynamic features consider placement of an intra-aortic balloon pump and try reduction of afterload with sodium nitroprusside or GTN and/or use of dobutamine, dopamine or levosimendan. In selected cases, placement of a left ventricular assist device may also be considered.

## Long-term management of chronic heart failure

1 Modify cardiovascular risk factor profile, e.g. cigarette smoking, obesity. Arrange once only pneumococcal vaccination and regular immunisation against influenza.

2 Underlying causes should be treated, e.g. anaemia, hypertension, valvular disease.

3 If this proves inadequate or when there is no treatable underlying cause, diuretics should be given. The type of diuretic and dose depends on severity of failure.

4 All patients without contraindication who have heart failure resulting from left ventricular systolic dysfunction should be treated with an ACE inhibitor, to improve symptoms further (if still present), to delay worsening heart failure and to reduce major morbidity and mortality.

5 All patients without contraindication who have heart failure due to left ventricular systolic dysfunction should be treated with a beta-blocker, to improve symptoms, to delay worsening heart failure and to reduce major morbidity and mortality.

6 In patients with persisting symptoms and/or signs of congestion, add either an ARB or spironolactone to improve symptoms and reduce major morbidity and mortality.

7 Digoxin currently remains the drug of choice for the control of ventricular rate in patients with atrial fibrillation and heart failure (these patients should usually be treated with warfarin as well).

8 In patients with persisting symptoms several strategies can be adopted:
- If evidence of cardiac dys-synchrony (e.g. broad QRS on ECG) consider cardiac resynchronisation therapy.

- Add digoxin.
- An increase in diuretic dose.
- Ensure that the patient is on the maximally tolerated dose of ACE inhibitors.
- If arterial pressure is still elevated add hydralazine and an oral nitrate or a long-acting dihydropyridine calcium antagonist (amlodipine, felodipine).
- If angina is present add a nitrate, nicorandil or a long-acting dihydropyridine calcium antagonist (amlodipine, felodipine).
- If marked oedema is present increase loop diuretic or add a thiazide diuretic or metolazone (careful monitoring of blood chemistry required).

- In resistant cases patients may be admitted for intravenous diuretic therapy. If this fails, haemodynamic monitoring may be considered. Although empirical vasodilator therapy is not of proven benefit, observational experience suggests that vasodilator therapy tailored to optimise haemodynamics may be beneficial. Haemodynamic investigation often reveals overzealous diuretic therapy with too low a filling pressure to be the cause of the patient's symptoms.

9 Patients with atrial fibrillation should be considered for warfarin therapy.

10 Consider specialist referral for comment for cardiac support or transplantation.

# Chapter 7

# Antimicrobial therapy

## Aim

The aim is to control infection without damage to the patient.

## Principles of drug treatment

One of the greatest of all therapeutic advances was the introduction of drugs to treat bacterial infections in man. The introduction of sulphonamides in 1936 and penicillin in 1941 dramatically reduced mortality from infections. During the decades since then there has been a vast increase in the number of antimicrobial agents available for clinical use. This ready availability of drugs has enhanced the likelihood that a suitable agent can be found for a particular infection, but it has also resulted in a confusing range of choice and a readiness to prescribe antimicrobial agents even when the presence of bacterial infection is poorly documented. Moreover, the increasing rate of resistance of micro-organisms to antimicrobial agents is now limiting the choice of effective therapy. The newer antibiotics are expensive and not necessarily better than established agents: they should be prescribed only after careful consideration of the issues identified in Table 7.1.

## The patient

### Documentation of infection

Whenever possible the clinical suspicion of infection should be supported by laboratory diagnosis. Appropriate specimens, e.g. sputum, urine, pus, blood, etc., should be obtained before treatment is commenced.

### Age

Drug kinetics are influenced by age-dependent changes in pathways of elimination (Chapter 3). Clinically important examples involving antimicrobial agents include:

1 Relative deficiency of hepatic glucuronyl transferase in neonates, leading to an accumulation of chloramphenicol with a likelihood of cardiovascular collapse if serum concentration exceeds 25 mg/l.

2 Physiological decrease in renal function with age, leading to an accumulation of aminoglycosides in the elderly with a likelihood of toxicity: dose modification is necessary. Other antimicrobials contraindicated in specific age groups are:

- Sulphonamides in the neonate (displacement of bilirubin, leading to kernicterus)
- Tetracyclines in growing children (tooth discoloration)

Table 7.1 General principles of antimicrobial therapy.

| Patient | Organism | Drug |
|---|---|---|
| Document infection | Culture | Absorption |
| Factors altering kinetics: age, renal/hepatic function | Identification | Tissue distribution |
| Typing | | Route of elimination |
| | Adverse reactions | |
| Previous drug sensitivity | Drug interactions | |
| General health (resistance to infection) | Antimicrobial susceptibility | |
| Pregnancy | | |

## Renal and hepatic function

Many commonly used antimicrobials are eliminated by the kidney while a few undergo hepatic metabolism. Dose modification is likely to be necessary if renal function is moderately or severely impaired (see 'Influence of impaired renal function', Chapter 3) (Table 7.2). Drug level monitoring is mandatory for antimicrobials with concentration-related toxicity.

## Drug sensitivity

Always ask about previous exposure to drugs. Penicillins and cephalosporins are the antimicrobials most frequently associated with sensitivity reactions and there is a 5–10% cross-sensitivity between these two drug groups because they both contain the β-lactam ring. Minor sensitivity reactions to penicillins, such as rash, should not prevent prescription of a cephalosporin, but a life-threatening allergic reaction to penicillin is an absolute contraindication to the use of cephalosporins.

## Diminished resistance to infection

Patients with malignant disease or who are receiving cytotoxic or immunosuppressant drugs are

Table 7.2 Antimicrobials for which dose modification is required in mild, moderate or severe renal failure and in liver disease.

| Renal failure | | | |
|---|---|---|---|
| Mild | Moderate | Severe | Liver disease |
| Aminoglycosides | Metronidazole | Co-trimoxazole | Clindamycin |
| Amphotericin B | Ticarcillin | Penicillins | Isoniazid, cephalosporins, rifampicin, ethambutol |
| | Aciclovir | | *Avoid*: Erythromycin estolate, pyrazinamide |
| Flucytosine | | | |
| Vancomycin | | | |
| *Avoid*: Cephalothin, cephaloridine, nalidixic acid, nitrofurantoin, tetracyclines | | | |

susceptible to infections with commensal bacteria as well as less common organisms, e.g. some viruses, yeasts, fungi and protozoa. In particular, granulocytopaenia (less than $500 \times 10^6/l$) is accompanied by a high risk of septicaemia. Fever in such patients must be assumed to have an infective aetiology and should be treated aggressively before a definitive bacteriological diagnosis is available.

## Pregnancy

Penicillins and cephalosporins are not harmful to the fetus. Fetal damage has been associated definitely with streptomycin and the tetracyclines. Possible adverse fetal effects have been ascribed to gentamicin, kanamycin and cotrimoxazole (see 'Effect of drugs on the fetus', Chapter 4). In general, there is little data on possible teratogenic effects of newer agents.

*Comment.* The patient's age, sex and general state of health must be considered when choosing both the drug and its dose.

## The organism

### Bacteria

#### Sensitivity

Bactericidal drugs kill the organisms against which they are effective. Bacteriostatic drugs do not kill the organism but inhibit its ability to replicate. Use of a bacteriostatic drug assumes that body defences can destroy the organisms whose replication has been prevented. Testing *in vitro* is available for most antibacterial drugs. Application of *in vitro* findings to the patient assumes that adequate drug concentrations are achieved at the site of infection.

#### Resistance

Some bacteria have always been resistant to the effects of certain drugs, while others have developed resistance in the course of repeated exposure to antimicrobials. The two major mechanisms by which resistance is produced are gene mutation and DNA exchange between bacteria. Resistance may take three main forms:

1 An alteration in the bacterial component on which the drug acts, e.g. changes in the 30S ribosomal subunit in organisms developing resistance to aminoglycosides.

2 The drug might be destroyed by the organisms, as in the case of penicillins that are inactivated by β-lactamases produced by resistant bacteria. Bacteria have evolved a complex armamentarium of β-lactamases, such as extended spectrum β-lactamases that are able to degrade recently developed drugs such as third-generation cephalosporins (e.g. cefotaxime).

3 Cell membrane permeability to drugs is reduced, as in resistance to tetracyclines.

The development of resistance can be reduced if antimicrobials are not given indiscriminately. Additionally, the use of drug combinations should limit the appearance of resistant organisms in conditions such as tuberculosis (TB) where prolonged treatment is necessary.

### Viruses and fungi

The range of effective drugs is more limited and in many cases treatment is still experimental. Consequently, information about sensitivity or resistance to treatment is far less complete than for bacteria.

*Comment.* Antimicrobial treatment must take appropriate account of the organism's susceptibility to drugs and the patient's intrinsic ability to combat infection.

## The drug

### Absorption

Certain antimicrobials, e.g. the aminoglycosides, can only be given parenterally because absorption from the gastrointestinal tract is negligible. Where a choice exists between oral and parenteral drug formulations, the decision must rest on the severity of the illness and the need to achieve high tissue concentration. In severely ill patients, absorption of drugs from the gut may be unreliable necessitating use of intravenous preparations. However, when gut function recovers a switch to an oral

**Table 7.3** Antimicrobials for which high concentrations are achieved.

| CSF | Bile | Urine |
|---|---|---|
| Chloramphenicol | Penicillins | Penicillins |
| Erythromycin | Cephalosporins | Cephalosporins |
| Isoniazid | Erythromycin | Aminoglycosides |
| Pyrazinamide | | Sulphonamides |
| Rifampicin | | Nitrofurantoin |
| Flucytosine | | Nalidixic acid |
| | | Ethambutol |
| | | Flucytosine |

preparation reduces the risk of catheter-associated infection and is generally cheaper.

## Tissue distribution

The principles determining drug distribution are described in Chapter 1 (see 'Principles of pharmacokinetics', p. 7). In addition to these general considerations of blood concentration, protein binding, lipid solubility, etc., a further factor influencing antimicrobial distribution is the presence of inflammation, which tends to improve tissue penetration. However, it must not be assumed that the presence of inflammation greatly transforms the penetration of drugs. For example, gentamicin and vancomycin cross poorly into the cerebrospinal fluid (CSF) even in the presence of meningitis. Table 7.3 indicates those agents with high penetration to CSF, bile and urine.

## Route of elimination

This is usually renal or hepatic metabolism (or rarely biliary excretion); see Chapter 3 and the section above on renal and hepatic function.

## Adverse effects

These are of two general types:
1 Hypersensitivity reactions that are either immediate or delayed. The former produce anaphylaxis while the latter manifest themselves in various ways, the most common being rashes. Hypersensitivity reactions usually occur with no prior warning and are most commonly seen with penicillins, cephalosporins and sulphonamides.
2 The other type of adverse reaction is usually predictable in being concentration related; aminoglycoside ototoxicity is an example. Fortunately, the toxic concentrations of most antimicrobials in common use greatly exceed the required therapeutic concentrations. Where this is not the case, e.g. gentamicin, drug level monitoring is mandatory. Adverse reactions to antimicrobials are summarised in Table 7.4 and discussed in more detail under specific agents.

## Drug interactions

These can be either kinetic, e.g. enzyme induction or inhibition, or dynamic, e.g. two drugs adversely affecting the same organ. Examples include the following:
1 Aminoglycosides and frusemide have an additive nephrotoxic effect.
2 Rifampicin induces the same enzymes that metabolise the contraceptive pill and can cause failure of contraception.
3 Sulphonamides inhibit the enzymes that metabolise phenytoin and can cause phenytoin toxicity.
4 Tetracyclines form insoluble complexes in the gut lumen with both antacids and iron, leading to treatment failure.
5 Quinolones may trigger side effects of theophylline as a result of its decreased elimination.
6 Amphotericin B and aminoglycosides or vancomycin display increased nephrotoxicity and ototoxicity.

## Antimicrobial prophylaxis

Antimicrobial agents are sometimes given to people who do not have an infection but who are considered to be at risk from a specific organism. Examples include the use of rifampicin or ciprofloxacin in close contacts of patients with

**Table 7.4** Major adverse reactions of antimicrobial drugs.

| Organ system | Drug | Comment |
|---|---|---|
| Kidney | Aminoglycosides | Concentration–related |
| | Cephalosporins | Mainly earlier drugs of this group |
| | Sulphonamides | |
| | Methicillin | Other penicillins rarely |
| | Amphotericin B | |
| | Polymyxins | Limits use |
| Bone marrow suppression | Antiviral agents | |
| | Amphotericin B | |
| | Flucytosine | |
| | Chloramphenicol | |
| | Sulphonamides | Rare |
| Haemolytic anaemia | Sulphonamides | Two distinct mechanisms: immune and glucose-6-phosphate deficiency |
| | Nitrofurantoin | |
| | 4-Fluoroquinolones | |
| | Penicillins | Rare |
| | Cephalosporins | Rare |
| Thrombocytopenia | Sulphonamides | Rare |
| | Cephalosporins | Rare |
| | Latamoxef | Dose–dependent |
| | Rifampicin | Intermittent therapy |
| Neutropenia | Penicillins | Rare: mainly ampicillin, carbenicillin |
| | Cephalosporins | Rare |
| | Sulphonamides | Rare |
| | Chloramphenicol | |
| Neurological eighth nerve | Aminoglycosides | Concentration-related |
| | Vancomycin | |
| Optic nerve | Ethambutol | |
| Peripheral neuropathy | Isoniazid | Prevented by pyridoxine |
| | Metronidazole | Prolonged treatment |
| | Nitrofurantoin | |
| Convulsions | Penicillins | Large intrathecal or massive intravenous doses |
| | Cephalosporins | Large intrathecal doses |
| | 4-Fluoroquinolones | Large doses |
| Benign intracranial hypertension | Tetracyclines | |
| | Penicillins | |
| | Nalidixic acid | |
| Neuromuscular blockade | Aminoglycosides | |

*(Continued)*

**Table 7.4** (Continued)

| Organ system | Drug | Comment |
|---|---|---|
| *Gastrointestinal system* | | |
| Liver | Isoniazid | More often slow acetylators |
| | Rifampicin | Usually mild—worse in alcoholics/preceding damage |
| | Tetracyclines | Massive doses |
| | Erythromycin estolate | |
| | Nitrofurantoin | |
| Transient rise in transaminases | Penicillins, especially flucloxacillin | |
| | Cephalosporins | |
| Diarrhoea | Penicillins | Specially ampicillin |
| | Tetracyclines | |
| | Clindamycin and other broad-spectrum antibiotics | Pseudomembranous colitis (*C. difficile*) |
| *Other adverse reactions* | | |
| Hypersensitivity | Penicillins | 10% cross-sensitivity |
| | Sulphonamides | |
| Stevens–Johnson syndrome | Sulphonamides | |
| | Penicillins | |
| Bone development/tooth staining | Tetracyclines | Contraindicated in childhood and pregnancy |
| Pulmonary fibrosis | Nitrofurantoin | |
| Rashes | Commonly penicillins and sulphonamides but virtually any drug can cause rashes | |

meningococcal meningitis, the administration of penicillin before and following dental procedures in people at risk of endocarditis and the long-term use of amoxicillin in children with repeated urinary tract infections and evidence of vesicoureteric reflux. Perioperative prophylaxis in certain types of surgery where the risk of infection is high (e.g. colorectal) or the consequences of infection are life-threatening (e.g. open heart) is now standard practice, e.g. cefotaxime and metronidazole or ciprofloxacin and metronidazole.

*Comment.* An antimicrobial agent might be quite ineffective, or even dangerous, unless its clinical pharmacology is viewed in relation to the whole clinical situation. The drug chosen must reach the site of infection, in an effective concentration, without producing toxicity or adversely influencing any concurrent therapy. In many circumstances an antibiotic must be chosen before results of culture are available. Some guidelines

for empirical therapy of a variety of infections are shown in the Table 7.5.

# Antibacterial drugs

## Penicillins

### Mechanism

Penicillins have a bactericidal action. They inhibit cell wall synthesis by preventing the formation of peptidoglycan cross-bridges in actively multiplying bacteria.

### Pharmacokinetics

**Oral absorption**

*Not absorbed*: carbenicillin, ticarcillin

*Moderately absorbed*: benzylpenicillin (penicillin G), ampicillin

**Table 7.5** Empirical antibiotic therapy.

| Source of infection | Antibiotic |
|---|---|
| Urinary tract infection | Trimethoprim |
| | *or* Co-amoxiclav |
| Pyelonephritis | Ciprofloxacin |
| | *or* Ceftriaxone + gentamicin |
| Cellulitis | |
|    Mild | Flucloxacillin |
| | *or* Clindamycin (penicillin allergy) |
|    Severe | Flucloxacillin + benzylpenicillin |
| | *or* Clindamycin ± gentamicin (penicillin allergy) |
| Community-acquired pneumonia | |
|    Mild | Amoxycillin |
|    Severe | Co-amoxiclav + clarithromycin |
| Exacerbation of COPD | Amoxycillin |
| | *or* Clarithromycin (penicillin allergy) |
| Hospital-acquired pneumonia | Ciprofloxacin |
| Aspiration pneumonia | Co-amoxiclav *or* |
| | Ceftriaxone + metronidazole |
| Suspected staphylococcal pneumonia | Add flucloxacillin *or* vancomycin to above regimes |
| Gastroenteritis | No antibiotic usually required. If invasive disease suspected, ciprofloxacin |
| Biliary sepsis | Ceftriaxone + metronidazole *or* |
| | Tazocin + gentamicin |
| Meningitis | Ceftriaxone |
| Severe sepsis—uncertain origin | Ceftriaxone + gentamicin |

*Well absorbed*: phenoxypenicillin, amoxicillin, flucloxacillin

Even relatively well-absorbed penicillins are destroyed to some extent by gastric acid and should therefore be given at least 30 min before meals.

## Distribution

The penicillins have good penetration to most tissues but poor entry to CSF. However, meningeal inflammation increases CSF penetration allowing the use of these agents in the treatment of meningitis. Giving large doses when treating meningitis also increases CSF delivery.

## Elimination

Penicillins undergo enterohepatic circulation: drug is excreted via bile and reabsorbed. The major route of elimination after reabsorption is active secretion in the renal tubules. This tubular secretion can be blocked by probenecid with doubling of penicillin blood levels. Dose modification is necessary in severe renal failure (Table 7.6).

## Adverse effects

### Immediate hypersensitivity

This occurs in 0.05% of patients with manifestations ranging from urticaria or wheezing to a life-threatening anaphylactic response.

### Delayed hypersensitivity

This occurs in <5% of patients, mainly as rashes. Rare manifestations are hemolytic anaemia, interstitial nephritis (mainly reported with methicillin), and leucopenia. Cross-sensitivity with cephalosporins occurs in around 10% of patients.

### Toxicity

Convulsions follow large (>15 mg) intrathecal (no longer used) or very high intravenous doses of

**Table 7.6** Doses of penicillins.

> **1** Benzylpenicillin: intramuscular 300–600 mg two to four times daily (children 10–20 mg/kg daily); intravenous up to 14.4 g daily; intrathecal 6–12 mg daily
> **2** Phenoxymethylpenicillin: oral dose 250–500 mg 6-hourly (children, 125–250 mg 6-hourly)
> **3** Ampicillin: oral dose 250–1000 mg 6-hourly; intravenous or intramuscular 500–1000 mg 6-hourly (children, half doses)
> **4** Amoxicillin: oral 250–500 mg 8-hourly (children, half dose)
> **5** Carbenicillin: intravenous (rapid infusion) 5 g 4- to 6-hourly (children, 250–400 mg/kg daily divided doses); intramuscular 2 g 6-hourly (children, 50–100 mg/kg divided doses)
> **6** Ticarcillin: intravenous infusion (rapid) or intramuscular 15–20 g daily divided doses
> **7** Azlocillin: 2 g 8-hourly by intravenous injection; up to 5 g 8-hourly by infusion
> **8** Flucloxacillin: oral 250 mg 6-hourly
> **9** Co-amoxiclav: oral 1–2 tablets (of 250 mg amoxicillin, 125 mg clavulanic acid) 8-hourly

penicillin. Patients with renal insufficiency can develop cation overload following large doses of potassium penicillin or sodium carbenicillin. Diarrhoea is commonly reported, particularly with ampicillin (20%). Ampicillin has a unique adverse effect comprising a rash in up to 90% of patients with infectious mononucleosis or chronic lymphocytic leukaemia.

## Drug interactions

Ampicillin can lead to oral contraceptive failure. This is probably because of diminished enterohepatic circulation. The anticoagulant effect of warfarin is potentiated.

## Antibacterial spectrum

The major factor limiting efficacy is the production by certain organisms of enzymes (β-lactamases or penicillinases) that destroy the β-lactam ring of the penicillin molecule. This structure is essential to the antibacterial action of penicillins. Several synthetic penicillins incorporate side chains that protect the β-lactam ring against these enzymes. An alternative approach has been to combine amoxicillin with clavulanic acid, which itself has very little antibacterial activity but inhibits β-lactamase activity.

## Penicillinase-sensitive penicillins

Benzylpenicillin and phenoxypenicillins are active against streptococci, pneumococci, gonococci and meningococci, *Treponema pallidum*, *Actinomyces israelii* and most anaerobic organisms that are found in the mouth and upper gastrointestinal tract, but not below the diaphragm such as *Bacteroides fragilis*.

Ampicillin has a broader spectrum and is effective against some strains of *Escherichia coli*, *Proteus mirabilis*, *Shigella*, *Salmonella*, *Haemophilus influenzae* and various enterococci; amoxicillin is better absorbed but has the same antibacterial spectrum. The main indications are acute exacerbations of chronic bronchitis and urinary tract infection.

Carbenicillin and ticarcillin are active against *Pseudomonas aeruginosa* and *Proteus* sp. At least *in vitro*, ticarcillin is more effective than carbenicillin and azlocillin is more effective than ticarcillin against *P. aeruginosa*. All three drugs must be given parenterally. Drug resistance is encountered in some strains.

## Penicillinase-resistant penicillins

Cloxacillin, flucloxacillin and methicillin are indicated only in the treatment of infections caused by penicillinase-producing staphylococci. Flucloxacillin is better absorbed from the gut than cloxacillin. More cases of interstitial nephritis have been reported following methicillin therapy than with any other penicillin.

## Co-amoxiclav

The amoxicillin/clavulanic acid combination is used in treating urinary tract infections caused by β-lactamase-producing coliforms, as well as in severe community-acquired pneumonia.

## Tazocin

This combination of piperacillin with tazobactam is used mainly in the treatment of patients with impaired host defences (e.g. following bone marrow transplantation) where infection with β-lactamase-producing coliforms is suspected. It is also used extensively in severely ill patients in intensive care units.

## Imipenem

This β-lactam is a carbapenem with a very broad spectrum of activity against many Gram-negative, Gram-positive and anaerobic organisms. It is partially inactivated within the kidney and is thus co-formulated with cilastatin, which blocks this renal metabolism. It is indicated for the treatment of severe infections, particularly those that are resistant to other antibiotics. In addition to the side effects of all penicillin-like drugs, imipenem does lower seizure threshold. The closely related drug meropenem is thus preferred in patients with epilepsy.

## Cephalosporins

### Mechanism

Cephalosporins are bactericidal. They contain a β-lactam ring and their mechanism of action is similar to penicillins.

### Pharmacokinetics

Six cephalosporins are effective orally: cefalexin, cefradine (cephradine), cefaclor, cefixime, cefadroxil and cefuroxime. They distribute widely. A range of intravenous cephalosporins is also available, such as cefotaxime and ceftriaxone. This latter agent has a long half-life allowing once-daily dosing, of considerable benefit in managing administration of a parenteral antibiotic to outpatients. Cephaloridine does not cross the blood–brain barrier. The drugs are eliminated renally, partly by glomerular filtration and partly by tubular secretion, with the contribution of each route varying with individual cephalosporins. Doses of cephalosporins are shown in Table 7.7.

### Adverse effects

Hypersensitivity is the main adverse effect, with around 10% cross-reactivity with penicillin-sensitive patients. Cephaloridine can cause renal tubular necrosis, particularly in doses above 6 g/day. Cephalosporins can reduce prothrombin concentration and bleeding has been described. Several cephalosporins, including those commonly used orally, cause false positive urinalysis tests for glucose, as measured by reducing substances.

### Drug interactions

The nephrotoxicity of cephaloridine is potentiated by loop diuretics and aminoglycoside antibiotics.

### Antibacterial spectrum

The early cephalosporins were broad spectrum but with limited activity against Gram-negative organisms. Cephamandole and cefuroxime are more resistant to β-lactamases and are effective against a number of Gram-negative bacilli. Cefotaxime is more effective than cephamandole or cefuroxime against Gram-negative bacilli but less effective against Gram-positive organisms. Ceftazidime is active against *P. aeruginosa*. Cefoxitin is closely

**Table 7.7** Doses of cephalosporins.

| Oral | |
|---|---|
| Cefalexin ad cefradine: 250–500 mg 6-hourly (children, 25–50 mg/kg daily in divided doses) | Cefuroxime: 1.5 g 6-hourly (children, 30–100 mg/kg daily in divided doses) |
| | Cephamadole: 500–2000 mg 6-hourly (children, 50–100 mg/kg daily in divided doses) |
| Cefaclor: 250 mg 8-hourly (children, 20–40 mg/kg daily in divided doses) | Cefsulodin: 1–4 g daily in divided doses (children, 20–50 mg/kg daily). |
| Cefadroxil: 0.5–1.0 g 12-hourly | Cefotaxime: 1 g 12-hourly to 3 g 6-hourly, depending on severity (children, 100–200 mg/kg daily in divided doses) |
| *Intravenous* | |
| Cefradine: 500–1000 mg 6-hourly (children, 50–100 mg/kg daily in 6-hourly doses) | Cefoxitin: 1–2 g 8-hourly (children, 80–160 mg/kg daily in divided doses) |
| Ceftazidime: 1–2 g 8- to 12-hourly | |
| Cefazolin (cephazolin): 500–1000 mg 6-hourly (children, 125–250 mg 8-hourly) | Ceftriaxone: 1.0–1.2 g daily (children 20–50 mg/kg daily as a single dose) |

related to the basic cephalosporin structure and is active against Gram-negative and anaerobic bacteria. Ceftriaxone provides excellent Gram-negative cover as well as modest anti-staphylococcal activity.

*Comment.* The newer intravenous cephalosporins are expensive, but increasingly have become drugs of choice for severe and hospital-acquired infections.

## Aminoglycosides

### Mechanism

Aminoglycosides are bactericidal. They bind to the 30S subunit of bacterial ribosomes, leading to misreading of mRNA codons.

### Pharmacokinetics

Oral absorption is negligible. They have poor penetration into CSF and only moderate penetration into bile. Otherwise, there is good entry to inflamed tissue. Elimination is mainly by glomerular filtration. Traditionally, gentamicin is administered 8-hourly, but recent evidence shows that better antimicrobial killing is achieved by administering the drug once daily. Bacterial eradication is faster the higher the level of gentamicin is in the blood, leading to a more rapid clearance of microbes with once-daily dosing and lower chance of emergence of resistant organisms. Doses of aminoglycosides are shown in Table 7.8.

**Table 7.8** Doses of aminoglycosides.

*Gentamicin*: if renal function is normal, the intramuscular dose is 2–5 mg/kg daily given at 8-hourly intervals. Various nomograms and formulae are widely available for calculating dose modifications in renal impairment. A rough guide, based on creatinine clearance, is: >70 ml/min 8-hourly; 30–70 ml/min 12-hourly; 10–30 ml/min 24-hourly; 5–10 ml/min 48-hourly.

Increasingly, once-daily dosage regimens of gentamicin are used at 7 mg/kg, adjusted according to renal function. These give better antimicrobial killing and are not associated with increased toxicity. It must be emphasized that rules of thumb are not a substitute for drug level monitoring.

*Tobramycin*: 3–5 mg/kg daily given in divided doses 8-hourly. Modify dose in renal failure.

*Amikacin*: 15 mg/kg daily in 12-hourly doses. Modify dose in renal failure.

*Netilmicin*: 4–6 mg/kg daily in divided doses.

## Adverse effects

There are two major adverse reactions, both concentration related: nephrotoxicity and oto-toxicity. The renal lesion consists of tubular destruction. Eighth nerve damage can be mainly vestibular (streptomycin, gentamicin) or mainly auditory (kanamycin).

The severity of these reactions is related to aminoglycoside serum concentration, which in turn is related to dose and rate of elimination. Accumulation of drug occurs when glomerular filtration is decreased by renal disease or at the extremes of age. Doses must be modified in these situations and drug concentration monitoring is mandatory. Aminoglycosides cross the placenta and can cause eighth nerve damage in the fetus. An uncommon effect of aminoglycosides is neuromuscular blockade occurring after rapid intravenous injection; this is marked in patients with myasthenia gravis.

## Drug interactions

Nephrotoxicity is enhanced by co-administration with cephaloridine. Similarly, ototoxicity is enhanced by loop diuretics. The neuromuscular blockade of curare-like drugs can be prolonged by aminoglycosides.

## Antibacterial spectrum

Gentamicin is the most widely used aminoglycoside and is active against most aerobic Gram-negative rods, including *Pseudomonas* and *Proteus* spp., and also against staphylococci. Most streptococci are resistant because gentamicin cannot penetrate the cell. However, penicillin and aminoglycosides have synergistic effect against some streptococci. All anaerobic organisms are resistant. Tobramycin is two to four times more active against pseudomonas but is otherwise very similar to gentamicin. Amikacin is resistant to most of the bacterial enzymes that inactivate gentamicin, but is more toxic than gentamicin and is thus only indicated for infections caused by aerobic Gram-negative rods against which gentamicin is no longer effective. Netilmicin has a similar antibacterial spectrum to gentamicin, but is claimed to be less ototoxic: confirmatory evidence is limited. Neomycin is given orally to decrease the bacterial content of the colon in liver failure or before bowel surgery. If there is severe liver or renal failure or inflammatory bowel disease, sufficient neomycin can be absorbed to cause ototoxicity. Streptomycin is effective against tubercle bacilli and is discussed later.

*Comment.* The major role of aminoglycosides is the parenteral treatment of serious infection caused by sensitive organisms. These drugs are popular for the initial management of life-threatening septicaemia of uncertain aetiology. In this situation an aminoglycoside is usually combined with metronidazole and/or an extended spectrum penicillin.

# Sulphonamide–trimethoprim combinations

## Mechanism

These drugs are bactericidal. Co-trimoxazole contains a sulphonamide, sulphamethoxazole (sulfamethoxazole), and trimethoprim in the ratio 5:1. The basis of the action of sulphonamides is that bacterial cells are impermeable to folic acid and so they must synthesise their own from *p*-aminobenzoic acid, with which sulphonamides have a strong similarity. Thus, competitive inhibition of folic acid synthesis occurs. Trimethoprim blocks the next synthetic step, from folic acid to tetrahydrofolate, by inhibiting the enzyme dihydrofolate reductase.

## Pharmacokinetics

Co-trimoxazole is well absorbed following oral administration and is also available for intravenous use. There is wide tissue distribution and elimination is by renal excretion.

## Adverse effects

The sulphonamide component can cause rashes and, much less commonly, Stevens–Johnson syndrome, renal failure and blood dyscrasias.

Trimethoprim can also cause rashes and impaired haemopoiesis and can produce gastrointestinal symptoms. The trimethoprim component has been implicated in teratogenesis. In the newborn, sulphonamides can displace bilirubin from protein-binding sites and cause kernicterus.

## Drug interactions

The sulphonamide component competes for hepatic enzyme-binding sites and can decrease the clearance of phenytoin, tolbutamide and warfarin sufficiently to produce phenytoin toxicity, hypoglycaemia and enhanced anticoagulation, respectively. Displacement of methotrexate from protein-binding sites can also lead to toxicity.

## Antibacterial spectrum

These drugs have a broad spectrum, including Gram-positive cocci, *Neisseria gonorrhoeae*, *H. influenzae*, *E. coli*, *P. mirabilis*, *Shigella* sp., *Salmonella* sp., *Pneumocystis carinii* and *Brucella* sp..

**Dose**
Co-trimoxazole: 960 mg (two tablets of 400 mg sulphamethoxazole, 80 mg trimethoprim) 12-hourly for oral or intravenous administration (children, 120–480 mg 12-hourly depending on age).
*Comment.* Although an effective antibiotic, the risk of severe reactions such as Stevens–Johnson syndrome has limited the use of this drug. It remains the drug of choice in treating pneumonia caused by the opportunist pathogen *P. carinii* (now renamed *P. jiroveci*), a common infection in patients with AIDS.

## Trimethoprim

Trimethoprim alone is also used in treating urinary tract and respiratory tract infections. Dose: 300 mg daily or 100 mg daily for prophylaxis.

## Tetracyclines
### Mechanism

Tetracyclines are bacteriostatic, binding to the 30S ribosomal subunit with consequent misreading of information needed for protein synthesis.

### Pharmacokinetics

Tetracyclines are adequately absorbed following oral administration. Tissue distribution is good and the drugs are eliminated mainly unmetabolised by biliary excretion. Doxycycline has a long half-life and can be administered once daily.

### Adverse effects

Tetracyclines bind to calcium in bones and teeth, leading to impaired bone growth and discoloration of teeth during active mineralisation (up to 7 years). Tetracyclines cross the placenta and are contraindicated in pregnancy. Following large doses, both hepatic necrosis and renal failure have been reported. Except for doxycycline and minocycline, these drugs are contraindicated in renal failure because they impair protein synthesis and so enhance the effects of catabolism. Many patients develop diarrhoea on tetracycline therapy.

### Drug interactions

Milk, antacids, calcium, magnesium and iron form insoluble complexes with tetracyclines in the gut lumen, leading to treatment failure, the exception being minocycline.

### Antibacterial spectrum

The tetracyclines are effective against a wide range of bacteria but resistance is increasing, and they should no longer be considered useful broad-spectrum antibiotics. The importance of tetracyclines is based on their efficacy against Chlamydia (e.g. non-specific urethritis, psittacosis), rickettsia (e.g. Q fever, typhus, Rocky Mountain spotted fever), mycoplasma, brucella and cholera. Tetracyclines are also useful adjuncts to the treatment of acne by preventing the growth of *Propionibacterium acnes* in the blocked sebaceous ducts.

## Dose

Tetracycline and oxytetracycline: 250–500 mg 6-hourly. Minocycline: 200 mg, then 100 mg 12-hourly. Doxycycline: 200 mg loading dose, then 100 mg daily.

## Other antibacterial drugs

### Metronidazole

Metronidazole was initially used in protozoal infections, but was later found to be very effective against anaerobic bacteria, including *B. fragilis*. It is currently popular in treating serious anaerobic infections. In addition, metronidazole is often combined with gentamicin in treating serious mixed infections or septicaemia of uncertain aetiology. The other major uses are in treating trichomonal vaginitis, amoebiasis and giardiasis. Metronidazole is often combined with gentamicin or ciprofloxacin as prophylaxis in abdominal surgery. The only major adverse effects are peripheral neuropathy following prolonged therapy and seizures following high doses.

### Dose

For severe infections, intravenous infusion of metronidazole is given at the rate of 500 mg every 8 h in adults and 7.5 mg/kg 12-hourly in children for 7 days.
Oral: 200 mg 8-hourly for 7 days for trichomoniasis and 2 g daily for 3 days in amoebiasis and giardiasis. If appropriate, suppositories can be used in circumstances where intravenous infusion might be considered: similar blood levels but much cheaper. Dose: 1 g 8-hourly.

### Macrolides

Erythromycin was the first of these drugs to be used; newer agents include clarithromycin and azithromycin. They have an antibacterial spectrum similar to penicillin and often are suitable second-line drugs for patients allergic to penicillin. The use of erythromycin is frequently associated with nausea and vomiting; these side effects are much less prominent with clarithromycin and azithromycin. Clarithromycin is currently the drug of choice for *Legionella pneumophilia* and mycoplasma infections. It is also used in chlamydial non-specific urethritis and campylobacter enteritis. Azithromycin has an extremely long half-life of 68 h allowing once-daily dosing and short courses of treatment; it is currently very expensive. It has a broader spectrum of activity than erythromycin, including enhanced activity against *H. influenzae*, a common pathogen in infectious exacerbations of chronic pulmonary disease. It is useful in the treatment of gonococcal and non-gonococcal urethritis, and pelvic inflammatory disease, where single-dose therapy ensures complete patient compliance. It will treat effectively community-acquired pneumonia in patients with previously normal lung function as well as those with chronic pulmonary disease; cheaper alternatives for both are available.

### Dose

Erythromycin:
Oral: 250–500 mg 6-hourly for adults, 125–250 mg 6-hourly for children. Intravenous: 300 mg by infusion 6-hourly for adults, 30–50 mg/kg daily in divided doses 6-hourly for children.
Clarithromycin:
Oral: 500 mg 12-hourly for adults. Intravenous: 500 mg 12-hourly.
Azithromycin: For non-gonococcal urethritis/cervicitis 1 g single dose. For respiratory tract infections, 500 mg loading dose first day, then 250 mg daily for 4 days.

### Fusidic acid

This drug has a narrow spectrum and is indicated in combination with another anti-staphylococcal drug only in serious penicillin-resistant staphylococcal infections, e.g. those of bone.

### Dose

Fusidic acid is given at a dose of 500 mg 8-hourly by intravenous infusion or orally.

## Clindamycin

Clindamycin is effective against penicillin-resistant staphylococci and many anaerobic organisms. It is indicated only in serious conditions where other agents are contraindicated, or ineffective, notably staphylococcal bone and joint infections. However, an adverse effect is pseudomembranous colitis caused by toxigenic strains of *Clostridium difficile*. In practice, this complication is unfortunately common with the use of all widely used broad-spectrum antibiotics. Clindamycin is well absorbed by mouth and penetrates into tissues such as bone.

### Dose

Oral: Up to 450 mg every 6 hours. Intravenous: 0.6–2.7 g clindamycin daily is given in two to four divided doses by slow intravenous infusion; children, 15–40 mg/kg daily in divided doses.

## Nitrofurantoin

Nitrofurantoin, an orally administered drug that achieves antibacterial concentrations only in urine, is effective against many organisms infecting the urinary tract. However, it is a second-line drug for this indication because of frequent adverse effects, including gastrointestinal symptoms and rashes. It precipitates haemolytic anaemia in glucose-6-phosphate deficiency and can cause peripheral neuropathy and pulmonary fibrosis.

## Vancomycin

Vancomycin is effective against *C. difficile* and can be used to treat pseudomembranous colitis. It is also used intravenously in the prophylaxis and treatment of endocarditis caused by Gram-positive cocci. Increasingly vancomycin treatment is necessary in the treatment of catheter-associated infections resulting from coagulase-negative staphylococci. Because of possible nephrotoxicity, serum levels need to be monitored.

### Dose

Intravenous: 1 g 12-hourly.

## Teicoplanin

Teicoplanin is an alternative to vancomycin. Serum levels need not be monitored.

## Quinolones

Nalidixic acid, the first quinolone, has been available for 30 years. Administered orally, it achieves low tissue concentrations and its use is restricted to the treatment of uncomplicated urinary tract infections. Chemical modifications have produced a series of improved drugs and the most recent are the 4-fluoroquinolones; ciprofloxacin is the first agent in this group available in the United Kingdom.

## Ciprofloxacin

### Mechanism

Bactericidal in action, ciprofloxacin inhibits DNA-gyrase activity by binding to chromosomal DNA strands. This interferes with DNA replication and prevents supercoiling within the chromosome.

### Pharmacokinetics

It is well absorbed after oral administration and is distributed rapidly into body tissues. Most of the drug is eliminated unaltered by the kidneys; the remainder is excreted by hepatic metabolism or unchanged in the faeces.

### Adverse effects

The most frequently reported side effects are minor gastrointestinal upsets; severe systemic adverse reactions are rare. However, central nervous system disturbances such as insomnia, confusion and convulsions have been reported. As it can cause damage to cartilage in young animals, ciprofloxacin is contraindicated in children and growing adolescents.

### Drug interactions

Its absorption is reduced significantly by the co-administration of aluminium and magnesium antacids. It interferes with the metabolism of theophylline, caffeine and warfarin and so the toxic effects of these drugs may be encountered if they are given along with ciprofloxacin.

### Antibacterial spectrum

It is active against aerobic Gram-negative bacteria, including *P. aeruginosa*, and less active against Gram-positive bacteria: staphylococci are more sensitive than streptococci. Anaerobes, in general, are resistant. Ciprofloxacin is particularly useful for pseudomonas infections where oral therapy is preferred, such as respiratory tract infection in patients with cystic fibrosis. It is very effective in gastrointestinal infections ranging from traveller's diarrhoea to typhoid fever.

### Dose

Oral: 250–750 mg 12-hourly; intravenous: 200–400 mg 12-hourly.

## Levofloxacin

Similar spectrum to ciprofloxacin but with much greater activity against *Streptococcus pneumoniae*.

### Dose

Oral and intravenous: 500–750 mg once daily.

## Antituberculous drugs

### Isoniazid

#### Mechanism

Isoniazid inhibits a step in the biosynthesis of essential fatty acids within mycobacteria.

### Pharmacokinetics

Isoniazid is well absorbed following oral administration and is widely distributed throughout the body, including the CSF where concentrations equal those in blood. Isoniazid is inactivated in the liver by pathways including genetically dependent acetylation. The same metabolic pathway is involved in the acetylation of hydralazine, procainamide and dapsone (see 'Principles of drug elimination', Chapter 1). About 50% of Caucasians are slow acetylators but the proportion varies widely in other populations, and slow acetylation is very uncommon in people of Asian ethnic origin.

### Adverse effects

Peripheral neuropathy occurs mainly in slow acetylators and can be prevented by co-administration of pyridoxine (20 mg/day). Hepatotoxicity occasionally occurs and is more frequent in the elderly and those with a large alcohol intake. Very high doses of isoniazid can lead to psychosis, convulsions or coma.

### Drug interactions

Isoniazid inhibits enzymes that metabolise phenytoin and warfarin; thus, phenytoin concentrations and anticoagulation level should be carefully monitored.

### Dose

Oral: 3 mg/kg adults or 6 mg/kg daily in children, i.e. children require more on a weight basis; for tuberculous meningitis, 10 mg/kg daily. Also available for parenteral use.

### Rifampicin

#### Mechanism

It is bactericidal, and inhibits the DNA-dependent RNA polymerase of *Mycobacterium* sp.

## Pharmacokinetics

Rifampicin is well absorbed following oral administration and widely distributed, including the CSF. It is deacetylated in the liver and eliminated by biliary excretion.

## Adverse effects

There is often a transient elevation of liver enzymes but serious hepatotoxicity is uncommon. The risk of liver damage is increased by alcoholism and pre-existing liver disease. Intermittent treatment is associated with more frequent and serious adverse effects, including renal failure and thrombocytopaenia. Rifampicin causes red urine, tears and sputum.

## Drug interactions

Rifampicin induces hepatic enzymes and hence, because of increased clearance, can cause treatment failure with oral contraceptives, sulphonylureas, warfarin, steroids and barbiturates.

**Dose**
Rifampicin is given at a dose of 10 mg/kg daily before breakfast.

## Ethambutol

### Mechanism

The mechanism is uncertain but bacteriostatic.

### Pharmacokinetics

Ethambutol is well absorbed following oral administration. It has poor penetration of CSF but otherwise is adequately distributed. Excretion of unchanged drug is mainly renal.

### Adverse effects

The most important reaction is retrobulbar neuritis with loss of visual acuity and colour vision. This is largely preventable by using doses below 25 mg/kg daily. The visual defect usually reverses over several months after stopping the drug.

## Drug interactions

Aluminium hydroxide can decrease absorption.

**Dose**
A daily dose of 15 mg/kg is given.

## Pyrazinamide

### Mechanism

Pyrazinamide is bactericidal.

### Pharmacokinetics

It is well absorbed following oral administration and has good penetration to CSF. It is eliminated by renal excretion.

### Adverse effects

Pyrazinamide causes hepatotoxicity and arthralgia. Dose modification is required in patients with renal impairment.

**Dose**
A daily dose of 1.5 g (<50 kg) to 2 g (>50 kg).

**Second-line drugs**
Streptomycin is now infrequently used. It is an aminoglycoside that is eliminated by the kidneys. Ototoxicity is the main adverse reaction. Streptomycin could particularly be considered for use in patients with liver disease. Several other agents are available for use in situations of bacterial resistance or adverse reactions to first-line drugs, e.g. capreomycin, cycloserine, ethionamide and *p*-aminosalicylic acid.

*Comment.* *Mycobacterium tuberculosis* multiplies slowly and the long periods of treatment required encourage the emergence of resistant strains. Combination chemotherapy is thus the basis of treatment. Because of increasing drug resistance, initial treatment is now usually started with four drugs: isoniazid, rifampicin, ethambutol and pyrazinamide, administered for 8 weeks. Subsequently, isoniazid and rifampicin are given, as long as cultures indicate that the organism is susceptible, or, if the organism is not grown, that drug resistance is considered unlikely. Six months of treatment with this regimen is adequate for pulmonary TB. If other drugs are used, 9 months of therapy is necessary. If TB occurs elsewhere, or if intermittent therapy is used, 12–18 months may be required.

# Antifungal drugs

## Amphotericin B

### Mechanism

Amphotericin B combines with sterols in the plasma membrane, with a resulting increase in permeability and cell death.

### Pharmacokinetics

Absorption is negligible following oral administration. In practice it is usually given intravenously. It is highly protein-bound with apparently poor penetration to tissues and body fluids. It is not removed by haemodialysis. The mode of elimination is unknown but it is not influenced by renal function. Newer formulations consist of liposomal amphotericin.

### Adverse effects

These are very common. Most patients develop fever, chills and nausea. Nephrotoxicity (distal tubular destruction and calcification) usually occurs during prolonged treatment at or above 1 mg/kg daily and manifests as hypokalaemia, loss of concentrating ability and renal tubular acidosis; nephrotoxicity may reverse if detected early. Liposomal amphotericin has much less renal toxicity; it is much more expensive.

### Drug interaction

It is additive with other nephrotoxic drugs. Concurrent digoxin therapy can become toxic if hypokalaemia develops.

### Antifungal spectrum

It is currently the drug of choice for most systemic mycoses: active against *Cryptococcus*, *Candida* and other yeasts, *Aspergillus*, *Coccidioides* and other fungi.

### Dose

A dose of 1.0–1.5 mg/kg daily depending on disease severity and appearance of nephrotoxicity, infused over 2–4 h. Hydrocortisone can reduce febrile reactions and chlorpromazine can reduce nausea. Loading the patient with normal saline before administering the drug may limit nephrotoxicity. Liposomal amphotericin requires higher doses of 3–6 mg/kg.

*Comment.* Amphotericin B is an example of the need to carefully weigh the risks and benefits of treatment. It is highly toxic but untreated systemic mycoses are invariably fatal.

## Flucytosine

### Mechanism

It is deaminated inside the fungal cell to 5-fluorouracil, which inhibits nucleic acid synthesis with cell death.

### Pharmacokinetics

It is well absorbed following oral administration and is widely distributed, including the CSF. Elimination is mainly renal. Clearance is decreased in patients with renal impairment.

### Adverse effects

Concentration-related bone marrow suppression is the only major problem. This can usually be avoided by drug level monitoring.

### Antifungal spectrum

It is only active against yeasts; efficacy is limited by rapid emergence of resistance.

**Dose**

A dose of 150–200 mg flucytosine is given daily in divided doses.

*Comment.* Although much less toxic than amphotericin, flucytosine is of limited value because of its narrow spectrum and the existence of resistant organisms. It is usually administered together with amphotericin B. This combination is the therapy of choice for cryptococcal meningitis.

## Imidazoles and related compounds

### Mechanism

Imidazoles increase permeability by preventing ergosterol formation in cell membranes. They also produce cell necrosis by inhibiting peroxidative enzymes.

### Miconazole, clotrimazole, econazole

**Pharmacokinetics**

These drugs are poorly absorbed following oral administration and are usually restricted for topical use.

**Antifungal spectrum**

They are active against a wide range of yeasts and fungi. Their main use is topical, e.g. athlete's foot or vaginal candidiasis.

### Fluconazole, itraconazole, ketoconazole, voriconazole

**Pharmacokinetics**

Following oral administration these drugs are widely distributed; adequate CSF levels are obtained with the exception of ketoconazole. Fluconazole is eliminated by the kidneys; itraconazole, ketoconazole and voriconazole are metabolised by the liver.

**Antifungal spectrum**

They are active against a wide range of yeasts and fungi; fluconazole is particularly effective against yeasts and itraconazole and voriconazole additionally against filamentous fungi, e.g. *Aspergillus*.

**Adverse effects**

Hepatotoxicity is associated particularly with ketoconazole, which requires monitoring of liver function. Voriconazole commonly produces a number of reversible visual disturbances that do not require cessation of the drug.

**Doses**

Fluconazole: 100–400 mg orally or by i.v. infusion, daily single dose.
Itraconazole: 100–200 mg orally, daily single dose.
Ketoconazole: 200–400 mg orally, daily single dose.
Voriconazole: 200 mg orally b.d. An i.v. preparation is also available.

### Nystatin

Nystatin is used topically in the treatment of yeast infections of the skin and mucous membranes. It is not used parenterally because of high toxicity.

### Griseofulvin

Griseofulvin is active only against dermatophytes and is given orally in the treatment of skin or nail infections. It is fungistatic and so must be given for weeks or months. It diminishes the anticoagulant effect by enzyme induction. Barbiturates lead to griseofulvin treatment failure by enzyme induction. Griseofulvin can precipitate porphyria.

### Caspafungin

Caspafungin is a member of a novel family of antifungal drugs, the echinocandins. It acts as a noncompetitive inhibitor of the synthesis of 1,3-ß-glucan, a polysaccharide in the cell wall of many pathogenic fungi. Glucans are essential in maintaining osmotic integrity of the fungal cell wall, and hence inhibition of their synthesis leads to fungal cell death. Caspafungin is highly active against many *Candida* sp. and *Aspergillus* spp. It is available as an intravenous formulation for the treatment of serious infections caused by these organisms.

## Antiviral drugs

These are the least developed as a group of antimicrobial agents: viruses use the biochemical system of their host cells, and it is therefore difficult to prevent viral multiplication without seriously damaging the patient. However, effective therapy is now available for a number of virus infections of clinical importance.

## Aciclovir, valaciclovir and famciclovir

### Mechanism

The pharmacological effect of aciclovir depends on its conversion to an active metabolite by a herpes simplex coded enzyme, thymidine kinase. It is phosphorylated only in herpes-infected cells and normal cellular processes are unaffected. The resulting aciclovir triphosphate inhibits herpes-specified DNA polymerase, preventing further viral DNA synthesis. The herpes genome in latently (non-replicating) infected cells is not altered during antiviral therapy. Aciclovir is active against herpes simplex virus 1 and 2 as well as varicella zoster. Valaciclovir is an orally administered prodrug of aciclovir, which is much better absorbed than aciclovir and is converted into aciclovir by first-pass metabolism in the liver. Famciclovir is a prodrug of penciclovir, an agent with very similar structure and antiviral activity to aciclovir.

### Pharmacokinetics

Aciclovir is absorbed orally in patients with normal gut function, but with a bioavailability of only 15–30%. It is eliminated by renal clearance involving glomerular filtration and tubular secretion. Aciclovir penetrates the blood–brain barrier passively to enter CSF. The prodrugs valaciclovir and famciclovir have a much higher oral bioavailability of 50–80%, and are thus preferred for oral therapy.

### Adverse effects

Renal impairment occasionally follows intravenous administration.

### Drug interactions

No clinically important interactions have been observed yet.

### Clinical use

Aciclovir is indicated for herpes simplex and varicella zoster infections of the skin and mucous membranes, the brain and in lung disease and in prophylaxis against herpes infections in immunocompromised hosts. An intravenous route is required for serious disease manifestations and in immunocompromised patients.

**Dose**
Aciclovir
For herpes simplex: oral, 200 mg five times per day for 5 days; intravenous, 5 mg/kg over 1 h, repeated every 8 h (10 mg/kg in herpes encephalitis). A dose modification is necessary in renal failure. For varicella zoster: oral, 800 mg five times per day for 7 days; intravenous, 10 mg/kg 8-hourly.
Valaciclovir
For herpes simplex: oral, 500 mg b.d. for 5 days.
Famciclovir
For herpes simplex: oral, 750 mg once daily for 7 days.

## Idoxuridine

Idoxuridine is a thymidine analogue that inhibits DNA synthesis. It is highly toxic when given systemically and is therefore only used topically in the treatment of herpes simplex infections of the eye, as an aqueous solution.

## Amantadine

Amantadine (including its analogue, rimantadine) prevents entry of influenza A to host cells and is used predominantly in prophylaxis and also in the treatment of infections caused by this virus. Influenza B virus is not susceptible. Amantadine can produce neurological side effects but usually only if high concentrations are achieved, e.g. in renal failure.

## Zanamivir and Oseltamavir

Zanamivir and oseltamavir are sialic acid analogues that potently inhibit influenza A and B neuraminidases, an activity that is essential for viral release and spread within the respiratory tract. These drugs shorten the clinical symptoms in influenza infection when administered within 2 days of onset. However, they only shorten the disease by about 1 day. They are also effective in prophylaxis of infection, for example in susceptible high risk patients such as nursing home residents exposed to infection. Routine immunisation of such populations is, however, more cost-effective.

## Ribavirin

Ribavirin inhibits a number of DNA and RNA viruses. Its antiviral action has been demonstrated *in vitro* and *in vivo* against a number of important viruses, including respiratory syncytial virus (RSV), influenza A and B viruses, parainfluenza 1 and 3 Lassa fever virus and hepatitis C. The mechanism of action is not completely understood but involves the action of ribavirin triphosphate interfering with the binding of viral messenger RNA to ribosomes. It is predominantly used in the form of a nebulised aerosol in the treatment of bronchitis in infancy as a consequence of RSV infection and in combination with α-interferon in the treatment of chronic hepatitis C.

## Interferon-α

Interferons are natural antiviral proteins produced by humans in response to viral infection. They are active *in vitro* against a wide range of viruses, but their main clinical use is in the treatment of chronic hepatitis B and C,

the latter in combination with ribavirin. Interferons have numerous side effects, including an 'influenza-like' syndrome, leucopenia, thrombocytopenia, depression, renal impairment, arrhythmias and thyroiditis. They are only active when administered parenterally, usually by subcutaneous injection. Modification of interferons by addition of a polyethylene glycol side chain, 'pegylation', prolongs the half-life significantly without altering the antiviral activity, and is the preferred form for treatment of chronic hepatitis.

## Zidovudine (azidothymidine)

### Mechanism

Retroviruses such as human immunodeficiency virus (HIV) require a viral enzyme, reverse transcriptase, to copy the viral RNA genome into DNA. Azidothymidine (AZT) is a nucleoside reverse transcriptase inhibitor that is phosphorylated in both infected and uninfected cells by thymidine kinase and subsequently by other kinases to triphosphate, which is a chain terminator in DNA synthesis by HIV reverse transcriptase. It is a potent inhibitor of HIV replication. However, when administered as monotherapy, resistance to the drug rapidly appears. In combination with other anti-HIV drugs, AZT has proven to be a very useful agent in HIV treatment and prophylaxis. This combination of drugs is known as highly active antiretroviral therapy (HAART).

### Pharmacokinetics

It is well absorbed from the gut; CSF levels are 50% of plasma levels. It is eliminated by glucuronidation.

### Adverse effects

There is serious haematological toxicity: anaemia and neutropenia are seen in up to one third of patients treated with AZT.

## Clinical use

AZT is indicated in:

**1** Serious manifestations of HIV infections in patients with acquired immunodeficiency syndrome (AIDS) or AIDS-related complex, as well as asymptomatic patients with evidence of high levels of viral replication and/or significant depression of CD4 T-lymphocytes in blood. AZT is always administered with other anti-HIV drugs, most commonly with another nucleoside reverse transcriptase inhibitor, as well as one other drug from a different class, such as a protease inhibitor or non-nucleoside reverse transcriptase inhibitor. These are considered further below and in Table 7.9. It has been shown to prolong life in these groups of patients.

**2** As part of combination chemotherapy in preventing transmission of HIV infection from mother to child during delivery, and in those exposed to HIV-infected blood following accidental needle-stick injury.

### Dose

300 mg twice daily.

Dose modification is required in anaemia, myelosuppression, renal and hepatic impairment, pregnancy and the elderly.

## Antiretroviral drug therapy

As outlined above, AZT is now one of many effective drugs against HIV. When used in combination, these agents significantly prolong life in patients infected with HIV. The details of the drugs and their side effects are shown in Table 7.9. Many of these agents have very significant interactions with other drugs that are beyond the scope of this chapter. Some of these interactions are therapeutically valuable, e.g. ritonavir inhibits the hepatic cytochrome P450 system, dramatically increasing the levels of some co-administered protease inhibitors. This can boost their levels significantly, such as used in the combination of lopinavir with ritonavir (Kaletra).

## Lamivudine

This nucleoside reverse transcriptase inhibitor is active against HIV (see Table 7.9) but also has activity against the reverse transcriptase essential for the replication of the hepatitis B virus. When given as monotherapy in hepatitis B it gives good suppression of viral replication, although viral production tends to return to pre-treatment levels on discontinuing the drug. However, when administered for prolonged periods, e.g. 1 year, a sustained antiviral response can be seen in up to 20% of patients.

## Ganciclovir and valganciclovir

### Mechanism

Ganciclovir is an acyclic analogue structurally related to aciclovir. It acts as a substrate for viral DNA polymerase and as a chain terminator aborting virus replication. Valganciclovir is a ganciclovir prodrug that has excellent oral bioavailability.

### Pharmacokinetics

It is excreted primarily unchanged in the kidneys and is largely unbound in plasma. Renal impairment leads to altered kinetics.

### Adverse effects

Neutropenia occurs in 40% of patients but is usually reversible. It occurs after 1 week of induction therapy. There is occasional rash, nausea and vomiting.

### Drug interactions

No drug interactions have been observed as yet.

### Clinical use

Ganciclovir is indicated for life-threatening cytomegalovirus (CMV) infections in immunocompromised individuals, particularly with AIDS or

**Table 7.9** Antiretroviral drugs.

| Class of Drug | Mechanism of action | Drug | Side effects | Usual adult dose |
|---|---|---|---|---|
| *Nucleoside/nucleotide reverse transcriptase inhibitors* | Selective inhibition of HIV reverse transcriptase | All | Lactic acidosis; most common with AZT, ddl and d4T | |
| | | Zidovudine (AZT) | Anemia, neutropenia | 300 mg b.d. |
| | | Didanosine (ddl) | Pancreatitis, peripheral neuropathy | 400 mg o.d. |
| | | Zalcitabane (ddC) | Peripheral neuropathy | 0.75 mg t.d.s. |
| | | Stavudine (d4T) | Peripheral neuropathy, pancreatitis, lipoatrophy | 40 mg b.d. |
| | | Lamivudine (3TC) | Minimal | 300 mg o.d. |
| | | Abacavir | Hypersensitivity reaction: fever, rash, GI symptoms, dyspnoea | 300 mg b.d. |
| | | Tenovovir | Minimal | 245 mg o.d. |
| | | Emtricitabine | Minimal | 200 mg o.d. |
| | | Combivir (AZT + 3TC) | As AZT and 3TC | 1 tablet b.d. |
| | | Trizivir (AZT + 3TC + abacavir) | As AZT, 3TC and abacavir | 1 tablet b.d. |
| *Protease inhibitors* | Inhibition of HIV-encoded protease required for maturation of virus proteins | All | Lipodystrophy with hyperglycemia, fat redistribution, hyperlipidemia Hepatitis | |
| | | Amprenavir | GI intolerance, rash, oral parasthesias | 1200 mg b.d. |
| | | Atazanavir | Benign increase in unconjugated bilirubin, GI intolerance, prolongation of $QT_c$ | 400 mg o.d. |
| | | Fosamprenavir | Rash | 1400 mg b.d. |
| | | Indinavir | GI intolerance, renal stones, benign increase in unconjugated bilirubin | 800 mg t.d.s. |
| | | Lopinavir/Ritonavir (Kaletra) | GI intolerance | 3 caps b.d. |

*(Continued)*

**Table 7.9** *(Continued)*

| Class of Drug | Mechanism of action | Drug | Side effects | Usual adult dose |
|---|---|---|---|---|
| | | Nelfinavir | Diarrhoea | 1250 mg b.d. |
| | | Ritonavir | GI intolerance | 600 mg b.d. |
| | | Saquinavir (Fortovase) | GI intolerance | 1.2 g t.d.s. |
| *Non-nucleoside reverse transcriptase inhibitors* | Inhibit HIV reverse transcriptase | | | |
| | | Delaviridine | Rash, hepatitis | 400 mg t.d.s. |
| | | Efavirenz | Disturbed sleep, abnormal dreams, rash, hepatitis | 600 mg o.d. |
| | | Nevirapine | Rash, hepatitis | 200 mg o.d. for 14 days, then 200 mg b.d. |
| *Fusion inhibitor* | Prevents HIV membrane fusing with cell membrane preventing viral entry | | | |
| | | Enfuvirtide | Site reactions, bacterial pneumonia | 90 mg subcutaneous b.d. |

transplanted organs, and in the treatment and prevention of CMV retinitis in these patients.

**Dose**

Intravenous: Induction, 5 mg/kg over 1 h every 12 h for 14–21 days. Maintenance, 5 mg/kg daily. Oral: Valganciclovir—Induction 900 mg b.d. for 21 days then 900 mg daily for maintenance therapy. Dose reduction is required in patients with impaired renal function.

## Antimalarial drugs

### Quinine

#### Mechanism

Quinine is an alkaloid derived from the bark of the South American Cinchona tree. It is effective against the asexual blood stages of all four *Plasmodium* sp. that can produce malaria in humans. Its mechanism of action is unclear. It is inactive against the exoerythrocytic forms of the parasite, including the dormant hepatic forms of *P. ovale* and *P. vivax* which can produce recurrent malaria, for which primaquine provides effective eradication. Many areas of the world now report some degree of quinine resistance so that therapy is usually combined with another agent.

#### Pharmacokinetics

Quinine salts are well absorbed by the oral route. The drug is extensively protein-bound. It is metabolised by the liver and excreted renally, with a half-life of 11 h; this increases in severe infection.

## Adverse effects

Quinine has a low therapeutic index and most patients will experience one or more of the following side effects: tinnitus, poor hearing, nausea, vomiting and disturbed vision. It may exacerbate the hypoglycaemia of *P. falciparum* infection. It may precipitate hemolysis in those with G6PD deficiency, although this should not preclude its use in severe malaria. By the intravenous route, it can produce a variety of arrhythmias.

## Drug interactions

Increased risk of arrhythmias with amiodarone and flecainide. Increased risk of ventricular arrhythmias with terfenadine. It increases the concentration of digoxin and its own metabolism is inhibited by cimetidine, leading to increased drug concentrations.

## Dose

Oral: 600 mg quinine salt every 8 h for 7 days. If quinine resistance is known or suspected (which in practice means most patients), combine with doxycycline 200 mg o.d. for 7 days or pyrimethamine with sulphadoxine (Fansidar) three tablets as a single dose.

Intravenous: For seriously ill patients, loading dose of 20 mg/kg (max. 1400 mg) infused over 4 h (unless received mefloquine or quinine in the preceding 24 h) and then after 8 h maintenance dose of 10 mg/kg (max. 700 mg) infused over 4 h every 8 h. Patients receiving intravenous quinine should have continuous ECG monitoring. Once oral absorption is reliable, switch to oral quinine plus doxycycline or pyrimethamine/sulphadoxine as above.

## Chloroquine

### Mechanism

Chloroquine is active against most strains of *P. vivax*, *P. ovale and P. malariae* but resistance is now virtually universal in *P. falciparum*. Its mechanism of action is unclear. It remains the drug of choice for treating non-falciparum malaria, although incidence of resistance is increasing, especially in Brazil, India and Indonesia. It is also used in combination with proguanil as prophylaxis against malaria infection in some areas of the world.

## Pharmacokinetics

Chloroquine is well absorbed following oral ingestion (90%). It is about 50% protein-bound. It has a long half-life of 4–6 days. Excretion is principally via the kidneys, although its half-life is so long that poor renal function does not alter levels achieved in the treatment of acute malaria. When used in prophylaxis, dosage must be reduced in renal impairment.

## Adverse effects

GI disturbance, visual disturbance, pruritis, depigmentation or loss of hair. Retinal damage can be permanent in overdose. Can precipitate convulsions.

## Drug interactions

Chloroquine increases concentrations of digoxin and ciclosporin. Increased risk of arrhythmias with amiodarone. Cimetidine increases chloroquine levels.

## Dose

Treatment: For non-falciparum malaria, initial dose of 600 mg (base), then a single dose of 300 mg after 6–8 h and then 300 mg daily for 2 days. For *P. vivax* and *P. ovale*, radical cure to destroy dormant liver forms that can produce relapse is required with primaquine (see below).

Prophylaxis: 300 mg (base) weekly in conjunction with proguanil 200 mg o.d. Treatment should begin 1 week before travel and 4 weeks after return.

## Primaquine

Primaquine is used to eliminate the liver stages of *P. ovale* and *P. vivax*. It is given orally for 14 days. It often produces hemolysis in those with G6PD deficiency, so levels must be measured before starting

therapy. A once-weekly dose for 8 weeks is usually safe in such patients.

## Other antimalarials

A number of other drugs are available for the prophylaxis and treatment of malaria. They are summarised in Table 19.4 in the chapter on travel medicine.

# Chapter 8

# Respiratory disease

## Introduction

The most frequently encountered respiratory diseases in a general medical setting are chronic obstructive pulmonary disease (COPD), asthma, respiratory tract infection, lung cancer, bronchiectasis, interstitial lung disease and pulmonary embolic disease. Respiratory tract infections including pneumonia are discussed in Chapter 7.

## Asthma

The main features of asthma are:

wheeze, variable breathlessness, cough; reversible airflow obstruction (>15% reversibility to inhaled bronchodilator or >15% variability in mean peak flow).

The disease is characterised by:

respiratory tract inflammation with increased eosinophils and mast cells; damage to the airway epithelium; and in chronic disease, remodelling of the airway wall with increased smooth muscle mass and matrix deposition.

Therapy is aimed at minimising symptoms when patients are stable and treating acute exacerbations.

## COPD

The main features of COPD are:

Exercise-related breathlessness with relatively little day-to-day variability.

Fixed airflow obstruction with little or no reversibility to bronchodilator treatment.

Cough with sputum production is a variable feature but prominent in some patients. Histologically there may be destruction of the lung parenchyma (emphysema) and/or structural changes to the airway wall resulting in airflow obstruction.

Therapy is aimed at maximising any bronchodilator response that is present and treating acute exacerbations.

Greater than 90% of COPD is related to smoking. Lung function decline on average occurs 2–3 times more rapidly in smokers than in non-smokers and smoking cessation results in lung function decline reverting to the rate of non-smokers. Breathlessness is very variable and may not relate well to lung function with some patients having well-maintained exercise tolerance despite markedly reduced FEV1 values. In addition to the pharmacological interventions listed below surgical intervention may improve symptoms in a small number of patients with severe air-flow obstruction who are suitable for lung volume reduction surgery or lung transplantation. Both asthma and COPD are common conditions and may co-exist.

## Guidelines on the management of asthma and COPD

National Guidelines exist in most countries on the management of asthma and COPD (e.g. see www.brit-thoracic.org.uk).

Because many of the drugs used are common to both asthma and COPD, these are considered below by class.

## Inhaler devices

There are two main ways of administering inhaled drugs:

As a suspension via a metered dose inhaler (MDI)

As a dry powder (DPI)

## Bronchodilators

### β₂-Adrenoceptor agonists

#### Mechanism of action

$\beta_2$-Adrenoceptor agonists act by stimulating the $\beta_2$-adrenoceptor present on airway smooth muscle and other structural cells in the airway. Stimulation of the $\beta_2$-adrenoceptor results in activation of adenylyl cyclase and subsequent elevation of intracellular cyclic AMP. This produces a range of downstream effects depending on the cell type, the most important of which is relaxation of airway smooth muscle which results in bronchodilation.

#### Pharmacokinetics

There are two main groups of $\beta_2$-adrenoceptor agonists, short-acting $\beta_2$ agonists (SABAs) and long-acting $\beta_2$ agonists (LABAs). A list of the most commonly prescribed drugs is given in Table 8.1.

These drugs are administered by the inhaled route or, in acute exacerbations of asthma or patients with severe chronic disease (asthma or COPD), via nebuliser. Intravenous infusion of salbutamol is also used in acute asthma. Onset of bronchodilation with SABAs is within 1–2 min and sustained for 4–6 h. Formoterol also has a rapid onset of action, whilst salmeterol, which is a partial agonist, has a slower onset of action of around 20 min. Both LABAs produce sustained bronchodilation over a 12 h period.

#### Adverse effects

$\beta_2$ agonists produce hypokalaemia (via $\beta_2$-receptor-mediated effects on sodium-potassium exchange), tachycardia (via direct effects on the heart) and tremor. These effects are dose-related and are more severe with intravenous administration compared with inhaled administration.

There has been concern over possible links between monotherapy with β agonists in asthma and increased exacerbations and (very rarely) death. SABAs should therefore be used on an as-required basis and LABAs should only be used in combination with an inhaled steroid (see below).

#### Interactions

The only clinically important interaction occurs when these drugs are used in conjunction with theophylline which may worsen tachycardia and rarely produce supraventricular or ventricular arrhythmias.

#### Clinical use

$\beta_2$-Adrenoceptor agonists are the mainstay bronchodilators used for symptom control both in asthma and COPD. Because of the reversible nature of bronchoconstriction (at least in most asthmatics), they are much more effective in asthma than in COPD. SABAs should be used as required to relieve symptoms although they may be taken in advance of exercise in those asthmatics prone to exercise-induced bronchoconstriction. Further guidance on usage can be found in the guidelines shown in the text boxes 'Main groups of drugs used to treat airflow obstruction' and 'Drug treatment of asthma'. Asthmatics requiring SABAs more than once a day on an average should also be prescribed inhaled steroids (see step 2 in guidelines). As mentioned above LABAs should not be prescribed as monotherapy.

**Table 8.1** β-Adrenoceptor agonists in asthma.

| SABAs | LABAs |
| --- | --- |
| Salbutamol (Albuterol) | Salmeterol |
| Terbutaline | Formoterol |
| Fenoterol | |

---

**Main groups of drugs used to treat airflow obstruction**

1 β-Adrenoceptor agonists, which increase cAMP in airway smooth muscle cells and mast cells
2 Theophylline and related methylxanthines, which also increase intracellular cAMP by inhibiting phosphodiesterase, the enzyme that breaks down cAMP (whether this is their main mode of action is less certain)
3 Antimuscarinic drugs, which inhibit cholinergic (vagal) bronchoconstriction
4 'Anti-allergy' drugs, which inhibit the production, release or effects of bronchoconstrictor or inflammatory mediators
5 Corticosteroids, which reduce the inflammatory response in asthma in particular; the precise mechanisms(s) underlying their action are unknown but reducing the release of inflammatory cytokines is probably important

---

**Drug treatment of asthma**

**Step 1** This is the use of an inhaled β$_2$-receptor agonist (one or two puffs a day) for patients with very mild or occasional asthma.
**Step 2** For patients needing more than one or two doses of an inhaled β$_2$-agonist per day, is the addition of inhaled prophylactic therapy, i.e. low dose of an inhaled steroid, sodium cromoglicate or nedocromil sodium. Inhaled steroids are the most effective of these prophylactic agents.
**Step 3** If symptoms persist a higher dose of an inhaled steroid or a long-acting β$_2$-agonist is given.
**Step 4** If symptoms still persist, a long-acting β$_2$-agonist, inhaled ipratropium or oral theophylline should be tried.
**Step 5** Despite the use of the above drugs, a small percentage of patients with severe chronic asthma will require in addition a daily maintenance dose of oral prednisolone.

---

### Doses

Salbutamol 200 μg inhaled as required; Terbutaline 250–500 μg inhaled as required; Salmeterol 50 μg inhaled twice daily; Formoterol 12/24 μg inhaled twice daily.

## Anticholinergics

### Mechanism of action

Anticholinergics act by preventing acetylcholine released upon vagal stimulation from contracting airway smooth muscle. The most frequently used drug is the non-selective anticholinergic ipratropium bromide. Recently, muscarinic M$_3$-receptor selective anticholinergics have been introduced into practice particularly for COPD (tiotropium).

### Pharmacokinetics

Ipratropium bromide produces bronchodilation over 4–6 h and is usually administered by inhalers or occasionally nebulisers. Tiotropium has a longer duration of action (18–24 h) and is given once daily.

### Adverse effects

Adverse effects with anticholinergic agents are rare although high doses of ipratropium may at least in theory worsen glaucoma or symptoms of bladder outflow obstruction.

### Interactions

There are no major interactions with this class of drugs.

### Clinical use

Ipratropium bromide and tiotropium are used as bronchodilators predominantly in the management of COPD although ipratropium bromide is also used in the management of acute asthma (see below).

### Doses

Ipratropium bromide: inhaler 20–40 μg four times daily inhaled, nebulised 250–500 μg up to four times daily. Tiotropium 18 μg inhaled once daily.

## Inhaled corticosteroids

### Mechanism of action

Corticosteroids activate the intracellular glucocorticoid receptor to produce anti-inflammatory effects either by directly altering gene transcription or by transrepression (i.e. interacting with other important transcription factors for pro- and anti-inflammatory genes).

### Pharmacokinetics

Corticosteroids should be administered wherever possible by the inhaled route and via a device that maximises lung distribution. The aim is to achieve the maximum anti-inflammatory effect in the lung whilst minimising systemic absorption and unwanted adrenal suppression. Twice-daily administration is usual. Nebulised steroids have been used in a small number of asthmatic patients although controlled trials are few. Oral steroid usage is discussed below.

### Adverse effects

Side effects are usually due to local deposition with inhaled devices (hoarse voice, oral candidiasis). With high doses of inhaled corticosteroids/nebulised corticosteroids some adrenal suppression may occur: concerns of increased risk of osteoporosis or reduced growth rate in children have been raised particularly with high-dose inhaled/nebulised corticosteroids although these remain to be fully substantiated.

### Interactions

There are no important interactions when corticosteroids are given through the inhaled route.

### Clinical use

Inhaled corticosteroids remain the mainstay anti-inflammatory treatment for the management of asthma except for very mild patients (i.e. those at step 1 on the BTS [British Thoracic Society] guidelines). Clinical use should be tailored to give the minimum dose in the long term which controls disease: the dose–response relationship for corticosteroids is relatively flat and whilst some benefit may be obtained by doubling doses administered in many patients the benefit is relatively small. A dose of 400–800 µg of beclomethasone equivalent is usually adequate to control disease in most patients with asthma. Inhaled corticosteroids have not been shown to have clinically useful effects on lung function decline in patients with COPD but do reduce exacerbation rates and should be prescribed for patients experiencing more than one exacerbation per year.

There are a range of inhaled corticosteroids available including beclomethasone, budesonide, fluticasone and ciclesonide. Whilst there are theoretical differences between each steroid, both in pharmacokinetics and in the devices available for administering the drugs, in practice these differences are not large and the choice of drug is often determined by cost and patient preference.

### Doses

Beclomethasone, budesonide: start at 200 µg twice daily, increase to a maximum of 2000 µg per day if necessary. Fluticasone: fluticasone is roughly twice as potent as beclomethasone and is usually used at 125–250 µg twice daily. Chlorofluorocarbons (CFC)-free inhaled steroids have different distribution characteristics and beclomethasone administered through a CFC-free inhaler can be given at half the dose to achieve the same lung deposition. In practice CFC-free preparations are packaged so that the same number of doses (1–2 puffs twice a day) can be administered as with CFC-containing inhalers.

## Cys leukotriene receptor antagonists

### Mechanism

Leukotriene D4 (LTD4) is the major bronchoconstrictor mediator in the leukotriene synthesis pathway and brings about airway smooth muscle contraction via activation of the Cys leukotriene 1 receptor. A number of drugs have been developed to interfere either with synthesis of LTD4 or with its receptor. Whilst there have been clinical studies with 5-lipoxygenase inhibitors, the most frequently used leukotriene modifier drugs are antagonists of the Cys leukotriene 1 receptor. These drugs produce modest amounts of bronchodilation and in addition have some anti-inflammatory properties.

## Pharmacokinetics

All of the currently used Cys leukotriene receptor antagonists are administered by the oral route. There are differences in rates of absorption and metabolism between drugs in this class: montelukast is used once daily whereas zafirlukast is used twice daily.

## Adverse effects

In general Cys leukotriene receptor antagonists are well tolerated. Initial concerns regarding increased incidence of Churg Strauss syndrome have largely resolved.

## Interactions

Zafirlukast has been reported to enhance the anti-coagulant effect of warfarin in some individuals.

## Clinical use

Cys leukotriene receptor antagonists are generally used as add-on therapy at step 3 for management of asthma. In the United States in particular these agents are sometimes used as first-line anti-inflammatory therapy instead of inhaled steroids. Their use has also been suggested in individuals with mild to moderate asthma who are unable to take inhaled steroids for other reasons (e.g. severe oropharyngeal side effects). The potential use of these agents in COPD remains to be evaluated.

## Doses

Montelukast 10 mg once daily orally; Zafirlukast 20 mg twice daily orally.

## Theophyllines

## Mechanism

Although theophyllines were amongst the first drugs to be developed for the treatment of asthma and COPD, the precise mode of action remains contentious. The major possibilities include non-selective phosphodiesterase inhibition, antagonism of effects of adenosine and possible effects on muscle fatigue. Theophylline is a methylxanthine used orally, while aminophylline is the intravenous equivalent. Because of the belief that theophylline may work by phosphodiesterase inhibition, there are a number of drugs in development which target specific phosphodiesterase isoforms (especially PDE4).

## Pharmacokinetics

Theophylline has a narrow therapeutic window (therapeutic serum levels 10–20 mg/l). Metabolism is via cytochrome P450 1A2 and 3A4 and hence can be influenced by other drugs metabolised via cytochrome P450 (important examples include macrolide antibiotics such as erythromycin, antifungals including fluconazole, the oral contraceptive pill, cimetidine and verapamil, all of which potentially can increase serum theophylline levels). Serum theophylline levels can also be increased by heart failure, by viral infections, in the elderly and in patients with cirrhosis. Serum theophylline levels may be reduced, as a consequence of enzyme induction, in individuals taking anticonvulsants, in those with a history of alcohol abuse and in smokers.

## Adverse effects

The major limiting factor with theophylline is gastrointestinal side effects and especially nausea (around 10% of individuals). Toxicity may be associated with tachyarrhythmias and seizures: both are most frequently seen when aminophylline is used intravenously and because of this, general intravenous administration of aminophylline has been phased out in many centres. It is potentially dangerous to use intravenous aminophylline in a patient taking oral theophylline preparations unless a recent serum theophylline level is available.

## Interactions

See 'Pharmacokinetics' above.

## Clinical use

Oral theophylline is used as add on therapy at step 3 of the BTS guidelines in the management of asthma and is also effective in some patients with COPD. Intravenous aminophylline has been largely discontinued due to the lack of evidence of efficacy in acute asthma and/or COPD and the risk of tachyarrhythmias and/or seizures. It is still used in some patients with difficult asthma or severe COPD: its use should be limited to a high dependency unit or ICU setting where appropriate monitoring is available. Intravenous aminophylline should be given by slow infusion and not by bolus injection.

### Doses

Theophylline: various slow-release preparations are available and are the best way to administer the drug, the total dose administered usually being around 400 mg per day. For intravenous aminophylline the infusion rate is adjusted depending on the serum level (if known) and clinical setting: the usual dose is 0.5 mg per kg per hour. For patients not previously on oral theophyllines a loading dose of 5 mg per kg over 20 min may be given.

## Other drugs used in the treatment of asthma

### Sodium cromoglicate

Cromoglicate derivatives were amongst the first anti-inflammatory drugs developed for the management of asthma and rhinitis. They have limited efficacy and their use has been largely superseded by inhaled steroids. The precise mode of action is unclear although it has long been hypothesised that stabilising effects on mast cell degranulation or effects on sensory nerve endings may be important.

### Magnesium sulphate

Magnesium sulphate ($MgSO_4$) is used intravenously (8 mmols over 20 min) in the management of life-threatening asthma. This produces some bronchodilation: the mechanism of action is unclear.

### Anti-IgE therapy

A humanised monoclonal antibody against IgE has recently been approved for the management of chronic persistent asthma. Administration is subcutaneously on a monthly basis. Use is limited by patient's weight (dose to be administered being calculated in part from body weight and in part by total IgE levels). Currently as of the time of writing, patients with very high IgE levels are not being considered for therapy partly because of the dose that would need to be administered and partly because of potential concerns over immune complex formation. The use of anti-IgE therapy should be limited to specialist centres. Because anti-IgE therapy is much more expensive than other routinely used asthma medications, a cost-benefit analysis should be considered in each patient for whom therapy is suggested.

### Prednisolone

Prednisolone remains the mainstay anti-inflammatory agent used for chronic asthma unresponsive to high-dose inhaled steroid or for severe COPD although its use in this setting should be reserved for those patients in whom there is clear evidence of steroid responsiveness. Short courses of high-dose prednisolone are also used in the management of acute asthma and exacerbations of COPD. In addition high-dose prednisolone is effective in interstitial lung disease (see below), although prolonged courses (typically 40–60 mg per day for 4 weeks then gradually reducing) are frequently required.

Patients requiring long-term oral steroid usage should have bone density measurements (typically every 3 years) and be considered for bone protection (e.g. with a bisphosphonate) if at high risk of osteoporosis (see Chapter 11).

### Steroid-sparing agents in severe asthma

A small number of patients with chronic asthma require long-term treatment with prednisolone. Because of the potential for adverse effects related to high-dose steroid therapy (osteoporosis, avascular necrosis, steroid-induced diabetes, weight gain, adrenal suppression), there have been a number of trials of steroid-sparing agents in this setting. Reasonable evidence exists for efficacy with low-dose methotrexate, cyclosporin and azathioprine. These drugs should be used only in the setting of a specialist clinic with experience in this area.

## Management of acute asthma

Acute asthma is a medical emergency that requires rapid assessment and treatment. Typically, patients present with worsening of symptoms, deterioration in peak flow, increased respiratory rate, an inability to complete sentences in one breath and tachycardia (>110). Life-threatening features include a silent chest, cyanosis, confusion or coma, peak flow <33% predicted, oxygen saturations <92% predicted, hypoxia, acidosis or hypercapnoea on arterial blood gases.

Pharmacological management consists of:

• High flow rate oxygen (initially 40–60%)

• Nebulised salbutamol (5 mg in oxygen) repeated at 15- to 20-min intervals if necessary, also ipratropium 500 µg nebulised in oxygen 4-hourly if failure to respond to nebulised salbutamol

• Prednisolone 30–40 mg stat then continued for a minimum of 5 days: use i.v. hydrocortisone (100 mg q.d.s.) if life-threatening attack or if the patient is unable to take prednisolone orally (Note: it can take up to 6 h for steroids to have their initial effect)

• $MgSO_4$ 8 mmol over 20 min by slow intravenous infusion if the attack is life-threatening.

• If patients fail to respond to the above i.v. salbutalmol, i.v. aminophylline (see notes above) and ICU referral should be considered.

## Management of acute exacerbations of COPD

Exacerbations of COPD usually present with worsening breathlessness, cough and sometimes sputum production. Treatment consists of the following:

• Oxygen: initially 28% (see section on 'Oxygen therapy' below)

• Nebulised salbutamol (5 mg) and ipratropium (500 µg) 4–6 times per day

• Prednisolone 30 mg daily for 7–10 days

• Antibiotics (e.g. doxycycline 200 mg first day followed by 100 mg daily) if evidence of infection.

Patients failing to respond to the above measures sometimes respond to i.v. aminophylline. Non-invasive ventilation—usually BiPAP (Bilevel Positive Airway Pressure)—benefits some patients and may avoid the need for intubation in patients for whom this is being considered.

## Other therapy for respiratory diseases

### Smoking cessation

Because of the disease-modifying effects of smoking cessation (see above) in COPD and the increased risk of exacerbations in smoking asthmatics, smoking cessation remains an important part of the management of these and other conditions. Potential interventions that have been explored include non-pharmacological approaches (smoking support advice, acupuncture, etc.), nicotine replacement therapy (usually with transdermal patches or chewing gum) and oral administration of bupropion. Bupropion was originally developed as an antidepressant but has been shown to increase rates of smoking cessation in motivated individuals. The exact mode of action of the drug is uncertain although bupropion is a noradrenaline reuptake inhibitor with some additional effects on dopamine reuptake. Side effects may be related to antimuscarinic activity (dry mouth, AV block, tachycardia and gastrointestinal side effects); there is also a potential to increase seizure frequency. Insomnia may also be a problem. There are many important potential interactions because of inhibition of cytochrome P450 activity. The recommended dose is 150 mg daily for 6 days followed by 150 mg twice daily for a maximum of up to 9 weeks.

### Oxygen: acute use

Use of oxygen in hospitals is often poorly supervised. Oxygen should be prescribed in order to ensure that patients receive appropriate concentrations: this is particularly important in patients dependent upon hypoxic drive to maintain ventilation (especially patients with severe COPD and type II respiratory failure). In such patients the concentration should not initially exceed 28% via a Venturi mask: some patients may tolerate higher concentrations but repeat monitoring of arterial blood gases is required to ensure hypoxic drive is not reduced. In contrast, in acute asthma high flow rates of oxygen are safe and appropriate.

## Assessment for long-term oxygen therapy

Patients with chronic respiratory disease who are hypoxic at rest often benefit symptomatically from long-term oxygen therapy. Some studies have shown a survival advantage for patients with a $PaO_2 < 7.3$ kPa and who use $O_2 > 16$ hours per day. Long-term oxygen therapy (LTOT) should only be recommended for individuals with resting hypoxia, which improves on LTOT (initially 24% $O_2$ via a concentrator) without a concomitant rise in $PaCO_2$ (in general $PaCO_2$ must rise by $<1$ kPa to allow LTOT). Formal assessment is required before LTOT therapy can be recommended and because of the obvious risk of explosion, patients should not still be smoking. Installation of tubing within the patient's accommodation allows movement between rooms for patients who are still ambulant.

## Short-burst oxygen therapy

Some patients who do not fulfil the criteria for long-term oxygen therapy may benefit from short-burst oxygen therapy. In general these are patients who desaturate markedly on exercise despite having resting $PaO_2$ values above the recommended threshold for consideration for LTOT. Short-burst oxygen therapy can be administered using bottled or liquid oxygen.

## Notes on other respiratory diseases

### Bronchiectasis

Bronchiectasis is a chronic inflammatory condition where there is saccular dilatation of the terminal airways and/or thickening of the segmental bronchi. Patients usually present with productive cough with or without haemoptysis and may have variable amounts of airflow obstruction. There are a number of causes including previous pneumonia, tuberculosis, cystic fibrosis (see below), obstructed major airway

(e.g. inhaled foreign body), fibrotic lung disease (traction bronchiectasis), immunodeficiency and ciliary dysfunction syndromes. Management is aimed at treating infection and reversing airflow obstruction if possible. Patients with immunodeficiency syndromes (e.g. common variable hypogammaglobulanaemia) may also benefit from immunoglobulin replacement therapy although this will not reverse structural damage that has already occurred. Colonisation with pseudomonas is a particular problem that may require specialist microbiological input to determine the most appropriate antibiotic regimen.

## Cystic fibrosis

Cystic fibrosis presents with early onset bronchiectasis. Advances in specialist care with early treatment of infection, avoidance of colonisation, regular postural drainage and treatment of pancreatic insufficiency have meant that the prognosis has improved markedly over the last 20 years such that patients frequently survive into their early forties. Treatment should be in a specialist centre and as with bronchiectasis is aimed at treating infection and airflow obstruction: additional attention to pancreatic supplementation is also required.

## Interstitial lung disease

A wide range of systemic inflammatory conditions can cause interstitial lung disease (e.g. sarcoidosis, vasculitis): treatment is aimed at controlling the underlying disease process usually with high-dose immunosuppression. There is also a group of specific inflammatory conditions affecting predominantly or exclusively the lung, including extrinsic allergic alveolitis, cryptogenic fibrosing alveolitis (now subdivided into a range of overlapping conditions) and a number of rarer conditions. Treatment is with high-dose immunosuppression, initially using high-dose oral prednisolone and then introducing steroid-sparing agents (e.g. azathioprine). The prognosis depends upon the underlying disease process: this may be good if the disease process is characterised by an acute inflammatory response, but treatment response is likely to be limited at best in patients with long-standing fibrotic changes. Lung transplantation remains an option for selected patients.

## Pulmonary hypertension

Pulmonary hypertension may be primary or secondary, the latter usually due to chronic respiratory disease, cardiac disease or thromboembolic disease. Secondary pulmonary hypertension may respond in part to reversing underlying causes (e.g. right to left shunts in the heart) although by the time of presentation often little improvement is possible. LTOT is the most useful treatment in this situation, together with treating any underlying element of heart failure.

Primary pulmonary hypertension is a rare condition that most frequently affects middle-aged females. In addition to LTOT, pulmonary artery pressure can potentially be reduced by the use of prostacylin analogues (iloprost, epoprostenol), voltage-dependent calcium channel antagonists and the endothelin 1 receptor antagonist bosentan. Treatment should be in a specialist centre with experience of the use of these agents.

# Chapter 9

# Drugs and inflammatory joint disease

## Aims

In inflammatory joint disease, the aims are as follows:

1 To reduce pain.

2 To reduce stiffness and improve mobility.

3 To prevent chronic deformity by minimising the inflammation that results in synovial membrane proliferation and bone erosions.

## Relevant pathophysiology

Anti-inflammatory analgesic drugs are used to relieve the painful symptoms of joint diseases, including those listed below.

| Joint diseases | |
|---|---|
| Rheumatoid arthritis | Gout |
| Osteoarthritis | Reactive arthritis (including Reiter's syndrome) |
| Psoriatic arthritis | Arthritis associated with SLE |
| Ankylosing spondylitis | |

The aetiology of these diseases is varied and in most cases not entirely clear, but with the exception of gout and possibly osteoarthritis (OA), there seems to be a disturbance in immune responses. In rheumatoid arthritis (RA), for example, activated T-cells and cytokine release from macrophage result in a cascade of events that result in proteolytic enzyme release which damage cartilage, while prostaglandins promote synovial vasodilatation and exacerbate pain. Thus, there are a number of areas where an anti-inflammatory drug might be effective:

1 Immunosuppression

2 Inhibition of cell migration

3 Inhibition of enzyme release

4 Inhibition of prostaglandin synthesis

5 Inhibition of pro-inflammatory cytokines.

## Principles of drug treatment

The chronicity of inflammatory joint disease such as RA necessitates long-term follow-up and management within a multi-dimensional framework aimed at preserving the patient's quality of life. This is achieved by attempting to improve functional ability, mental and social health and vocational status, and reduce disease activity. While drugs are an important part of the treatment of patients with inflammatory joint disease, other non-pharmacological aspects demand careful consideration. These include rest, exercise and psychological management.

## Rest

Inflammatory arthritis is typically a disease of exacerbation and remission. During an acute attack it may be necessary to recommend bedrest and splinting of the affected joints.

## Exercise

After an acute attack, carefully graded exercises in the form of physiotherapy and hydrotherapy are required to ensure an early return to normal activities. Exercise also has psychological goals. It can enhance a feeling of well-being and provide active recreation. Excessive exercise, however, can be harmful. Assessing activities of daily life is an important role for occupational therapists.

## Psychological management

Psychological factors are implicated in pain perception. The intensity of pain is in part related to patients' beliefs in their ability to cope with or control the effect of their disease. Counselling about employment is also important, as the patient's self-esteem often depends on useful and purposeful work. The development of support groups for various inflammatory arthritides has an important role in improving patients' education, and these 'group therapies' encourage self-management behaviour and better adaptation to a chronic, incurable disease, often leading to psychological, social and perhaps financial well-being.

Various physical aids are available to allow those with disabilities to maintain independence while protecting the affected joints.

The traditional treatment of inflammatory arthritis is represented by a pyramid starting with non-steroidal anti-inflammatory drugs (NSAIDs) and progressing to disease-controlling antirheumatic therapies (DCARTs) such as antimalarials, sulphasalazine (sulfasalazine), gold, D-penicillamine, methotrexate, leflunomide, azathioprine and other immunosuppressive agents. Over the past decade, there has been an increasing use of DCARTs, especially in the early course of the disease, together with an NSAID because

the majority of patients who develop joint damage do so in the first 2 years, thus inverting the pyramid.

## Symptom modifying antirheumatic therapies

### Simple analgesics

Simple analgesics such as paracetamol may be used to supplement other therapy, but they are relatively ineffective when used alone in RA. They do not retard the progress of the disease and cannot provide adequate pain relief. They may be adequate in the management of some patients with OA.

## Non-steroidal anti-inflammatory drugs

NSAIDs act in a variety of ways but their prime mode of action is via the inhibition of cyclooxygenase (Cox), which exists in two isoforms—Cox-1 and Cox-2. It is now known that Cox-1 is the constitutive form and Cox-2 is the inducible form of the enzyme. Most currently available NSAIDs primarily inhibit Cox-1 but there are now several highly selective Cox-2 inhibitors available. Although lysosome-stabilising effects and inhibition of cellular migration have also been demonstrated, the clinical significance of this observation is unclear. The available NSAIDs come in a variety of chemical classes (Table 9.1). Differences in physicochemical characteristics may influence their pharmacokinetics and give rise to differences in their efficacy and adverse effects.

## Aspirin and related salicylates

Aspirin is the longest established and most traditional of the anti-inflammatory drugs and is relatively cheap. However, in the United Kingdom, its role has been supplanted by other NSAIDs. Benorilate (benorylate) is a compound in which aspirin is linked with paracetamol, and diflunisal is a difluorophenyl salicylic acid derivative.

**Table 9.1** Examples of the principal groups of NSAIDs.

| Drug | Dose* (mg) | Dosage interval (h) |
|---|---|---|
| *Salicylates* | | |
| Aspirin | 900 | 4† |
| Diflunisal | 500 | 12 |
| Benorilate (benorylate) | 4000 | 12 |
| *Pyrazolones* | | |
| Phenylbutazone | 100 | 8 |
| Azapropazone | 300 | 8 |
| *Indoles* | | |
| Indometacin (indomethacin) | 50 | 8 |
| Sulindac | 200 | 12 |
| Etodolac | 400 | 8 |
| *Fenamates* | | |
| Mefenamic acid | 500 | 8 |
| Flufenamic acid | 200 | 8 |
| *Propionates* | | |
| Ibuprofen | 400 | 8 |
| Naproxen | 250 | 8 |
| Ketoprofen | 50 | 6 |
| *Phenylacetates* | | |
| Diclofenac | 50 | 8 |
| *Oxicams* | | |
| Piroxicam | 20 | Daily |
| Tenoxicam | 20 | Daily |
| Meloxicam | 7.5–15 | Daily |
| *Other* | | |
| Nabumetone | 1000 | Daily |
| *Cox-2 inhibitors* | | |
| Celecoxib | 200 | Daily |
| Etoricoxib | 60–90 | Daily |
| Valdecoxib | 10–20 | Daily |

* These doses are near the upper limit and therapy should be commenced with approximately half doses.
† Adjust according to serum concentration.

## Pharmacokinetics

The pharmacokinetics of aspirin are complex and when used in relatively high doses for long periods of time, plasma levels should be monitored. Aspirin is readily absorbed from the gastrointestinal tract and is given orally. Elimination normally follows first-order kinetics, but after very large doses the enzymes that metabolise aspirin become saturated.

## Adverse effects

1 Gastrointestinal effects. Nausea and vomiting follow high doses of aspirin. Dyspepsia, gastric irritation and occult or frank blood loss are common adverse effects, particularly when aspirin is associated with alcohol ingestion. Blood loss results from superficial gastric erosions or peptic ulceration. Inhibition of prostaglandin synthesis is probably responsible because some prostaglandins increase gastric mucosal blood flow and have other protective effects. Gastrointestinal blood loss occurs even with parenteral aspirin or aspirin by suppository. However, fewer erosions and ulcers are found with these and more recent enteric-coated formulations. Newer NSAIDs have been claimed to cause less gastric irritation. These comparisons have not usually been made with enteric-coated aspirin. At present, there appears to be a dose-dependent relationship between anti-inflammatory analgesic effect, prostaglandin synthetase inhibition and the frequency of gastric irritation. Less active analgesics cause less gastric irritation.
2 Prolonged bleeding time may result from the inhibition of thromboxane synthesis and impaired platelet aggregation (Chapter 5) or reduced hepatic clotting factor synthesis.
3 Bronchospasm, urticaria or hay fever may rarely occur in sensitive individuals and appear to result from release of immune mediators secondary to prostaglandin synthesis inhibition.
4 Tinnitus, dizziness and deafness are dose and plasma level related adverse effects. Vomiting and tachypnoea may also occur.
5 In overdose, confusion, convulsions and hyperpyrexia are seen. Forced diuresis may speed elimination of aspirin in cases of poisoning (Chapter 20).

## Dose

Aspirin tablets of 300–900 mg are given 4- to 6-hourly. In RA, up to 4.5 g/day may be required in divided doses.

## Phenylbutazone

This belongs to the pyrazolone class and has analgesic, antipyretic and potent anti-inflammatory actions. However, unfortunately, it can cause serious and sometimes fatal marrow depression. Its use is now limited to ankylosing spondylitis and is available on hospital prescription only.

## Azapropazone

Azapropazone is chemically related to phenylbutazone but it does not apparently give rise to the marrow depression that led to the severe restrictions on the use of phenylbutazone. In addition to acting as a non-steroidal anti-inflammatory agent, it has a uricosuric effect and is used in the treatment of gout. In the treatment of OA, RA and ankylosing spondylitis, dosage in elderly patients with a creatinine clearance of less than 60 ml/min should not exceed 300 mg twice daily. If creatinine clearance in these patients is greater than 60 ml/min, dosage may be increased to 900 mg daily. In younger patients who have normal renal function, the standard dose is 1200 mg daily.

## Drug interactions

Azapropazone increases plasma concentrations of phenytoin and combined use should be avoided. It also potentiates the action of warfarin and should not be used with this anticoagulant. It should be used with great caution, if at all, with any other oral anticoagulants. Combination with oral hypoglycaemics may result in excessively low blood sugars, and again, its concurrent use should be avoided if possible.

## Adverse effects

Skin rashes, fluid retention, angioneurotic oedema, dyspepsia and gastrointestinal bleeding have been reported.

## Indometacin and related drugs

Indometacin has been widely used in inflammatory and non-inflammatory joint diseases for years. It is given by mouth or by suppository, and is generally very effective. Gastric adverse effects are a predictable problem, but headache, mental confusion and dizziness may also present problems. Salt and water retention with oedema may aggravate cardiac failure or hypertension and reduce the efficacy of antihypertensive drugs. Rectal administration may be associated with pruritus, discomfort and bleeding. Sulindac is chemically related to indometacin and is a prodrug, reversibly metabolised by the liver into its active metabolite. This might explain its relatively lower incidence of gastric side effects. Etodolac, another member of this group, is extensively metabolised and excreted in both urine and bile. The kinetics of etodolac are unchanged in the elderly and in renal impairment.

## Dose

*Indometacin*: Oral, 25–50 mg two to three times daily. The 75-mg sustained release capsule is designed to deliver 25 mg of the drug immediately and the remaining 50 mg over the next 8–12 h. Rectal suppository, 100 mg at night; this may be repeated in the morning.

The recommended dose for sulindac is 200 mg twice daily and that of etodolac, 600 mg slow release once a day.

## Propionic acid derivatives

A large number of agents from this group of drugs have been marketed. They are well absorbed orally and have fewer gastric adverse effects than plain aspirin. This has led some rheumatologists to favour them as first-line therapy. This group consists of the drugs listed below.

| Propionic acid derivatives | |
| --- | --- |
| Ibuprofen | Flurbiprofen |
| Fenoprofen | Fenbufen |
| Ketoprofen | Tiaprofenic acid |
| Naproxen | |

Note that fenbufen is a prodrug with no direct effect on the stomach. None of these propionic acid derivatives has been shown to interact significantly with oral anticoagulants, and if a patient must also receive warfarin, this group of drugs is preferable.

## Phenylacetic acid derivatives

Diclofenac is very similar to the propionic acid derivatives. It may sometimes cause hepatitis.

## Fenamates

The long-established mefenamic acid and flufenamic acid are mildly effective in inflammatory joint disease, but they share the problems of salicylates to which they are chemically related. Thus, they share the gastric adverse effects but, in addition, they cause diarrhoea, a dose-related phenomenon for which the basis is not clear.

## Piroxicam and related oxicams

Piroxicam is an anti-inflammatory agent that is chemically unrelated to other drugs. It does, however, share their propensity to cause gastrointestinal adverse effects, and potentiates the effect of oral anticoagulants. It is contraindicated in asthmatic patients who cannot tolerate aspirin. It may cause fluid retention, a particular hazard in the elderly. Tenoxicam is reported to have less gastric toxicity and meloxicam has some Cox-2 selectivity.

## Nabumetone

This is a non-acidic compound and a poor inhibitor of prostaglandin synthesis. After absorption, it is metabolised rapidly by the liver into an acidic metabolite that has effective anti-inflammatory actions. In comparison to other NSAIDs, nabumetone is less gastrotoxic. The recommended dose is 1000 mg daily.

*Comment.* This group of drugs forms the first-line and mainstay of treatment aimed at symptom modification in inflammatory joint disease. There is now a bewildering array of strongly promoted agents. Despite this, no drug has been shown to be clearly superior to the remainder in terms of symptomatic relief, disease suppression or toxic effects. It is important that a constant vigilance is maintained for side effects and drug interactions, particularly in elderly patients. It is advisable to become familiar with a few drugs and restrict use to them. Unfortunately, individual response to a particular drug is unpredictable and the choice of drug is inescapably empirical.

## Cox-2 inhibitors

There are now several Cox-2 inhibitors available for the treatment of RA and OA. They have been shown to reduce gastrotoxicity with a decrease in perforations, ulcers and bleeds, but some such as rofecoxib, celecoxib and valdecoxib may also increase the incidence of cardiovascular events such as stroke and myocardial infarction. Rofecoxib has been withdrawn from the market and the others should only be used in patients with no cardiovascular risk factors. Etoricoxib is a long-acting Cox-2 inhibitor that has not been implicated to date in patients with an increased cardiovascular risk, although the possibility of a class effect has not been ruled out.

## Disease-controlling antirheumatic therapies

DCARTs are used in the management of inflammatory arthritis to achieve disease remission and slow down the progression of joint erosions. These antirheumatic agents comprise a group of widely different chemical entities, including hydroxychloroquine, sulphasalazine, gold, D-penicillamine, immunosuppressant drugs (methotrexate, leflunomide, azathioprine, cyclophosphamide, chlorambucil and ciclosporin) and corticosteroids. Mechanisms of action of these drugs are not clear. There is a lag between starting therapy and observing an effect. They are indicated in the earlier years of the disease. It is usual to continue with conventional anti-inflammatory drugs. Unlike NSAIDs, DCARTs may influence the underlying disease process. For example, in RA, decreasing erythrocyte sedimentation rate and rheumatoid factor titre will be associated with an increase in haemoglobin in patients who respond and a slowing down of the rate of radiological progression. There is evidence that combination therapy with several DCARTs, e.g. methotrexate, sulphasalazine and hydroxychloroquine, is more effective than using single agents alone.

## Chloroquine and hydroxychloroquine

These drugs, originally developed as antimalarials, have been used to treat RA and systemic lupus erythematosus (SLE) since the 1950s, and responses in RA are similar but somewhat less than those observed with other DCARTs except for auronofin (oral gold). However, they have a major advantage in their lack of life-threatening toxicity compared to other DCARTs and are being increasingly used early in the course of disease and in combination regimens with other DCARTs. The mechanisms of action of these preparations may be by lysosome stabilisation and inhibition of phagocytic functions.

They are well absorbed orally, taken up by many tissues and then very slowly excreted in the urine. The most disturbing toxic effect (although rare) is a retinopathy as a result of gradual accumulation of the drug in the retina and is dose-dependent. Irreversible retinal damage with permanent blindness has been reported in patients taking high doses of chloroquine. Rashes and marrow toxicity are rarely seen. Neuropathies and myopathies have been reported.

## Clinical use

Hydroxychloroquine employed in the usual doses is less likely to be associated with adverse effects and has largely superseded chloroquine in clinical practice. Initially, 400 mg is given daily and this dose can be reduced after 6–12 months depending on response. Careful ophthalmological screening at baseline and after 2 years should be done to identify retinal damage, which is reversible if

diagnosed early, although this complication is rare provided dosage is kept below 6.5 mg/kg.

## Sulphasalazine

Sulphasalazine is an effective and relatively safe antirheumatic drug in RA and also in ankylosing spondylitis and HLA-B27 related arthropathies such as reactive arthritis and psoriatic arthritis. It consists of 5-aminosalicylic acid joined to sulphapyridine (sulfapyridine) by an azo bond. In the gut, these two moieties are liberated following bacterial reduction of the azo bond. Sulphapyridine is thought to be the principal antirheumatic agent, while 5-aminosalicylic acid is the active anti-inflammatory moiety when sulphasalazine is used in the treatment of inflammatory bowel disease.

## Adverse effects

These include skin rashes, nausea, headache and occasional leucopenia, neutropenia and thrombocytopenia. The blood abnormalities usually occur early on in the course of treatment (within 6 months) and reverse if the drug is stopped. Other side effects are mentioned in Chapter 13.

## Clinical use and dose

Sulphasalazine ranks with antimalarials and auronofin as the best tolerated of the DCARTs. The oral dose is initially 500 mg daily, usually increased by 500 mg at 1-week intervals to a maximum of 2–3 g daily. Blood counts are performed fortnightly in the first 12 weeks, and 3-monthly thereafter.

## Gold salts

These have been used for over 40 years in the management of RA. Previously, gold salts were thought to act by reducing macrophage activity. A potentially important new finding is that gold salts affect the immune system by regulating gene expression and consequent protein synthesis. One-third of patients derive considerable benefit, one-third have only a modest response and one-third have adverse effects that require interruption of treatment.

## Adverse effects

1 Pruritic rashes are common and present in many forms, including mouth ulcers.
2 Proteinuria secondary to a membranous glomerulonephritis occurs in 10% of patients but it resolves on stopping gold treatment.
3 Vasodilatation with orthostatic hypotension may acutely follow drug dosing.
4 Neutropenia and thrombocytopenia may occur suddenly or develop slowly.

Recovery is usually assured provided no more gold is given. Aplastic anaemia is extremely rare now. Gold treatment is closely supervised with haematological checks before each dose. If it occurs, it has a high fatality rate.

## Clinical use and dose

An intramuscular injection of sodium aurothiomalate is given initially as a 10-mg test dose followed by 50 mg weekly for up to 6 months or until a response or toxic effects are observed. Dose frequency may be reduced to monthly and continued for years. An oral preparation (auronofin) is also available. It is safer and less toxic than injectable gold, but is commonly associated with diarrhoea and lower abdominal discomfort. It is also much less effective than other DCARTs. Gold therapy is no longer as commonly used as in the past.

## D-Penicillamine

First introduced as a copper-chelating agent in Wilson's disease, D-penicillamine modifies the formation of immunoglobulin. It has a similar action to gold salts but relapse may occur with continuing therapy.

## Adverse effects

These are similar to those with gold. Cross-toxicity with gold has been reported but is disputed.
1 Skin rashes are common.

2 Taste disturbance is usually transient.
3 Proteinuria, as with gold.
4 Marrow toxicity is similar to gold, consisting of thrombocytopenia and neutropenia. As these changes develop gradually, routine fortnightly haematological monitoring is essential during the initial stages of therapy.
5 Immunological effects. Up to 50% of patients develop positive antinuclear antibodies. Rarely, SLE or myasthenia gravis may be precipitated.

## Clinical use and dose

D-Penicillamine is given as a 125-mg dose initially followed by monthly increments of 125 mg until response is satisfactory or a dose of 1000 mg is achieved. It is now rarely used as a first-line DCART.

## Cytotoxic drugs

Methotrexate, azathioprine, cyclophosphamide and chlorambucil are used in inflammatory arthritis. Their use as immunosuppressants is discussed in Chapter 10. In rheumatic diseases, these drugs are indicated in resistant inflammatory joint disease, and commonly used together with corticosteroids in the presence of potentially serious extra-articular disease involvement, systemic vasculitis and connective tissue diseases such as SLE and dermatomyositis.

## Methotrexate

Methotrexate is currently considered by many as the DCART of choice after NSAIDs, especially in early aggressive inflammatory joint disease. It works quickly and significant improvement in the disease is observed within the first 4–6 weeks. It shares similar side effects with other cytotoxic agents. In addition, hypersensitivity pneumonitis is seen in 2–6% of patients. This can be serious but if detected early, it is reversible on stopping the drug. Liver toxicity leading to raised transaminase levels is common and reversible on reducing the dose or stopping the drug, although progressive hepatic fibrosis can occur rarely.

## Clinical use and dose

Methotrexate is given by a weekly oral pulse regimen, starting at 7.5 mg and increasing by 2.5 mg every 6 weeks to 15–25 mg weekly depending on disease response. Lower doses should be used in the frail elderly or if there is significant renal impairment. Folic acid 5 mg given 3 days after each dose may reduce the incidence of toxicity, in particular oral ulceration. Cotrimoxazole should be avoided in patients taking methotrexate.

## Leflunomide

This drug is increasingly used as a second-line DCART in patients who do not respond to methotrexate, sulphasalazine or hydroxychloroquine. It is a pyrimidine synthesis inhibitor and shares the side effects of immunosuppressive agents but diarrhoea and hepatotoxicity can be a problem. It must be used cautiously in renal impairment.

## Clinical use and dose

Leflunomide is given as a loading dose of 100 mg daily for 3 days and then maintenance at 10–20 mg thereafter.

## Azathioprine, cyclophosphamide and chlorambucil

A number of controlled trials have shown these drugs to be effective in inflammatory arthritis. Azathioprine is a prodrug that is metabolised to its active form, 6-mercaptopurine. The starting dose is usually 50 mg/day orally, with increments of 25 mg every 3 months depending on disease response, or until a maximum recommended dose of 2.5 mg/kg per day (about 175 mg) has been reached. Cyclophosphamide is usually reserved for more life-threatening conditions such as systemic vasculitis and SLE because of its toxicity. It can be given orally or intravenously, and either as regular daily doses or as weekly/monthly pulses. One of the most serious complications of cyclophosphamide therapy is haemorrhagic cystitis related to its metabolite,

acrolein. The co-administration of mesna (mercaptoethane sulphonate) reduces acrolein urotoxicity (see 'Cytotoxic drugs and cancer chemotherapy', Chapter 10).

Chlorambucil has been used as an alternative to cyclophosphamide, but most clinicians regard it as an inferior drug for the majority of rheumatic conditions. In addition, chlorambucil appears to be associated with a higher incidence of leukaemia and other malignancies. These drugs are discussed in greater depth in Chapter 10.

## Combination therapy

Rheumatologists are now using selected DCARTs in combination with clinical evidence of a synergistic effect. Two combinations have been shown to be efficacious: (i) ciclosporin with methotrexate, and (ii) methotrexate with sulphasalazine and hydroxychloroquine. The incidence of side effects is not increased when these drugs are used in combination.

## Immunotherapy

### Ciclosporin

Ciclosporin is effective in improving inflammatory joint disease but is limited by its potential nephrotoxicity. New onset hypertension is a common side effect seen in about a third of rheumatoid and psoriatic patients, possibly requiring antihypertensive therapy.

Further details are given in Chapter 10.

## Corticosteroids

Corticosteroids have potent immunosuppressant activity (Chapter 10) and a range of other effects (Chapter 11). They are the most powerful anti-inflammatory drugs available.

In RA, there is little evidence that high doses are more effective than low doses. For chronic use, not more than 7.5 mg prednisolone per day (or on alternate days) or the equivalent can be given without the development of serious adverse effects. They should be used judiciously in view of the long-term risks of osteoporosis (see 'Glucocorticoids', Chapter 11). Steroids are particularly useful in SLE and are essential in polymyalgia rheumatica and giant cell arteritis.

Where one or two joints are particularly troublesome in an otherwise reasonably controlled patient, an intra-articular injection of corticosteroid is widely used.

## Anti-cytokine therapy

Three monoclonal antibodies etanercept, infliximab and adalumimab are now available for the treatment of RA and juvenile idiopathic arthritis. They both block the actions of the pro-inflammatory cytokine tumour necrosis factor alpha (TNF$\alpha$) and have been shown to be of clinical benefit and to delay joint damage as measured by X-ray. Etanercept is given by twice-weekly subcutaneous injections, adalumimab by fortnightly subcutaneous injections and infliximab by one or two monthly intravenous infusions. They should be avoided in patients with a past history of serious infections or a history of recent malignancy.

*Comment.* Inflammatory joint disease remains an important and difficult therapeutic challenge. The chronicity of the disease, its variable expression, with remissions and exacerbations, and its implications for the patient's life must all be considered. Therapeutic decisions must be tailored to individual patients at any particular time. The most logical approach to choosing a DCART is to work through the drugs available, continuously weighing the risk of serious toxicity against their benefits in terms of pain relief and minimisation of joint destruction and deformity, moving from one to the next only when there is convincing evidence of therapeutic failure.

## Drugs used in gout

It is important to distinguish the following:
1 Management of the acute attack
2 Long-term management.

## Management of the acute attack

An acute attack of gout is extremely painful and effective anti-inflammatory drugs should be given at once. The drugs used are:
1 NSAIDs such as indometacin, naproxen, diclofenac, piroxicam and etoricoxib in large doses for 24–48 h.
2 Colchicine: This drug can still be used in acute gout (orally or intravenously) or in the early months of treatment with allopurinol. Adverse effects—nausea, vomiting, abdominal pain and diarrhoea—can be less common with low-dose regimens.

## Long-term management

As the underlying mechanism in gout involves excess production of uric acid and/or reduced renal excretion of urate, long-term management aims at reducing uric acid in the body in two ways:
1 Inhibition of uric acid formation from purines by xanthine oxidase inhibition
2 Promotion of urate excretion in the urine.

## Xanthine oxidase inhibition

### Allopurinol

**Pharmacokinetics**
Allopurinol is well absorbed from the gastrointestinal tract and is rapidly cleared from the plasma with a half-life of 2–3 h. It is converted to alloxanthine and this metabolite in turn inhibits the metabolism of the parent drug. Alloxanthine is also a xanthine oxidase inhibitor.

**Adverse effects**
These are not common. Hypersensitivity reactions, which subside on withdrawing the drug, consist of a skin rash accompanied by fever, malaise and muscle pain. Rarely, leukopenia or leukocytosis with eosinophilia occur.

**Drug interactions**
Drugs depending on xanthine oxidase for their metabolic conversion should be given with

caution in association with allopurinol. This applies to 6-mercaptopurine and azathioprine. Inhibition of warfarin metabolism may also occur; anticoagulant control should be monitored closely in circumstances such as these.

### Clinical use and dose

Allopurinol must not be used in an acute attack of gout because this will be prolonged. Initially, 100 mg allopurinol is given daily as a single dose, increasing to about 300 mg daily depending on serum uric acid levels. The aim is to keep serum uric acid levels in the bottom half of the normal range. Colchicine or indometacin may be given concurrently over the first 2 months to prevent acute gout.

Allopurinol should be considered in:

1 Urate overproduction, primary or secondary
2 Acute uric acid nephropathy (tumour lysis syndrome)
3 Nephrolithiasis of any type
4 Renal impairment (dose 100 mg/day per 30 ml/min glomerular filtration rate)
5 24 h urinary uric acid >0.42 g
6 Intolerance or allergy to uricosuric agents
7 Chronic tophaceous gout.

## Uricosuric drugs

### Probenecid

Probenecid inhibits the transport of organic acids across lipid membranes, including the renal tubule. Whereas this leads to an increase in the plasma concentration of a number of acidic drugs, the uric acid concentration falls because its reabsorption from tubular fluid is inhibited.

*Pharmacokinetics*

Probenecid is well absorbed from the gastrointestinal tract and peak concentrations are achieved in 2–4 h. Metabolism and renal excretion result in a half-life of about 9 h; a large proportion of the parent drug is actively secreted by the proximal tubules.

*Adverse effects*

About 25% of patients experience dyspepsia and this limits its use in peptic ulceration. Hypersensitivity reactions occur occasionally as skin rashes. Drug-induced nephrotic syndrome has been reported.

*Drug interactions*

The uricosuric effect of probenecid may be inhibited by large doses of salicylates. Aspirin should therefore be avoided in patients receiving probenecid.

*Dose*

A 250-mg dose of probenecid is given twice daily initially, increasing to a maximum of 2 g daily over 2–3 weeks, depending on serum uric acid concentrations.

### Sulphinpyrazone (Sulfinpyrazone)

Sulphinpyrazone inhibits the tubular reabsorption of uric acid when given in sufficient dose. Like probenecid, it reduces the renal tubular secretion of many other organic acids.

*Pharmacokinetics*

Sulphinpyrazone is well absorbed from the gastrointestinal tract. It is strongly bound (98–99%) to plasma albumin; 90% is excreted unchanged in the urine; 10% is metabolised to the N-p-hydroxyphenyl metabolite, itself a potent uricosuric.

*Adverse effects*

Ten to fifteen per cent of patients receiving sulphinpyrazone develop gastrointestinal symptoms; as a rule it should be avoided in patients with a history of peptic ulceration. Rarely, it causes skin rashes and fever.

*Drug interactions*

As with probenecid, salicylates inhibit the uricosuric effect of sulphinpyrazone and more than occasional doses of aspirin should be avoided. Decreased excretion of oral hypoglycaemic agents may lead to hypoglycaemia and sulphinpyrazone may enhance the effect of warfarin.

*Dose*

A 100- to 200-mg dose of sulphinpyrazone is given daily, increasing over 2–3 weeks to about 600–800 mg daily, depending on serum uric acid concentrations.

**Azapropazone**

Azapropazone has a uricosuric effect and is used in acute attacks of gout and in long-term prophylaxis.

*Dose*

During the first 24 h of an acute attack, 2400 mg azapropazone is given in divided doses and then 1300 mg daily until acute symptoms subside, followed by 1200 mg daily until symptoms have disappeared. In chronic gout, 600 mg twice daily is given unless the patient is elderly (over 65 years of age; see above).

*Comment.* The management of gout aims to reduce uric acid formation prophylactically by xanthine oxidase inhibition with allopurinol and thus prevent arthritis and renal damage. If acute arthritis occurs, it should be managed symptomatically with high doses of NSAIDs and allopurinol therapy begun after symptoms subside. The uricosuric drugs are now used less commonly and indicated mainly in patients who are intolerant to allopurinol. They are ineffective in patients with poor renal function and contraindicated in renal failure and in patients with uric acid stones or a history of uric acid stones.

# Chapter 10

# Cytotoxic drugs and immunopharmacology

Drugs that modify the growth of cells are used in the treatment of cancer, in the control of immune responses after organ transplantation and in the management of autoimmune diseases.

## Cytotoxic drugs and cancer chemotherapy

### Aims

Drug therapy is used in patients with cancer to:
1 Eradicate the disease
2 Control the disease: induce a remission
3 Control symptoms.

In most situations, the drugs used to treat cancer are cytotoxic agents, i.e. drugs that kill cells. There are roughly 30–40 standard cytotoxic drugs in common usage. More recently, there has been an explosion in biological agents, which are the therapeutic fruits of 40 years of basic science research. These are specifically targeted at some of the anomalies in growth pathways that exist in tumour cells. This has taken the number of agents that might be used in oncology to well over 100; however, most of these agents are still finding their precise place in routine clinical practice. Cytotoxics remain the workhorse of medical oncology. These agents selectively damage cells that are rapidly dividing. Since tumour cells are normally in a state of rapid division, this explains the ability of these agents to reduce tumour growth and in some cases bring about tumour shrinkage. Some normal cells in the body are also dividing rapidly (for example bone marrow, gut epithelium and hair follicles). These cells are also killed by cytotoxics, which is the cause for most of the side effects of chemotherapy. One aims to kill more cancer cells than normal cells. This is called the 'therapeutic window' due to the cancer cells being more sensitive to cytotoxics than the normal cells. Without this, one kills the patient as quickly as one kills the cancer cells.

This therapeutic window exists because:
- Cancer cells tend to be cycling more quickly than most normal cells, and are thus more susceptible to toxic agents.
- Cancer cells by their very nature have abnormal growth regulatory pathways. This makes them less able to withstand cytotoxics, and perhaps more importantly, less able to repair themselves than normal cells after exposure to cytotoxic agents.
- Some cytotoxics specifically target pathways or enzymes that are more active in cancer cells than normal cells.
- Unfortunately, this therapeutic window is narrow.
- A way of widening it is to give the drugs repeatedly. Give a dose that the normal tissues (bone marrow) can recover from. Just when this occurs, give another dose of chemotherapy before the

cancer cells have fully recovered from the original insult.

• Hormonal agents can be used in some cancers (breast and prostate cancer).

• More recently, biological agents are becoming increasingly available. These are agents targeted at specific growth pathways that are overactive in cancer cells (anti-EGF receptor agents).

• Antibody treatments targeted at receptors overexpressed on cancer cells (anti-CD 20).

• Radiopharmaceutical agents either attached to antibodies or preferentially taken up at sites of active cancer. This delivers a dose of radiation specifically to the cancer cells.

• Differentiating agents, all–trans-retinoic acid, used in acute progranulocytic leukaemia.

## Relevant pathophysiology

Chemotherapy, or the use of drugs in the management of cancer, was introduced in the 1890s with non-specific cell poisons. More specific agents became available with the discovery in the 1940s of nitrogen mustard, an alkylating agent, and methotrexate, an antimetabolite.

Treatment was initially restricted to patients with leukaemia and lymphomas, but drugs are now used in patients with solid tumours, in adults and in children. Considerable progress has been made towards curative treatment of some of the childhood cancers and rarer solid tumours. Nevertheless, there are still many forms of cancer that are difficult to treat with chemotherapy. In order to obtain maximum therapeutic benefit, it is important to clearly define the aims of therapy at the outset. This often dictates the choice and duration of therapy. It may also dictate what potential adverse effects may be acceptable to patients.

Chemotherapy represents only one component of cancer management. Typically and historically, surgery has been the primary treatment modality. It is used to locally remove tumour that can be seen. Radiotherapy can also be used as primary treatment, without surgery (head and neck cancer), but more typically is used after surgery to control disease locally that cannot be seen. Chemotherapy has the potential to treat more widespread disease, whether it can be seen on imaging or not. One centimetre of tissue contains roughly $10^9$ cells. Thus, one millimetre of tissue, far too small to be significant in any form of imaging, will still contain $10^8$ cells. Thus with 'normal' scans, there may be large numbers of viable cancer cells present. Increasing use is made of 'combined modality therapy', or the integration of all three modalities to cancer treatment.

Drug therapy is used in patients with cancer to:

1 Eradicate macroscopic disease: primary radical treatment (lymphoma and teratoma).

2 Eradicate microscopic disease: adjuvant treatment. Chemotherapy after surgery or radiotherapy, used to eradicate microscopic disease and increase statistical chance of cure. Adjuvant treatment significantly prolongs survival for certain groups of patients with early breast, bowel and lung cancer (Table 10.1).

3 Facilitate radical treatment: neo-adjuvant treatment. Chemotherapy before surgery or radiotherapy to enable the radical treatment (bladder/oesophageal cancer).

**Table 10.1** Chemotherapy as part of combined modality treatment of primary tumours.

| Neo-adjuvant | Adjuvant | In combination with radiotherapy |
| --- | --- | --- |
| Oesophagus | Colon | Cervix |
| Nasopharynx | Breast | Head and neck |
| Bladder | Non-small-cell lung | Oesophagus |
| Locally advanced breast | Ovarian | Small-cell lung |
| | | Rectal |
| | | Anal |

**Table 10.2** Chemotherapy for the management of metastatic cancer.

| Curative | Prolongs survival | Useful palliation | Benefit unlikely |
|---|---|---|---|
| Testis | Ovary | Pancreas | Melanoma |
| Lymphoma | Small-cell lung | Cervix | Renal |
| Acute leukaemia | Chronic leukaemia | Head and neck | Mesothelioma |
| Certain childhood cancers | Myeloma | Brain: glioma | |
| Choriocarcinoma | Breast | | |
| | Colon/rectum | | |
| | Bladder | | |
| | Small-cell lung | | |
| | Non-small-cell lung | | |

**4** Control symptoms: palliative treatment: To improve survival, control symptoms and improve quality of life (most tumour types) (Table 10.2).

## Patient selection

It is not always possible, appropriate or sensible to treat all patients with cytotoxics even if they have an indication for treatment. Other considerations may affect drug selection or schedule. Physiological (as opposed to chronological) age is important; however, performance status is often the most significant factor. Obesity can affect planned doses due to its effect on body surface area. Typically, doses can be capped at a certain level irrespective of a patient's weight. Previous chemotherapy for a different or same disease can affect the body's capacity to tolerate further treatment. Previous chemotherapy for the same illness almost always significantly reduces the chance of the tumour responding to treatment. End organ function may preclude the use of certain drugs. Kidney, hepatic, bone marrow, cardiac or lung function must be checked prior to certain drugs.

## Principles of drug treatment

Although cytotoxics can be given as single agents, it is more common to use a combination of two to six drugs (see below). With a few important exceptions, combinations of drugs are more effective than single agents. In a palliative setting, it is often

---

**Drug combinations**

This is achieved by combining drugs:
**1** That are active when used alone.
**2** With different mechanisms of action.
**3** That have different toxicities.
**4** At doses close to their maximum tolerated levels.

---

more appropriate, when quality of life issues are perhaps more pressing, to use a sequence of single-agent drugs.

Most drug combinations have been developed empirically. Typically, they would have complimentary mechanisms of cytotoxicity disrupting a different point in the cell cycle or DNA synthesis. They would have different dose-limiting side effects: one might be highly myelosuppressive and the other neurotoxic so as to maximise their synergistic action. Using together two drugs that are both highly myelosuppressive means it is unlikely that they can be used at an adequate dose or frequency. When treating tumours with the aim of cure, be it in the radical or adjuvant setting, it is very important to attempt to maintain dose intensity.

Myelosuppression is the commonest dose-limiting toxicity of most cytotoxic agents. When chemotherapy is given at standard doses, treatment is usually given intermittently as pulses administered at 3- to 4-weekly intervals, allowing time for marrow recovery. The co-administration of haemopoetic growth factors (granulocyte colony-stimulating factor [G-CSF] and granulocyte–macrophage colony-stimulating factor [GM-CSF]) allows drugs to be given at significantly higher doses, or more frequently, by reducing the risk of significant neutropenia. Unfortunately, there is little evidence outwith haematological malignancies that this approach improves outcomes and so the place of growth factors in routine practice is not established.

Much higher doses of drugs such as cyclophosphamide, melphalan, etoposide and carboplatin have been used with the aim of eliminating the tumour completely. These high-dose chemotherapy regimens result in eradication of all the bone marrow's progenitor stem cells and so the patient must be rescued from total bone marrow failure by bone marrow transplantation or peripheral blood stem cell transfusion. Such treatment is used in the management of leukaemias and lymphomas. Trials into such treatment in solid tumours have till date been disappointing. When giving high-dose chemotherapy, it is essential that supportive measures, such as platelet transfusions, are available to deal with marrow failure, infection and bleeding.

Measurement of plasma concentrations (therapeutic drug monitoring) allows administration of agents at doses that could otherwise be lethal, e.g. methotrexate. Methotrexate is a potent but reversible inhibitor of the enzyme dihydrofolate reductase, a key enzyme for DNA synthesis. Enzyme inhibition and the toxic effects of methotrexate can be reversed by the subsequent administration of folinic acid. It is possible to give methotrexate in doses of 100–1000 times those used previously, to measure plasma methotrexate levels and to calculate the amount of folinic acid required for 'rescue'. This method of treatment may be of considerable therapeutic value in some situations.

Cytotoxics are almost always given intravenously; occasionally they are given orally and rarely they can be given in other ways:

1 Intrathecally, to achieve effective concentration in the cerebrospinal fluid. Most drugs do not readily cross the blood–brain barrier.

2 Intra-arterially into a limb, the head and neck or the liver.

3 Intraperitoneally or intrapleurally to increase the local concentration of drug, particularly where rapidly accumulating ascites or pleural effusions present clinical problems.

4 Topically onto lesions of the skin, vagina or buccal mucosa.

If a drug requires metabolic activation by the liver, e.g. cyclophosphamide or azathioprine, it is of little value to administer it locally, intraperitoneally or intrathecally.

## Cytotoxic drugs

The majority of cytotoxic drugs act by interfering with the synthesis and replication of DNA. The molecular basis of action of some widely used agents is shown in Fig. 10.1. Currently, much research is directed at identifying novel targets for cancer treatment such as intracellular signalling pathways.

## Mechanisms

Cytotoxic drugs can be classified as follows:

1 *Alkylating agents.* These include drugs such as nitrogen mustard, cyclophosphamide, chlorambucil and melphalan. These are highly reactive molecules when activated and bind irreversibly to macromolecules in the cell, notably DNA, RNA and proteins, thus disrupting normal growth.

2 *Antimetabolites.* These are analogues of the normal components of metabolism or DNA synthesis. They are taken up into the normal synthetic process, but then inhibit its continued normal function. These can be split into three classes: antifolates, pyrimidine analogues and purine analogues. Methotrexate inhibits folic acid metabolism, and the nucleotides (5-fluorouracil, gemcitabine, cytosine arabinoside, 6-mercaptopurine) inhibit DNA synthesis.

3 *Natural products.* A wide range of drugs has been developed from plants, bacteria, yeasts and fungi. Others inhibit DNA synthesis through intercalation into the helix itself.

• Mitosis inhibitors: During mitosis, spindles develop between the poles of the two potential

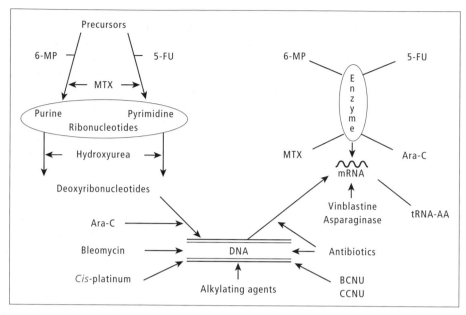

**Figure 10.1** Mechanism of action of cytotoxic drugs.

new nuclei. The chromosomes move along these spindles. Stopping either spindle formation or, perhaps less obviously, their normal breakdown will prevent two new daughter cells developing during mitosis. The vinca alkaloids (vincristine, vinblastine and vindesine) stop the mitotic spindle developing. The taxanes (taxol and taxotere) inhibit mitosis by stabilising the spindle and preventing its normal breakdown.

- Topoisomerase enzyme inhibitors: These enzymes are involved in the unbinding and loosening of the DNA supercoiled double helix, as well as the cutting of DNA strands to enable access into the DNA of the enzymes required for normal DNA replication. Part of these enzymes' normal function is to cause single- or double-strand DNA breaks. Drugs that stall or disrupt this process will leave DNA uncoiled and with DNA breaks. Topoisomerase 1 and topoisomerase 2 inhibitors disrupt this process in slightly different ways. Examples of these drugs are:

○ Topoisomerase 1 inhibitors—the camptothecins: topotecan and irinotecan

○ Topoisomerase 2 inhibitors—the podophyllotoxins: etoposide and teniposide

- Anthracyclines, such as doxorubicin, epirubicin and daunorubicin, intercalate into DNA and also form highly reactive free radicals. This disrupts normal DNA synthesis. However, their principal action appears to be as inhibitors of the enzyme topoisomerase 2.

- Antitumour antibiotics: Bleomycin binds to DNA to cause DNA strand breaks and may also form free radicals. Actinomycin D binds to DNA to inhibit RNA transcription.

**4** *Others.* Several drugs have been identified, often by random synthesis and screening, whose mechanism of action is not fully established but are thought to interact with DNA synthesis or replication. They include the hydroxycarbamide (hydroxyurea), dacarbazine, procarbazine, cisplatin and its analogue carboplatin.

**5** *Steroid hormones.* These are widely used in cancer management. They are particularly cytotoxic against lymphoid tumours but are also used in the treatment of symptoms such as anorexia and vomiting. The drug most commonly used is prednisolone.

*Targetted inhibition.* Increased understanding of the molecular faults in tumour cells has led to the development of relatively 'tumour-specific' treatments. The transmembrane tyrosine kinase receptor HER-2/neu was identified as an oncogene overexpressed by about 30% of breast cancers that are characteristically more aggressive. Trastuzumab is a monoclonal antibody specific for HER-2/neu, which has proven effective in management of metastatic HER-2/neu-overexpressing breast cancers as a single or combination agent. Many oncogenes are signal pathways that regulate normal cellular biochemistry and cell cycle. Kinases are a group of signal molecules now recognised to be crucial in oncogenesis. Imatinib mesylate is a kinase inhibitor that targets ABL, KIT and platelet-derived growth factor receptor. It has proven very effective in chronic myeloid leukaemia and recently in treatment of gastrointestinal stromal tumours.

For clinical purposes, cytotoxic drugs are generally grouped according to their mechanism of action as above, but they may also be classified according to their effect on the cell cycle, as demonstrated in tissue culture. Actively dividing cells pass through several phases. Mitosis is followed by a gap or delay (G1), then a synthetic phase (S), a second gap (G2) and mitosis again. Cells may cycle continuously or enter a quiescent phase. Some drugs act at all phases of the cell cycle; others exert effects specifically at certain phases of these cell cycles.

Class I drugs are non-specific and act on cells whether or not they are actively dividing, e.g. nitrogen mustard. Class II drugs act only at specific phases of the cell cycle, e.g. vincristine, methotrexate and cystosine arabinoside. Class III drugs act on cells in division and at all phases of the cycle, e.g. cyclophosphamide, actinomycin D and the nitrosoureas.

## Pharmacokinetics

Pharmacokinetic aspects of cytotoxic drugs may present drug-specific or general problems. Most cytotoxic drugs have a narrow therapeutic index: they are active only at doses close to those causing significant toxicity. This makes the administration of cytotoxics potentially lethal. The initial dose is typically not the same dose for all patients as is the case in most other clinical scenarios (i.e. antihypertensives or antibiotics), but rather is based on body surface area (mg/m$^2$), calculated from the patient's height and weight. This is a concept derived from animal studies.

Individuals' normal enzyme systems function at different levels; this is called pharmogenetics. So even in ideal circumstances, individual response to drugs may vary considerably. Some drugs are inactive on administration, but are activated in the liver or in the tumour. Cyclophosphamide is converted to an active metabolite in the liver. Similarly, inactive azathioprine is converted to the antimetabolite 6-mercaptopurine in the liver. If an individual's normal level of enzymes involved in these processes is low, then very little of the prodrug may be converted to active drug, thus making the process ineffective. Alternatively, body enzymes may inactivate the active drug. Drugs such as doxorubicin and vincristine are predominantly excreted via the biliary tract. In the presence of hepatic impairment, dose reduction of these drugs is recommended. Even with normal liver function, variable pharmogenetics means that active drug may be in the body longer than expected, leading to greater toxicity. Some cytotoxic drugs (cisplatin, carboplatin and methotrexate) are excreted unchanged by the kidney. When using these drugs in patients with renal impairment, dose modification is important. With carboplatin, dose-limiting thrombocytopenia is more common in patients with renal impairment and is related to an increase in the area under the concentration–time curve (AUC). As total body clearance of carboplatin is directly correlated with glomerular filtration rate (GFR), it is possible to relate drug exposure (AUC) to dose and GFR using the equation:

$$AUC = Dose/GFR. \qquad \text{(Eqn. 10.1)}$$

This equation, rearranged as

$$Dose = \text{'Target'} AUC \times GFR, \qquad \text{(Eqn. 10.2)}$$

is widely used to calculate carboplatin dose.

There are other clinical pharmacokinetic problems with cytotoxic drugs:

1 The problem of the 'third space'. Many patients with cancer have pleural effusions or ascites. Administration of a cytotoxic drug to such a patient may result in the sequestration of the drug into this compartment, with slow release back into the circulation. This may aggravate toxicity, most classically seen with methotrexate.

2 Sanctuary sites. Often cancer can be considered to be a systemic disease. It is therefore essential that the administered drug reaches all parts of the body. Most drugs do not cross the blood–brain barrier, certainly not to therapeutic levels, and therefore may not act on tumour cells in the brain. Patients with small-cell lung cancer who respond well to chemotherapy will receive prophylactic whole-brain radiotherapy to reduce the risk of relapse in this site (and improve the chances of overall survival). Another important sanctuary site appears to be the testes; lymphomas in particular may relapse there. Clinically, perhaps the most important sanctuary site in a large tumour is the core of the tumour itself where there is poor blood supply into which the drug cannot adequately penetrate. In teratoma, an exquisitely chemosensitive disease, any residual mass post-chemotherapy will be removed surgically.

## Adverse effects

Reactions to chemotherapy are secondary to cell death both in the tumour and in other rapidly dividing cells of bone marrow, gastrointestinal tract, germinal epithelium, etc. These can be divided into:

1 General adverse reactions to chemotherapy

2 Specific adverse reactions to individual agents.

### General adverse reactions

1 Nausea and vomiting may be severe with many, although not all, drugs and are related to the direct actions of cytotoxic drugs on the chemoreceptor trigger zone (see 'Nausea and vomiting', Chapter 13). Anticipatory vomiting can, rarely, be a problem in patients after repeated treatments. The selective $5HT_3$ receptor antagonists often in combination with steroids are highly effective in preventing acute emesis.

2 Alopecia is a common adverse effect of some, but not all, cytotoxic drugs. Hair re-grows after the course of chemotherapy has been completed.

3 Hyperuricaemia, with precipitation of clinical gout or renal failure, may complicate the treatment of highly chemosensitive tumours when there is rapid tumour lysis, e.g. leukaemias and lymphomas. Allopurinol, the xanthine oxidase inhibitor, may be used to prevent gout (Chapter 9) but care should be taken when azathioprine or mercaptopurine are given at the same time (see 'Drug interactions' below).

4 The gastrointestinal tract from mouth to anus has a fast turnover and thus can be susceptible to side effects. Mucositis can occur with some drugs, causing ulceration in the mouth or oesophagus. When there is co-existent neutropenia, there is increased risk of opportunistic infections: thrush, indigestion, abdominal cramps and diarrhoea all may occur.

5 Bone marrow depression. The bone marrow is particularly sensitive to many cytotoxic drugs (see 'Anticoagulant drugs', Chapter 14). Neutropenia is common, and opportunistic infections occur as a result of impaired humoral and cell-mediated responses. Unusual infection with fungi and protozoa, in addition to more common pathogenic bacteria and viruses, may occur. Thrombocytopenia may result in an increased risk of haemorrhage.

6 Neuropathy. Typically, the greatest effect is on the longest nerves, and thus peripheral neuropathy can occur. Classically with the spindle poisons: taxanes and vinca alkaloids. Most common effects are sensory, but can be motor and autonomic.

7 Infertility. Many cytotoxics cause sterility; this must be discussed prior to starting treatment and appropriate action undertaken. Conversely, treatment with chemotherapy is not a guarantee of birth control.

8 Secondary cancers. The incidence of this is hotly debated, but certainly is a real effect. Typically, they occur 10–15 years after treatment. The risks vary between agents but are the highest with alkylating agents.

**Table 10.3** Effects of cytotoxic drugs.

| Drug | Mechanism | Specific adverse effects | Indications |
| --- | --- | --- | --- |
| Cyclophosphamide | Alkylating agent | Haematuria, cystitis | Haematological malignancy, solid tumour |
| Doxorubicin | Anthracycline | Alopecia, cardiac failure, local tissue necrosis | Wide range of haematological and solid tumours |
| Cisplatin | Interacts with DNA | Neurotoxicity, nephrotoxicity, vomiting | Wide range of solid tumours, including lung, ovarian and testicular carcinoma |
| Bleomycin | Antibiotic | Pulmonary fibrosis, skin rashes | Lymphomas, testicular teratoma, squamous cell carcinoma |
| Methotrexate | Antimetabolite | Mucositis | Leukaemia |

## Specific adverse reactions

Specific effects of some of the more widely used cytotoxic drugs are shown in Table 10.3. Some have a specific pharmacological basis. Haemorrhagic cystitis with cyclophosphamide is a consequence of urinary excretion of the irritant metabolites, e.g. acrolein. Maintaining a high-fluid output can prevent this or by giving the drug mesna (mercaptoethone sulphonate) that conjugates these metabolites to promote safe excretion.

## Drug interactions

Drug interactions may occur between cytotoxics but more important are interactions with non-cytotoxic agents.

### Methotrexate and salicylates

As methotrexate is highly protein bound, it is readily displaced from the binding site by aspirin and other salicylates. This may increase the risk of adverse effects of methotrexate. Other acidic drugs that are highly protein bound may show similar effects.

### 6-Mercaptopurine and allopurinol

These two drugs are frequently used together. Allopurinol is a competitive inhibitor of xanthine oxidase (see 'Drugs used in gout', Chapter 9) and also inhibits the breakdown of 6-mercaptopurine.

The dose of 6-mercaptopurine must be halved at least or toxicity ensues. Azathioprine, which is metabolised to 6-mercaptopurine, should also be given in lower doses if used with allopurinol.

### Procarbazine and alcohol

Hot flushing may occur and patients should be warned of this before treatment. Procarbazine is a monoamine oxidase inhibitor, and tyramine-containing foods should be avoided (see 'Mood stabilising agents', Chapter 16).

*Comment.* Physicians who have experience and facilities for managing malignant disease and the problems associated with chemotherapy should give cytotoxic drugs. Haemorrhage and opportunistic infections secondary to marrow and immune suppression may shorten life rather than prolong it if they are not aggressively managed.

## Hormones and antihormones

### Oestrogens, progestogens and testosterone

Surgical removal of endocrine organs, such as the ovaries, testes, adrenals and pituitary gland, has been used for many years in the treatment of breast and prostatic cancer. These are tissues that are normally under some hormonal control. Treatment with hormones and antihormones aims to achieve the same effect of changing the hormonal environment. Hormonal effects are mediated by receptors on the cell surface or within the cell. These receptors, notably oestrogen and progesterone receptors, can be identified within tumours and allow a prediction of the response to endocrine manipulation in breast cancer. Patients whose breast cancer contains oestrogen receptors are treated with hormonal therapies. Patients whose tumour has neither oestrogen nor progesterone receptors do not receive hormonal therapies. A number of different hormonal treatment strategies exist:

1 *Stop gonadal hormone production.*
Ovarian or testicular ablation using surgery or radiotherapy.

2 *Stop hormone production.*
LHRH (luetinising hormone-releasing hormone) agonists: Goserelin or leuprorelin. This results in the down-regulation of the hypothalamus pituitary axis.
Aromatase inhibitors: These block the production of oestrogen in the adrenals and body fat and are used in post-menopausal women only.

3 *Block the action of the hormone on hormone receptors.*
SERMs (selective oestrogen receptor modifiers): Tamoxifen is widely used as an adjuvant treatment in breast cancer.
Anti-androgens: flutamide, cyproterone.

4 *Cause degradation of the hormone receptors.*
Fulvestrant.

In metastatic breast and prostate cancer, first-line hormone therapies have a median duration of action of roughly 18 months.

## Glucocorticoids

The corticosteroids cortisol, hydrocortisone and prednisolone are used with other drug combinations in the management of leukaemia and lymphomas. Dexamethasone is used in the management of raised intracranial pressure associated with intracerebral primary or secondary tumours, and is also a useful anti-emetic agent, often in combination with other agents.

Steroids can also be useful in stimulating appetite in patients with advanced cancer. Progestogens can also be used in this way and to improve the quality of life.

## Immunopharmacology

### Relevant pathophysiology

The immune system is a host defence network of different cell types and molecules that protect against invasion by pathogens. Immune responses occur at different levels of specificity.

### Innate or natural immunity

Innate immunity is mediated by phagocytic cells (neutrophils and macrophages), eosinophils and natural killer cells together with complement proteins. It is a rapid response system. It does not rely on specific recognition of organisms and has no 'memory' of previous infecting agents. Microorganisms are recognised through pattern recognition molecules, e.g. the 'toll-like' receptors. Production of cytokines, such as interleukin (IL)-12, IL-15, IL-23 and IL-18, during innate responses is critical to efficient generation of subsequent acquired immunity.

### Acquired or adaptive immunity

Acquired (adaptive) immunity is mediated by lymphocytes and their secreted products, notably cytokines and antibodies. Acquired immunity is highly specific and re-exposure to a previously encountered antigen produces a greatly augmented and more efficient immune response. T-lymphocytes are of primary importance in regulating acquired immune responses. CD4$^+$ T-inducer/helper (Th) cells initiate and define the nature of the subsequent response and as such represent important therapeutic targets. T-cells possess highly specific cell-surface receptors that recognise foreign proteins only after they have been broken into peptide antigens and attached to major histocompatibility complex (MHC) molecules expressed on the surface of specialised antigen-presenting cells, e.g. dendritic cells. Th cells may be functionally subdivided into two distinct populations—Th1 cells produce interferon-$\gamma$ and thereby promote a *cell-mediated immune response*; Th2 cells produce IL-4 and IL-5 and promote B-cell maturation into plasma cells, leading to antibody formation and thus *humoral responses*. CD8$^+$ T-cells function predominantly as cytotoxic effector cells able, for example, to kill virus-infected cells or tumours. A critical role of the immune system is to distinguish self-proteins from those belonging to invading micro-organisms—this process is called *tolerance*. Tolerance is mediated via thymic selection of developing lymphocytes (*central tolerance*) or via suppression/deletion of lymphocytes post-emergence from the thymus (*peripheral tolerance*). There are a variety of immunological diseases in which the immune system inflicts damage on normal cells and body tissues, representing a 'breach' of tolerance.

Immune responses have historically been classified according to the principal effector mechanism responsible.

### Type I: Immediate hypersensitivity

Antigen binds to antibody (IgE) attached to mast cells or basophils and provokes release of inflammatory mediators such as vasoactive amines, proteases and prostaglandins. This results in increased vascular permeability, smooth muscle contraction and local inflammation. The clinical manifestations, especially in atopic individuals are:

1 Allergic asthma
2 Hay fever
3 Eczema.

In extreme cases anaphylactic shock may result.

### Type II: Antibody-mediated hypersensitivity

Autoreactive or cross-reactive antibodies (IgG and IgM) bind to antigens found on cells or tissues and cause damage by activating complement or recruiting inflammatory cells. This may result in tissue- or organ-specific autoimmune diseases (e.g. pernicious anaemia, autoimmune haemolytic anaemia or thrombocytopenic purpura and glomerulonephritis). Alternatively, antibodies directed against cell-surface receptors may

either stimulate or block target cell function (e.g. anti-TSH receptor antibodies in Graves disease and anti-acetylcholine receptor antibodies in myasthenia gravis). Antibody-mediated cytotoxicity is also responsible for hyperacute (immediate) organ allograft rejection in sensitised renal transplant recipients who have preformed anti-donor antibodies.

### Type III: Immune complex-mediated hypersensitivity

Circulating antibody–antigen complexes are deposited in tissues where they produce local activation of complement and leucocytes. Immune complex deposition occurs mainly in the glomeruli resulting in nephritis but other tissues may also be affected. Administration of large amounts of protein antigen intravenously may result in serum sickness.

### Type IV: Cell-mediated hypersensitivity

CD4$^+$ effector T-cells release pro-inflammatory cytokines (particularly interferon-$\gamma$, i.e. Th1 type) and recruit activated macrophages to produce a delayed-type hypersensitivity (DTH) reaction. DTH is responsible for contact sensitivity after topical exposure to chemicals. T-effector cells are suspected of causing several autoimmune diseases (e.g. insulin-dependent diabetes mellitus, multiple sclerosis and rheumatoid arthritis). This form of hypersensitivity is responsible for causing acute rejection of organ allografts and is also likely to be important in organ-specific autoimmunity.

## Drugs that suppress immune responses

Excess immune activity has clinical importance in several areas, particularly transplantation and autoimmune disease (Table 10.4). Until recently, immune suppressive drugs have comprised mainly *small chemical agents* that have been 'borrowed' from the chemotherapeutic area. Most immunosuppressive drugs currently in use are therefore relatively non-specific and therefore increase the risk of both opportunistic and conventional infections. They may also increase the risk of

**Table 10.4** Immunosuppressive drugs used to prevent graft rejection.

| Induction/maintenance of immunosuppression | Treatment of rejection |
|---|---|
| Ciclosporin (cyclosporin) monotherapy | High-dose prednisolone |
| or | or |
| Ciclosporin + prednisolone | Polyclonal/monoclonal antibody |
| or | |
| Ciclosporin + prednisolone + azathioprine (triple therapy) | |
| or | |
| Polyclonal/monoclonal antibody + ciclosporin + prednisolone + azathioprine (quadruple therapy) | |

lymphoproliferative disorders and of solid tumours. In addition to the problem of non-specific immunosuppression, individual agents have drug-specific side effects.

The immune modulator class now also includes *biologic agents*. These represent a new class of drugs comprising either monoclonal antibodies or protein receptor complexes that are delivered by parenteral routes. They are highly specific for molecular targets in the immune system, including cytokines and cell-surface receptors.

## Small chemical agents that modify immune response

A variety of small chemical drugs have been adapted to immunosuppressive use. For example, antimetabolites and alkylating agents are used as immunosuppressives but given at lower doses than when used in cancer chemotherapy. They inhibit actively dividing cells and at low doses are relatively selective for activated lymphocytes. Other agents found to be effective in treatment of inflammatory disease do so through means as yet poorly understood. The following agents are used in a variety of immunological conditions.

### Azathioprine

This pro-drug is metabolised in the liver to 6-mercaptopurine, a purine nucleotide analogue, which inhibits DNA and RNA synthesis. It is widely used in organ transplantation and in several autoimmune diseases. Side effects include leucopenia and thrombocytopenia.

### Mycophenolate mofetil

This new drug appears more selective than azathioprine and may find a use in organ transplantation. It inhibits inosine monophosphate dehydrogenase, the rate-limiting enzyme for the *de novo* pathway of purine synthesis. Because lymphocytes have no salvage pathway for purine synthesis, they are selectively inhibited.

### Methotrexate

Methotrexate is used as prophylaxis for graft vs. host disease following bone marrow transplantation and increasingly as a disease modifying antirheumatic drug for rheumatoid arthritis, psoriasis and psoriatic arthritis. It is not used directly in organ transplantation.

### Sulphasalazine

Sulphasalazine is used in the treatment of rheumatoid arthritis, psoriatic arthritis (useful for joint but not skin disease) and inflammatory bowel disease. Its precise mechanism of action is unclear but likely includes inhibition of the pro-inflammatory transcription factor NF-$\kappa$B.

### Hydroxycholoroquine

Originally derived as an antimalarial agent, hydroxycholoroquine is a useful disease-modifying agent used widely in the treatment of rheumatoid arthritis and systemic lupus erythematosis (SLE). It acts in part via inhibition of phagolysosome function in macrophages and dendritic cells.

### Cyclophosphamide and chlorambucil

These drugs are used to treat some types of glomerulonephritis, e.g. complicated SLE or systemic vasculitis, and occasionally other types of autoimmune disease but are not used in organ transplantation.

## T-cell targeting agents

### Ciclosporin

*Mechanism*

Ciclosporin acts predominantly on T-helper cells. It selectively impairs production of cytokines, particularly IL-2, and inhibits IL-2 receptor expression, thereby blocking T-cell growth. This prevents T-cell activation and stops the generation of the cell-mediated immune responses responsible for allograft rejection, or tissue damage in autoimmune diseases.

*Pharmacokinetics*

Ciclosporin is poorly absorbed following oral administration but this problem has been reduced by a new microemulsion formulation. It is a highly lipophilic compound and is distributed widely in body tissues. It is metabolised in the liver and small bowel by the cytochrome P-450 system and then excreted in the bile. Because of variation between individuals in ciclosporin pharmacokinetics, measurement of whole blood ciclosporin levels is used as a guide to dose requirements.

*Side effects*

Nephrotoxicity is the major drug-specific side effect of ciclosporin. Other side effects include hypertension, convulsions, mild elevation of hepatic transaminases, anorexia, nausea, vomiting, hypertrichosis, gingival hyperplasia, tremor and paraesthesia. Toxicity is usually managed by lowering the dose.

*Drug interactions*

A large number of drug interactions with ciclosporin have been reported. There are two major types:

1 Drugs that are nephrotoxic themselves. Examples are the aminoglycosides and amphotericin, which may enhance the nephrotoxicity of ciclosporin.

2 Drugs that alter the pharmacokinetics of ciclosporin.

Cytochrome P-450 inhibitors such as erythromycin and ketoconazole lead to increased ciclosporin blood levels. Conversely, drugs that induce cytochrome P-450 such as carbamazepine, phenytoin and rifampicin reduce ciclosporin blood levels.

*Clinical use and dose*

The introduction of ciclosporin revolutionised organ transplantation, allowing greater than 80% 1-year graft survival for kidney, heart and liver transplantation. Nearly all immunosuppressive protocols for organ transplantation include ciclosporin, although treatment regimens vary widely between centres (Table 10.4).

The daily oral dose in the immediate post-transplant period is usually 10–15 mg/kg and this is gradually reduced to a maintenance dose of 3–5 mg/kg, guided by ciclosporin blood levels and clinical assessment. Ciclosporin is used in the prophylaxis and treatment of graft vs. host disease after bone marrow transplantation and increasingly in some types of autoimmune disease. It has been used either alone or in combination with methotrexate to treat severe rheumatoid arthritis.

### Tacrolimus

This fungal macrolide acts in a very similar way to ciclosporin, although it has a different structure. Its clinical role is not yet clear but it is sometimes used in organ transplantation as an alternative to ciclosporin. Drug-specific side effects are broadly similar to those of ciclosporin. Gingival hypertrophy and hypertrichosis are not seen but neurological side effects may occur.

### Sirolimus

This new drug is similar in structure to tacrolimus but acts at a different site within the lymphocyte. It may synergise with ciclosporin and has the potential advantage of reduced nephrotoxicity.

**Leflunomide**

Leflunomide inhibits the mitochondrial enzyme, dihydroorotate dehydrogenase (DHODH), involved in synthesis of pyrimidines. It thereby inhibits lymphocyte activation and growth. This drug has recently been shown to exhibit efficacy and disease-modifying activity in rheumatoid arthritis.

## Glucocorticoids

Prednisolone and other glucocorticoids have both anti-inflammatory and immunosuppressive properties (see 'Glucocorticoids', Chapter 11). They have many different effects on the immune system and interfere with the following:

1 Lymphocyte recirculation
2 T-cell activation
3 Generation of cytotoxic lymphocytes
4 Cytokine release
5 Macrophage and monocyte function.

Steroids are widely used as immunosuppressives but long-term use in high dose is associated with an unacceptable incidence of adverse effects, and it is therefore preferable to use low-dose steroids combined with other immunosuppressive agents.

## Antihistamines

These block classical histamine ($H_1$) receptors and interfere with the actions of histamine released in type I immune reactions.

They are used in hay fever, allergic rhinitis, urticaria and other acute allergic reactions. The vascular effects of histamine including flare, wheal and itch are prevented. They are of no use in asthma.

Older antihistamines like promethazine and diphenhydramine have sedative and anticholinergic side effects. These are less prominent with cyclizine and chlorphenamine (chlorpheniramine). New agents like terfenadine cause little or no sedation, have non-reversible antagonist properties and can be given once daily.

Antihistamines are also used to treat motion sickness and vestibular disease (Chapter 13). Combination with type II histamine receptor antagonists may be beneficial in some forms of urticaria.

## Drugs that block mediator release

Drugs that increase intracellular cyclic adenosine monophosphate (cAMP) stabilise the mast cell and prevent degranulation and mediator release. This reduces or attenuates the symptoms of IgE-mediated hypersensitivity reactions.

### $\beta_2$-Adrenoceptor agonists

Drugs like adrenaline, terbutaline or salbutamol (Chapter 8) increase intracellular cAMP, reduce mediator release and improve symptoms.

### Theophylline derivatives

These block phosphodiesterase, prevent cAMP breakdown, increase local levels and thus reduce mediator release.

### Disodium cromoglicate and ketotifen

These agents stabilise the mast cell membrane and reduce mediator release. The precise mechanism is unknown but it may be related to inhibition of phosphodiesterase.

### Non-steroidal anti-inflammatory drugs/Cox-2 selective inhibitors

Indomethacin and related agents block synthesis of eicosanoids, including prostaglandins and also leukotrienes. Non-steroidal anti-inflammatory drugs (NSAIDs) are useful in the management of some autoimmune diseases, particularly rheumatoid arthritis, but the interference with prostaglandin synthesis may interrupt normal homeostatic prostaglandin-dependent functions in the lung, kidney and gut. NSAIDs may provoke acute asthma in some sensitive individuals, promote nephrotoxicity or lead to gastrointestinal perforation.

Cyclo-oxygenase (Cox) exists in two isoforms—Cox-1 is primarily involved in normal homeostatic function, whereas Cox-2 is up-regulated during inflammatory responses. Agents that specifically inhibit Cox-2 have recently been developed that show efficacy in treating pain and arthritis (e.g. celecoxib, valdecoxib and etoricoxib), with improved gastrointestinal toxicity profiles. Effects on renal function may persist. There is now considerable concern that Cox-2 inhibitors may exacerbate cardiovascular risk. Rofecoxib has been withdrawn for this reason and it is probable that this will prove a class effect. Recent studies also implicate non-selective NSAIDs in increased vascular risk (except aspirin). NSAIDs and Cox inhibitors should therefore be used with caution in patients with vascular risk factors or history, and should be used at the lowest dose necessary and for limited periods if possible.

## Combination of drugs in treatment of immune-mediated disorders

The treatment of chronic inflammatory diseases, such as rheumatoid arthritis, and connective tissue diseases now often entails use of combinations of immune modulatory drugs. In rheumatoid arthritis, combination of methotrexate, sulphasalazine and hydroxycholorquine has proven superior to single therapy. Additional combinations shown to be beneficial include methotrexate/ciclosporin and methotrexate/sulphasalazine. Low-dose corticosteroids are often added to these combinations. It is unclear yet whether autoimmune diseases and chronic inflammatory disease should be treated with several drugs from outset with agents removed as disease improves (*step down therapy*) or whether disease should be treated by sequential addition of drugs until disease is in remission (*step up therapy*).

## Biological therapies

Biological therapies consist of antibodies or receptors that can specifically bind soluble or cell-bound molecules of demonstrable importance in pathological immune responses. They are usually developed following elucidation of pathophysiologically important pathways that appear amenable to immunomodulation. Broadly they can target cells mediating immune responses, or their soluble products, usually cytokines.

## Targeting cells, cell receptors and co-stimulatory molecules

Polyclonal anti-T-cell antibodies are raised by injecting animals (e.g. goats or rabbits) with human lymphocyte or thymocyte preparations. OKT3 is a mouse monoclonal antibody to the CD3 complex on T-lymphocytes. These antibody preparations are given intravenously and cause profound immunosuppression by depleting T-cells from the circulation. They are used in transplantation either as prophylaxis or to treat steroid-resistant acute graft rejection. Polyclonal antibody preparations often cause fever and thrombocytopenia and rarely serum sickness or anaphylaxis. OKT3 may result in the cytokine release syndrome (pyrexia, rigors, nausea, wheeze, diarrhoea and rash).

Several other monoclonal antibodies are currently being assessed for treatment of graft rejection and autoimmune disease. Monoclonal antibodies directed against CD4 and the IL-2 receptor are being tried in organ transplantation. Genetic engineering technology is being used to 'humanise' relevant mouse monoclonal antibodies to render them less immunogenic and therefore more effective. Several cell-targeted therapies are close to or already in clinical use.

### Rituximab

This is a chimeric (part mouse/part human protein) monoclonal antibody directed against CD20 which is a receptor expressed on B-cells. Rituximab is effective in treatment of lymphoma but has beneficial effects also in rheumatoid arthritis and probably also in SLE and immune thrombocytopenic purpura. It is given by intravenous infusion together with methotrexate and corticosteroid to achieve maximal benefit. Clinical improvement in rheumatoid arthritis can last at least 6 months after a single therapeutic course.

## Abatacept

This is a protein therapy that blocks co-stimulatory function. T-cells are activated upon receipt of two signals from a dendritic cell (*signal* 1 is mediated via the antigen receptor/MHC/peptide interaction and *signal* 2 comes from a co-stimulatory molecule such as CD28). CTLA-4 regulates the capacity of CD28 to mediated signal 2. If only one signal is received then the T-cell becomes anergic (unable to respond). Abatacept is a CTLA-4, immunoglobulin Fc fusion protein that can interfere with T-cell dendritic cell interactions. It has been shown to be effective in rheumatoid arthritis and psoriasis. It is given by subcutaneous injection. Benefit is noted within 3 months of starting therapy. Best effects may require co-prescription with methotrexate.

## Alefacept

A further essential co-stimulatory pathway for T-cells is that mediated via CD2 and LFA3. Alefacept is a fusion protein containing LFA3 together with an Fc protein segment. It interferes with interactions between T-cells and adjacent dendritic cells and macrophages. It has beneficial effects shown in psoriasis.

## Efalizumab

Blocking adhesion between leukocytes as they migrate into an inflammatory lesion and receive activatory signals represents an attractive approach to therapy exemplified in this antibody that blocks the adhesion molecule LFA-1. Efalizumab has been introduced for the treatment of psoriasis thus far.

## Targeting cytokines

Biologic agents that target cytokines have proven highly effective in the treatment of a variety of inflammatory diseases. A chimeric antibody (part mouse/part human immunoglobulin) against tumour necrosis factor (TNF) (infliximab) and a fully human antibody against TNF (adalimumab) have been successfully used to treat rheumatoid arthritis and Crohn's disease. Similarly, a soluble TNF receptor fused to the Fc portion of human immunoglobulin (etanercept) has similar efficacy in rheuma-toid arthritis. All three agents appear effective also in psoriasis. These agents induce significant clinical responses in up to 70% of patients. The risk of potential side effects, which theoreticallywill include infection and development of lymphoproliferative diseases or solid tumours, is as yet poorly defined although early clinical studies appear promising. Effects in other autoimmune diseases are variable with some benefits reported in ulcerative colitis, vasculitis and uveitis. Soluble decoy receptors to IL-1 (IL-1 receptor antagonist) are also being tested in patients with rheumatoid arthritis. Numerous other biological agents (monoclonal antibodies and soluble receptors) targeting cytokines, chemokines and pro-angiogenic factors implicated in autoimmune responses are in development.

## Infliximab

It is an anti-TNF antibody given by i.v. infusion every 8 weeks. Benefits onset within 4 weeks usually. It must be used in combination with methotrexate in rheumatoid arthritis with which it has synergistic benefit.

## Etanercept

It is a TNF receptor Fc fusion protein given by s.c. injection twice weekly. It has synergistic benefit when used with methotrexate in rheumatoid arthritis.

## Adalimumab

It is a fully human anti-TNF antibody given by s.c. injection every 1–2 weeks. It has synergistic benefit when used with methotrexate in rheumatoid arthritis.

Regardless of disease indication, before starting TNF blocking therapies, all patients should be screened for prior or current tuberculosis (usually CXR and skin testing), history of severe infection and malignancy. Live vaccines are contraindicated. No information is yet available about safety during pregnancy. Monitoring is not required but is advisable since patients are often on complex drug regimes and exhibit co-morbidities together with the underlying inflammatory disorder.

## Immunostimulatory and immunomodulatory agents

Effective strategies for stimulation of the immune system have proved elusive, although there has been some recent progress.

## Cytokines

Cytokines are soluble proteins produced by a wide variety of cells and act primarily in an autocrine or paracrine manner. They have many important and complex actions and play a particularly important role in the regulation of immune and inflammatory responses. Recombinant DNA technology has allowed the large-scale production of many cytokines and these are being used increasingly to modify the biological response to malignancy and infection. Interferon-$\alpha$ is an effective therapy for hairy cell leukaemia (a rare form of chronic leukaemia) and is useful for Kaposi's sarcoma in patients with acquired immunodeficiency syndrome (AIDS). Selected patients with chronic hepatitis B or C infection may also respond to interferon-$\alpha$ therapy. Interferon-$\alpha$ and IL-2 have been used in the treatment of metastatic renal carcinoma and malignant melanoma but response rates are disappointing and, in view of the cost of therapy and side effects, this is a controversial area. Interferon-$\beta$ has been employed successfully in multiple sclerosis. G-CSF and GM-CSF are being used to shorten the duration of neutropenia after cytotoxic therapy for non-myeloid malignancies, and also in bone marrow transplantation. The use of cytokines as biological response modifiers is at an early stage of development and holds much promise for the future. This may be of particular relevance in immune stimulation in patients with human immunodeficiency virus (HIV)/AIDS.

## Other immunostimulatory agents

Bacille Calmette–Guérin (BCG) and other agents, e.g. levamisole and *Corynebacterium parvum*, have been tried as immunostimulants in a wide variety of malignancies because of their potential ability to enhance cell-mediated immunity. Results have been disappointing and they are not in widespread use. Recently, adaptive transfer of live dendritic cells to recipients has been used to stimulate immune responses against tumours. These exciting studies remain at an early stage.

# Chapter 11

# Corticosteroids

Corticosteroids are usually given for one of the following three reasons:
1 Suppression of inflammation
2 Suppression of immune responses
3 Replacement therapy.

Corticosteroids are hormones synthesised from cholesterol by the adrenal cortex and have a wide range of physiological functions. Pharmacologically, they are divided according to the relative potencies of their physiological effects into:
1 Glucocorticoids that principally affect carbohydrate and protein metabolism (type II receptor)
2 Mineralocorticoids that principally affect sodium balance (type I receptor).

Production of the naturally occurring glucocorticoid, cortisol (hydrocortisone), is stimulated by the release of adrenocorticotropic hormone (ACTH) from the anterior pituitary. Production of the major naturally occurring mineralocorticoid, aldosterone, is controlled by other factors in addition to ACTH, including the activity of the renin–angiotensin system and plasma potassium. Synthetic steroids have largely replaced the natural compounds in therapeutic use as they are usually more potent, may be more specific with regard to mineralocorticoid and glucocorticoid activity and can be given orally. Prednisolone, betamethasone and dexamethasone are widely used as anti-inflammatory and immunosuppressant drugs.

## Glucocorticoids

### Cortisol and its derivatives

Glucocorticoids act primarily via binding to a cytosolic glucocorticoid receptor that in complex with glucocorticoid enters the nucleus and binds to glucocorticoid–response elements situated in the promoters of genes coding for proteins that regulate inflammation and immune responses (*transactivation*). The glucocorticoid receptor complex can also interfere directly with other transcription factor complexes and thereby further suppress inflammatory gene expression (*transrepression*).

### Pharmacological effects

1 Inflammatory response. Irrespective of the injury or the insult, corticosteroids interfere nonspecifically with all components of the inflammatory responses. This includes reduced capillary dilatation and exudation, inhibition of leucocyte migration and phagocytic activity and reduced fibrin deposition with diminution of subsequent scar formation (see 'Disease-controlling antirheumatic therapies', Chapter 9).
2 Immunological response. In high doses, lymphocyte mass and immunoglobulin production are reduced as are monocyte and macrophage function. This results in impaired immunological competence (see 'Immunopharmacology', Chapter 10).

3 Carbohydrate and protein metabolism. Steroids promote glycogen deposition in the liver and gluconeogenesis, an increase in glucose output by the liver and a decrease in glucose utilisation by peripheral tissues. There is a concomitant increase in protein catabolism with mobilisation of amino acids from peripheral tissues.
4 Fluid and electrolyte balance. Even glucocorticoids have some mineralocorticoid activity and can act on type I receptors. The principal effect is of enhanced sodium reabsorption from the distal tubule of the kidney, with an associated increase in the urinary excretion of potassium and hydrogen ions. Oedema is rare but moderate hypertension is not uncommon.
5 Lipid metabolism. Corticosteroids facilitate fat mobilisation by adrenaline and redistribution of body fat to 'centripetal' areas: face, neck and shoulders.
6 Mood and behaviour changes. Mild euphoria is quite common with higher doses.
7 Increase in the number of red cells, platelets and polymorphs, but a decrease in the number of eosinophils and lymphocytes. These effects may in part arise from altered cell migration.
8 Increased production of gastric acid and pepsin.
9 Reduction in bone formation: A decrease in calcium absorption from the intestine and an increase in calcium loss from the kidney. There is also reduced secretion of growth hormone and antagonism of its peripheral effects, and so there may be growth retardation in children.

## Adverse effects

The adverse effects of corticosteroids are largely predictable from the wide range of known physiological and pharmacological effects.
1 Metabolic effects. Patients on high-dosage steroid therapy quickly develop a characteristic appearance: a rounded, plethoric face (moon face), deposits of fat over the supraclavicular and cervical areas (buffalo hump), obesity of the trunk with relatively thin limbs, purple striae typically on the thighs and lower abdomen and a tendency to bruising. Disturbed carbohydrate metabolism

leads to hyperglycaemia and glycosuria and rarely proceeds to overt diabetes mellitus.
In addition to the loss of protein from skeletal muscle, patients also develop muscular weakness, which particularly affects the thighs and upper arms (proximal myopathy).
2 Fluid retention may be associated with hypokalaemic alkalosis and hypertension.
3 Increased susceptibility to infection.
4 Osteoporosis. It may cause compression fractures of the vertebral bodies and avascular necrosis of the head of the femur. UK national guidelines now dictate that osteoporotic prophylaxis be introduced in a proportion of patients destined to receive steroid treatment for prolonged periods; all patients starting steroids should be entered into prophylaxis algorithms and a bisphosphonate commenced if indicated.
5 Psychosis. A sense of euphoria frequently accompanies high-dosage steroid therapy and this may rarely proceed to overt manic psychosis. The increased sense of well-being leads to an improved appetite and contributes to weight gain.
Steroids may precipitate a depressive illness.
6 Cataract. This is a rare complication, usually in children, reflecting prolonged high-dosage therapy.
7 Gastrointestinal symptoms. Dyspepsia frequently accompanies high-dosage oral steroid therapy. Signs of peritonitis, which would complicate a perforated peptic ulcer, may be masked by the anti-inflammatory effect of steroids.

These predictable and serious adverse effects should lead to particular caution in the use of steroid therapy in patients who have pre-existing peptic ulceration, severe hypertension, congestive cardiac failure and osteoporosis.

## Adrenal suppression

The administration of exogenous corticosteroids results in negative feedback to the anterior pituitary, with inhibition of ACTH release and the consequent withdrawal of trophic stimulation to the adrenal cortex. In time, the adrenal cortex atrophies and when long-term steroid therapy is finally stopped it may be 6–12 months before normal pituitary–adrenal function recovers. An alternate-day steroid regimen may cause less adrenal suppression than daily treatment. Adrenal suppression has two consequences:

1 Impairment of patient's response to 'stress' (illness, injury, surgery) and susceptibility to infection. Chickenpox may be particularly severe: passive immunisation with varicella zoster immunoglobin should be given to non-immune patients.

2 The withdrawal of corticosteroid therapy must be slow and supervised.

Short-term therapy (4–6 weeks) can be reduced quickly and stopped abruptly without difficulty. Long-term therapy, particularly with more than 7.5 mg prednisolone daily, or equivalent, carries the risk of adrenal and hypothalamic–pituitary suppression. Withdrawal must be undertaken cautiously and gradually. Assuming that there is no flare-up of the systemic disease for which the steroid therapy was originally prescribed, the daily dose should be reduced by 5 mg of prednisolone, or equivalent, every 1–2 weeks until the total daily dose is at the physiological replacement level of 5 mg daily. This dosage should be converted to a single morning administration, and at intervals of 2 weeks, decrements of 1 mg should be made. The safety of this gradual withdrawal can be monitored by the endogenous plasma cortisol level; full recovery can be verified by a Synacthen (ACTH) test. All these patients require supervision and advice for 6 months after steroid withdrawal.

Patients on long-term steroid therapy, and particularly those undergoing steroid withdrawal, require a temporary increase in the dose of steroid during periods of stress because of the inability of the hypothalamic–pituitary–adrenal axis to respond normally with an increased production of endogenous corticosteroid, e.g. in times of intercurrent illness. Similarly, patients on steroid therapy who undergo surgery require an increased steroid dosage to enable them to withstand the stress of the operation. Such patients need to carry a steroid card (or bracelet/necklace) so that they can be identified as steroid dependent in the event of an accident/emergency. They should understand the need for uninterrupted treatment and report any problem (vomiting/diarrhoea) immediately. Patients on steroids are now specifically advised to avoid contact with people who have chickenpox or shingles and to see their doctor if such contact occurs. If travelling to remote areas, they should be instructed in the self-administration of intramuscular hydrocortisone and given the appropriate equipment and drugs.

## Topical therapy

Topically applied steroids are absorbed through the skin and in the case of very potent drugs, such as clobetasol or betamethasone, adrenal suppression and the toxic effects described above can occur. This usually happens only if recommended doses are exceeded, extensive areas of skin are covered or very prolonged administration is used.

Other effects peculiar to topical application are:
1 Worsening of local infections. This is particularly important in the eye, where ulcers caused by herpes simplex (dendritic ulcers) spread dramatically and dangerously following application of steroids.
2 Local thinning of the skin. This slowly resolves on stopping steroids, but some permanent damage may remain.
3 Atrophic striae. These are irreversible.
4 Increased hair growth.
5 The use of high doses of beclomethasone by aerosol inhalation can result in hoarseness or candidiasis of the mouth.

## Clinical use and dose

### Hydrocortisone

Hydrocortisone is used in three different situations:

1 Replacement therapy—when it is given orally in a dose of 20 mg in the morning and 10 mg in the afternoon. Body size needs to be taken into consideration ($12$–$15$ mg/m$^2$ surface area).
2 Shock and status asthmaticus—when it is given intravenously up to 200 mg 6-hourly.
3 Topical application—for example 1% cream or ointment in eczema; 100-mg dose as enema or foam in treating ulcerative colitis.

## Cortisone acetate

Cortisone acetate is metabolised to cortisol, although some patients may be deficient in the relevant enzyme.

## Prednisolone

Prednisolone is used orally in three types of condition:

1 Inflammatory diseases, e.g. rheumatoid arthritis, ulcerative colitis, chronic active hepatitis
2 Allergic diseases, e.g. severe asthma
3 Acute lymphoblastic leukaemia and non-Hodgkin lymphoma.

A single dose of up to 60 mg daily is given, depending on disease severity, reducing to a maintenance dose in the range 2.5–15 mg daily.

It is used topically in ulcerative colitis as a 20-mg enema.

## Prednisone

Prednisone is a synthetic steroid that is metabolised to prednisolone in much the same way as cortisone acetate is converted to cortisol.

## Beclometasone

Beclometasone is a fluorinated, and therefore polar, steroid that passes poorly across membranes. It is used topically in:

1 Asthma—when it is given by metered aerosol doses. About 20% reaches the lungs, and the rest is swallowed and destroyed by first-pass metabolism (Chapter 8).
2 Severe eczema—when it is used as 0.025% cream.

## Betamethasone

Betamethasone is used for:

1 Cerebral oedema caused by tumours and trauma; given either orally or intramuscularly in doses up to 4 mg 6-hourly. It is ineffective in cerebral oedema resulting from hypoxia.
2 Severe eczema; given topically as 0.1% cream.

## Dexamethasone

Dexamethasone is used in cerebral oedema.

## Triamcinolone

Triamcinolone is used for:

1 Local inflammation of joints or soft tissue; given by intra-articular injection in doses up to 40 mg depending on joint size.
2 Severe eczema; given topically as 0.1% cream.

## Clobetasol

Clobetasol is used topically in severe resistant eczema and discoid lupus erythematosus.

# Mineralocorticoids

## Pharmacological effects

These drugs produce retention of salt and water by the same mechanism as aldosterone on the distal renal tubule. Their main adverse effect is excessive fluid retention and hypertension.

## Clinical use and dose

Fludrocortisone is a fluorinated hydrocortisone with powerful mineralocorticoid activity and very little anti-inflammatory action. It is used in:

1 Replacement therapy in doses of 50–200 µg/day.
2 Congenital adrenal hyperplasia in doses up to 2 µg/day.
3 Idiopathic postural hypotension in doses of 100–200 µg/day.

*Comment.* Steroids are powerful drugs. Dramatic improvement in certain severe diseases is matched by equally dramatic ill health resulting from adverse effects when these drugs are used in mild inflammatory disorders for which they are not indicated.

Steroids should therefore be used only when other less toxic drugs have failed, or when the severity of the condition justifies aggressive treatment with steroids in high doses. Once control of the clinical state has been achieved, steroid dose should be reduced to the minimum necessary to maintain the desired effect and, if possible, stopped altogether.

# Chapter 12

# Drugs and the reproductive system

## Sex steroids

### Oral contraceptives

The use of combined hormonal contraception is safe for most women. Nevertheless, there are some situations (for example previous venous thromboembolism, migraine with aura or a smoker aged over 35 years) where the risks of using combined hormonal contraception outweigh benefits or pose an unacceptable health risk. Currently, in the United Kingdom, combined hormonal contraception can be administered orally as the combined oral contraceptive (COC) pill or transdermally via a patch.

### Composition

Both of the naturally occurring steroids, oestradiol (estradiol) and progesterone, are ineffective if taken orally because of extensive first-pass metabolism; thus, synthetic compounds are used in hormonal contraception. Combined hormonal contraception (pills, patch, vaginal ring) usually contains a synthetic oestrogen (ethinyloestradiol, EE). An alternative to EE mestranol is found in the COC (Norinyl-1) but its bioavailability compared to EE is unknown. Synthetic progesterones (called a progestogen) are mainly derivatives of 19-nortestosterone. Progestogens have

androgenic, estrogenic as well as progestogenic properties. Progestogens have been described as 'first-generation' (norethynodrel), 'second-generation' (levonorgestrel and norethisterone), 'third-generation' (desogestrel and gestodene) and 'fourth-generation' (drospirenone). The newer generations of progestogens have *in vitro* been shown to have progestational potency with low androgenicity.

### Mechanism

The COC is taken for 21 consecutive days; the first seven pills in the packet inhibit ovulation, while the remaining pills in the packet maintain anovulation. Most women follow 21 days of pill taking with 7 pill-free days known as the hormone-free interval. Some women use every day pills that have seven placebo hormone-free pills which are taken in week 4. One combined hormonal patch is used weekly for 3 weeks followed by a patch-free week. During the hormone-free week, due to the withdrawal of EE and progestogen, a complex series of events is triggered in the endometrium which allows it to shed, and a withdrawal bleed usually occurs. Contraceptive protection is maintained during the hormone-free interval as long as the previous and subsequent pills or patches are taken consistently and correctly.

## Progestogen-only contraception (pills, injectables, implant and intrauterine system)

The progestogen-only pill (POP) works by thickening cervical mucus so that it inhibits sperm penetration into the upper reproductive tract. With traditional POPs ovulation is inhibited in between 20 and 60% of cycles. A new desogestrel-containing POP (Cerazette) has been shown in randomised controlled trials to inhibit ovulation in up to 97% of cycles. All POPs should be taken every day without a pill-free interval.

The progestogen-only injectables (depot medroxyprogesterone acetate [DMPA] and norethisterone enanthate [NET-EN]) and the progestogen-only implant [Implanon] work by inhibition of ovulation in all women.

The levonorgestrel-releasing intrauterine system (LNG IUS) works by its effects on the endometrium, and in around 25% of women ovulation is also inhibited.

## Pharmacokinetics

Progestogens and EE are absorbed from the small intestine and are metabolised in the mucosa of the small intestine and liver 'first-pass metabolism'. After metabolism in the liver conjugates of EE, unaltered EE and progestogens are excreted into the bile and subsequently into the small intestine. In the large intestine, hydrolytic enzymes released from colonic bacteria break down inactive conjugates of EE. These active metabolites of EE can be reabsorbed again. This is called the *enterohepatic circulation*. There is no enterohepatic circulation for progestogens.

## Adverse effects

The most important, but not the most common, adverse reactions involve the effects of *oestrogen* on the cardiovascular system.

### Venous thromboembolic disease
1 The risk is increased by:

• Women using COC have an increased relative risk of venous thromboembolism (VTE). In absolute terms however, the risk is still very small. Women not using COC have a 5 per 100,000 woman-years of developing a VTE (deep vein thrombosis or pulmonary embolus).

The relative risk of VTE for women using a COC containing a second-generation progestogen (levonorgestrel and norethisterone) is increased 3- to 15-fold per 100,000 woman-years. However, this is still a very low absolute risk.

The relative risk of VTE is increased 5- to 30-fold per 100,000 woman-years with COCs containing third-generation progestogens (desogestrel and gestodene).

The risk of VTE also increases with increasing EE content, and COCs with more than 50 μg of EE are not in general use. Women using liver enzyme-inducing drugs may use a 50-μg COC; however, due to increased liver metabolism, this is clinically comparable to lower doses of EE.

• Major surgical procedures where the woman will be immobilised.

• Factor V Leiden and other hereditary thrombophilias.

2 The increased risk is confined to those actually taking the pill:
  • Develops within first month
  • Remains constant during use
  • Returns to normal within 1 month of stopping.

3 Pathogenesis:
  • Decreased antithrombin III
  • Decreased plasminogen activator in endothelium.

### Myocardial infarction and stroke (including subarachnoid haemorrhage)
1 The risk is increased by:
  • Age
  • Cigarette smoking
  • Exogenous oestrogen.

Age and cigarette smoking multiply, rather than add to, the risks of the oral contraceptives with regard to myocardial infarction and stroke. Most cases occur in women aged over 35 years who smoke. It is assumed that the risk is also enhanced by hypertension, diabetes, obesity and hyperlipoproteinaemia, but numbers are too small for statistical analysis.

2 The risk is not confined to those currently taking the pill, but persists after stopping.

3 Third-generation pills reduce the risk of arterial disease—users have one-third of the risk of myocardial infarction compared with second-generation pill users.

4 Pathogenesis:

- Acceleration of platelet aggregation
- Decreased antithrombin III
- Decreased plasminogen activator.

### Hypertension

1 Blood pressure rises by a small amount in all women using COC. There is a progressive rise with duration of use. In most cases, this increase in pressure is small and of little clinical significance. Less frequently there is a rise to levels at which treatment might ordinarily be considered. The best course of action in these cases is to stop the pill and observe for several months. Rarely, malignant hypertension occurs and should be treated as a medical emergency. Blood pressure should be checked before prescribing combined hormonal contraception and at each return clinic visit.

2 Blood pressure usually returns to normal 3–6 months after stopping the contraceptive pill.

### Oral contraceptives and cancer

This is a controversial area. Use of COC reduces the risk of ovarian and endometrial cancer by 50%. Cervical cancer has been identified more frequently in pill users than in women using an intrauterine contraceptive device. Interpretation of this finding is difficult because age at first intercourse and number of sexual partners are risk factors for cervical carcinoma and could differ substantially between these two groups. This increased risk appears to increase after 5 years of COC use. The suggestion that oral contraceptive use at a young age increases the risk of breast cancer remains unproven. Current evidence suggests that COC use is associated with either no increase or a very small increase in the risk of breast cancer.

This risk decreases after cessation and by 10 years after discontinuation, the risk is the same as for non-COC users.

### Glucose tolerance and lipid metabolism

There is a small decrease in glucose tolerance. Oestrogens increase, and progestogens decrease, high-density lipoproteins. The clinical relevance of these observations is unknown.

### Focal migraine and stroke

There is a very small increase in the absolute risk of stroke with COC use. This increased risk is further increased for COC users who have focal migraine.

## Other adverse effects

Common side effects of oral contraceptives include:

1 Irregular bleeding during the first few cycles
2 Headaches
3 Mood swings.

Less commonly, subjects may present with:

1 Cholestatic jaundice, particularly if a history of jaundice or pruritis in pregnancy.
2 Increased incidence of gallstones
3 Elevation of thyroid-binding globulin (does not affect analysis of free T4)
4 Precipitation of porphyria.

There is no good evidence that oral contraceptives containing low doses of oestrogen (reduce the quantity or quality of breastmilk) either impair established lactation or harm a breast-fed infant. Nevertheless, COC is not generally recommended if breastfeeding and less than 6 months post-partum.

## Drug interactions

Oral contraceptive failure resulting in unplanned pregnancy can be precipitated by enzyme induction (see below) resulting from the co-administration of drugs that induce hepatic microsomal enzymes (see 'Principles of drug elimination', Chapter 1).

This applies to oestrogen-containing and some progestogen-only contraceptives (POP and implants but not injectables or the LNG-IUS). If

---

**Hepatic microsomal enzyme inducers (some, not all, anti-epileptics, antiretrovirals, antibiotics)**

| | |
|---|---|
| Phenytoin | Primidone |
| Carbamazepine | Rifampicin |
| Phenobarbital (phenobarbitone) | |

---

long-term treatment with liver enzyme-inducing drugs is necessary (e.g. treatment of epilepsy) then a higher dose of COC should be used (at least 50 μg of EE) if oral contraception is the method of choice.

As mentioned on page 151, EE undergoes re-absorption via the enterohepatic circulation. The importance of this is unclear. Nevertheless, antibiotics that alter colonic bacteria may reduce reabsorption of EE and potentially reduce contraceptive efficacy. Pregnancies have been documented in women using COC with antibiotics. Failure of oestrogen-containing oral contraceptives can be precipitated by reduced absorption resulting from altered bowel flora caused by the co-administration of broad-spectrum antimicrobials. The mechanism depends on the fact that oestrogens undergo conjugation in the liver, but hydrolytic enzymes produced by gut bacteria cleave these conjugates and release free hormone, which is then reabsorbed. Broad-spectrum antimicrobials prevent this process by altering gut flora, and hormone absorption is decreased. When an antibiotic such as ampicillin is prescribed for a woman who is also taking an oral contraceptive, she should be advised to use additional contraception during and for 14 days after the course of antibiotic. Advice for women using COC is to use additional contraceptive protection, such as condoms, while taking the antibiotic and for at least 7 days after their discontinuation.

## Clinical use and dose

The dose of both oestrogen and progestogen should be kept as low as possible. Current advice is that for women starting COC for the first time, a COC with 30–35 μg of EE and levonorgestrel or norethisterone should be used, although other COCs can also be used.

1 Combined oral contraception (COC): One tablet daily for 21 days starting on day 1 (but new advice is up to and including day 5 of cycle) of the menstrual cycle and repeating after 7 pill-free days.

2 Combined contraceptive patch: Wear one patch for 7 days and replace every week for 3 weeks. Then have a patch-free week.

3 Phased formulations (biphasic or triphasic): These provide varying doses of EE and progestogen during the pill packet. Theoretically, these formulations should minimise deviations from normal metabolism; however, there are no proven benefits of biphasic and triphasic preparations compared to monophasic regimens.

4 Progestogen-only pill (POP): Continuous administration of one tablet daily starting on the first day of menstruation and taking the dose at the same time each day. A delay of more than 3 h risks loss of efficacy.

5 Desogestrel-only POP: Continuous administration of one tablet daily starting on the first day of menstruation and taking the dose at the same time each day. A delay of more than 12 h risks loss of efficacy.

6 Intramuscular DMPA: This is a long-acting progesterone derivative. Injections are given every 12 weeks. NET-EN is given every 8 weeks.

7 Progestogen-only implants: These implants provide a low daily etonorgestrel released from a rod placed in the subcutaneous tissue of the upper inner arm. They provide effective contraception for 3 years.

8 The levonorgestrel-releasing intrauterine system (LNG-IUS): It provides a high intrauterine dose of levonorgestrel with minimal systemic absorption. It can provide effective contraception for 5 years.

All hormonal methods are more than 99% effective if taken consistently and correctly. True method failures are low but user failure (due to missed pills) varies. Methods of hormonal contraception that avoid daily pill taking, such as the progestogen-only implant, are among the most effective methods of female contraception.

## Contraindications

These are summarised in Table 12.1.

Patients with established diabetes mellitus may use the combined pill with appropriate adjustment

**Table 12.1** Contraindications to the use of oral contraceptives.

| Absolute | Relative |
|---|---|
| History of thromboembolism | Diabetes |
| Moderate/severe hypertension | Cigarette smoking |
| Focal migraine | Mild hypertension |
| Active liver disease | Age >35 years |
| Age >35 years and cigarette smoker | |
| Porphyria | |
| Oestrogen-dependent tumour | |
| Impending major surgery | |
| History of jaundice in pregnancy | |
| Major haemoglobinopathy | |

of insulin requirements. Ideally, nobody with a relative contraindication should receive an oestrogen-containing oral contraceptive. However, real life is not ideal and pressure of social circumstances sometimes dictates that the risks of an unwanted pregnancy outweigh those accompanying the use of the contraceptive pill; the other forms of contraception are less reliable. The presence of two or more relative contraindications strengthens the case against using an oestrogen-containing contraceptive.

*Comment.* The widespread use of oral contraceptives is a testament to their popularity. Serious cardiovascular complications are clearly of concern and must be explained to a woman proposing to take the pill. However, they must be explained in the perspective that risk of myocardial infarction and stroke is concentrated largely in older women who smoke and that some, at least, of the morbidity in currently available statistics can still be ascribed to the use of now obsolete high-dose oestrogen preparations.

## Hormone replacement therapy

This is used for the alleviation of menopausal vasomotor symptoms and symptoms related to tissue atrophy, for example vasomotor symptoms and atrophic vaginitis. There is also good evidence that oestrogen administration will reduce postmenopausal osteoporosis. Recent large clinical trails have clarified the relationship between hormone replacement theory (HRT) use and cardiovascular disease. In a large American study of HRT, both 'oestrogen-only' HRT and a combination of oestrogen and progestogen increased the risk of stroke by approximately 8 per 10,000 woman-years. No convincing effect was seen on the incidence of coronary heart disease or in preventing colorectal cancer. In this study both HRT preparations reduced the incidence of hip fractures.

Natural oestrogens (estradiol, oestrone [estrone] and oestriol [estriol]) provide a more physiological effect for HRT than synthetic oestrogens (ethinylestradiol and mestranol). Oestrogen may be administered in various ways, for example tablet, transdermal patch, cream, gel, subdermal implant or intrauterine system. Oral oestrogens are subject to first-pass metabolism; therefore, subcutaneous or transdermal administration is more representative of endogenous hormone activity than other preparations.

Unopposed oestrogen can increase the risk of endometrial hyperplasia and malignancy. Therefore, a woman with a uterus should also be given one progestogen for at least 10–14 days of her cycle. Some HRT preparations contain cyclical progestogens and women have a regular withdrawal bleeding following the progestogen administration. Other HRT preparations have continuous combined oestrogen and progestogen and in women over 54 years, they can be used to prevent a cyclical bleed.

Studies indicate that there is an increased risk of breast cancer in women taking HRT. This risk is increased only after 5 years of HRT use. For women who have had a hysterectomy and oophorectomy, HRT replaces the endogenous hormone they would have had had they not undergone surgery. The risk of breast cancer increases only from the age of menopause (50 years). The increased risk is related to duration of use and the excess risk disappears within about 5 years of stopping. For example, for women over 50 years, the risk of developing breast cancer increases by 2 per 1000 in those taking HRT. In those women taking HRT for 15 years, this figure rises to 12 per 1000.

## Progestogens

1 Dysfunctional uterine bleeding (DUB). Cyclical progestogen is used to treat DUB secondary to anovulation. Side effects are mild but may include nausea, fluid retention and weight gain.
2 Progestogens are also used in the treatment of endometrial carcinoma only if unfit for surgery.

## Dopamine agonists

### Mechanism

Dopamine receptor agonists prevent the release of prolactin (PRL) by stimulating dopamine receptors in the pituitary. They increase growth hormone (GH) release in normal subjects but suppress GH release in acromegaly.

### Pharmacokinetics

Bromocriptine is effective orally and eliminated by liver metabolism followed by biliary excretion. Cabergoline has actions and uses similar to bromocriptine, but its duration of action is longer. Other similar drugs are pergolide, lisuride (lysuride) and terguride.

### Adverse effects

### Bromocriptine

Nausea and vomiting may limit dose increases. Postural hypotension can occur. Constipation is common. High doses (>20 mg/day) can produce a wide range of neuropsychiatric effects, including confusion, psychosis, dyskinesias and bizarre choreiform movements.

### Cabergoline

The pattern of side effects is different to bromocriptine. Therefore, patients intolerant of one drug may tolerate the other.

## Clinical use and dose

### Bromocriptine

Hyperprolactinaemia: up to 7.5 mg twice a day. Post-partum suppression of lactation: 2.5 mg twice a day for 2 weeks. Acromegaly: 5 mg 6-hourly. Parkinsonism: high doses up to 100 mg daily (see 'Migraine, other headaches and neuralgic pain', Chapter 17).

### Cabergoline

Hyperprolactinaemia: 500 mg weekly. Post-partum suppression of established lactation: 250 mg every 12 h for 2 days.

## Danazol

### Mechanism

Danazol inhibits pituitary gonadotrophin release, thereby reducing ovarian function and producing atrophy of the endometrium. It also blocks oestrogen and progesterone receptors but has some androgenic activity.

### Adverse effects

Avoid danazol during pregnancy; virilisation of female fetus has been reported.

Danazol is not an effective contraceptive and non-hormonal methods should be used during treatment. Acne, hirsutism and voice changes occasionally occur.

### Drug interactions

Danazol potentiates the action of carbamazepine and anticoagulants.

### Clinical use

Endometriosis, menorrhagia and occasionally for pre-menstrual syndrome, although it is not licensed for this indication.

## Gonadotrophin-releasing hormone analogues

### Mechanism

Gonadotrophin-releasing hormone (GnRH) is a decapeptide. It was isolated and characterised in 1971. GnRH analogues are produced by altering the amino acids in positions 6 and/or 10, resulting in compounds with high affinity for the GnRH receptor, and a long half-life as a result of their resistance to cleavage by endopeptidases. After an initial brief stimulation, the GnRH analogues paradoxically result in the suppression of the pituitary and therefore of ovarian activity.

### Adverse effects

The main disadvantages of GnRH analogues are secondary to the induced hypo-oestrogenic state, affecting the cardiovascular, skeletal and urogenital systems while producing vasomotor symptoms. Add-back therapy using oestrogens, progestogens or both may be used to negate their harmful effects.

### Clinical use

Their short-term use is of proven benefit in assisted reproduction and prior to endometrial resection or ablation. Long-term applications range from shrinking fibroids before surgery to the management of endometriosis, ovarian hyperandrogenism, the pre-menstrual syndrome (although not licensed for this indication), precocious puberty and DUB.

## Ovulation induction agents

### Anti-oestrogens

#### Mechanism

Clomiphene (clomifene) and tamoxifen are oestrogen receptor antagonists that prevent negative feedback of oestrogen at the hypothalamus, leading to increased secretion of FSH and LH.

### Clinical use and dose

Female subfertility: clomiphene 50 mg/day for 5 days starting within about 5 days of the onset of menstruation.

An important 'side effect' is the increased risk of multiple pregnancy, i.e. twins or occasionally triplets. There is a 7% chance of twins and a 0.5% chance of triplets. Recently, there has been a suggestion that clomiphene may be associated with an increased risk of ovarian cancer. Although this association is far from proven, it has been advised that clomiphene should not normally be used for more than six treatment cycles.

Tamoxifen: 20 mg/day starting on the second day of the cycle for 5 days.

### Additional use of tamoxifen

Tamoxifen competes with oestrogen at binding sites on oestrogen-dependent breast tumours in pre-menopausal women. Remission occurs in about 40% of patients (see 'Cytotoxic drugs and cancer chemotherapy', Chapter 10). Dose: 10 mg twice daily. Tamoxifen can cause hot flushes and uterine bleeding secondary to endometrial hyperplasia.

## Metformin

Metformin is a biguanide. It exerts its effect mainly by decreasing gluconeogenesis and by increasing peripheral utilisation of glucose. Studies of metformin in obese insulin-resistant women with polycystic ovarian syndrome (PCOS) have shown significant improvements in insulin sensitivity and hyperinsulinaemia. Also, the ovulatory response to clomiphene can be increased in obese women with PCOS by decreasing insulin sensitivity with metformin. It should be noted that metformin is not licensed for this use in the United Kingdom.

## Testosterone

### Mechanism

Testosterone is the major male sex hormone and is responsible for secondary sexual characteristics.

### Pharmacokinetics

Testosterone has an extensive first-pass metabolism; it is given either transdermally or by intramuscular injection.

### Drug interactions

Oral anticoagulant requirements are decreased by testosterone.

### Clinical effects

Testosterone is used as replacement therapy in hypogonadal or castrated men. In the normal male, it inhibits pituitary gonadotrophin secretion and depresses spermatogenesis. Menopausal women are also sometimes given implants of testosterone as an adjunct to hormone replacement therapy.

### Anti-androgens

Cyproterone acetate is a progestogen with antagonist properties at the androgen receptor. It can be used in low dose (2 mg) as part of a COC (Dianette) in the treatment of hirsutism. Dianette is licensed to be used in the management of moderate to severe acne and hirsuitism which has failed to respond to medical treatment. It should not be used solely as a contraceptive. If used, it should be discontinued 3–4 months after symptoms have improved or resolved. Higher doses (50 mg/day) can also be administered where more effective anti-androgen actions are required.

### Drugs adversely affecting sexual function

Several drugs can adversely influence sexual function and the more frequently used are listed in

**Table 12.2** Drugs that can adversely influence sexual function.

| Drug | Comment |
| --- | --- |
| Methyldopa | Impotence, failure of ejaculation, loss of sexual drive |
| Clonidine | Impotence Difficulty in achieving orgasm (women) |
| Tricyclic antidepressants | Delayed ejaculation |
| Phenothiazines | Difficulties in erection and ejaculation |
| Phenelzine | Delayed ejaculation |
| Cimetidine | Impaired spermatogenesis (reversible) Impotence |
| Isoniazid | Menstrual disturbance |
| Diuretics | Impotence and reduced libido: mechanism unknown |
| Guanethidine | Impotence, retrograde ejaculation |
| Sulphasalazine (sulfasalazine) | Impaired spermatogenesis (reversible) |

Table 12.2. Remember that patients might not volunteer information about an adverse effect which they consider embarrassing, and which they might not relate to their drug treatment.

## Drug treatment of impotence

### Sildenafil

Objective and subjective measures show that sildenafil improves rigidity and the number of erections in men with erectile dysfunction. The final common pathway for sexual arousal and stimulation leading to erection is the production in cavernosal tissues of cyclic guanosine monophosphate (cGMP) which relaxes the smooth muscle and permits swelling of the corpora with blood. Sildenafil is a potent and specific inhibitor of cGMP-specific phosphodiesterase type 5, the isoenzyme responsible for the breakdown of cGMP in the corpus cavernosum.

The most common side effects are headache, flushing, dyspepsia, nasal congestion and transient disturbance of colour discrimination. A very important drug interaction is the potentially dangerous potentiation of the haemodynamic effect of nitrates, specifically hypotension. This contraindication is important as erectile dysfunction is commonly associated with cardiovascular disease but also because amyl nitrates ('poppers') are drugs of misuse, particularly in the homosexual community.

# Chapter 13

# Drugs and gastrointestinal disease

## Peptic ulcer

### Aims

1 To relieve pain
2 To heal the ulcer
3 To prevent ulcer diathesis.

### Relevant pathophysiology

It is traditional to regard peptic ulceration as the result of an imbalance between aggressive and protective factors in the upper gastrointestinal tract. The principal aggressive forces are gastric acid and pepsin. The two most important factors disrupting the balance between acid/peptic attack and mucosal resistance are *Helicobacter pylori* infection and non-steroidal anti-inflammatory drugs (NSAIDs). *H. pylori* stimulates increased gastrin release and thereby increased acid secretion. In addition, it causes direct damage to the mucosa, thus further disrupting the physiological balance. NSAIDs impair mucosal resistance but do not alter acid secretion.

Almost all patients with duodenal ulcer (DU), and most patients with gastric ulcer (GU), have *H. pylori* infection. It is now clear that eradication of *H. pylori* infection is associated with prolonged remission from peptic ulceration, and perhaps with permanent cure. Recognition of the role of *H. pylori* infection in peptic ulcer and development of effective eradication treatments for it have had enormous impact on our approach to the patient with peptic ulceration.

## Drugs used in the treatment of peptic ulcer

1 Antacids
2 Drugs that inhibit gastric acid secretion:
   • H$_2$-receptor antagonists
   • Proton pump inhibitors
   • Synthetic prostaglandin analogues
3 Drugs that do not directly inhibit gastric acid secretion:
   • Chelated salts of bismuth
   • Sucralfate
4 Drug combinations to eradicate *H. pylori*.

## Antacids

*Mechanism*
These drugs are weak alkalis, so they partly neutralise free acid in the stomach. They may also stimulate mucosal repair mechanisms around ulcers, possibly by stimulating local prostaglandin release.

*Pharmacokinetics*
Most antacids (principally salts of magnesium or aluminium) are not absorbed from the alimentary tract to any appreciable extent. Some, such as sodium bicarbonate, are absorbed.

*Adverse effects*

Antacids that contain aluminium tend to cause constipation. Those containing magnesium have the opposite effect. Sodium bicarbonate in large quantities may alter acid–base status causing metabolic alkalosis and may promote the formation of phosphate-containing renal calculi. Absorbable antacids should not be administered in the long term. Antacids with a high sodium content should be avoided in patients with impaired cardiac function or chronic liver disease.

*Drug interactions*

Antacids may reduce the absorption of a number of different drugs from the gut. These include digoxin, phenothiazines and tetracyclines.

*Clinical use and dosage*

Antacids are mainly used for symptomatic relief in patients with peptic ulcer, gastro-oesophageal reflux disease or non-ulcer dyspepsia 'indigestion'. They can accelerate the healing of peptic ulcers but must be given frequently and in high doses.

Suitable antacids are:

Aluminium hydroxide 5–15 ml 6-hourly

Magnesium trisilicate 10–20 ml or 1–2 tablets as required.

## Drugs that inhibit gastric acid secretion

### $H_2$-receptor antagonists

Currently, there are four such agents available (cimetidine, ranitidine, nizatidine and famotidine). They are all competitive antagonists for histamine at the $H_2$-receptor found mainly on parietal cells.

*Mechanism*

By competing with histamine at the $H_2$-receptor, these drugs reduce acid secretion by the parietal cells, especially at night and in the fasting state. They are less effective in reducing food-stimulated acid secretion.

*Pharmacokinetics*

They are well absorbed following oral administration. They have relatively short half-lives and are excreted largely unchanged by the kidneys.

*Adverse effects*

These are rare and are usually of a minor nature. Cimetidine is weakly anti-androgenic in humans. It may cause impotence or gynaecomastia. Either cimetidine or ranitidine may cause reversible mental confusion, particularly in sick elderly patients. Some potentially serious cardiac dysrhythmias have occurred following intravenous injections of $H_2$-receptor antagonists.

*Drug interactions*

Cimetidine inhibits oxidative drug metabolism by the liver. It interacts with many drugs but only three are of clinical importance. These are phenytoin, theophylline and warfarin. These three drugs are metabolised in the liver and have narrow therapeutic indices; cimetidine will slow their metabolism and may induce toxicity.

To date, no clinically relevant drug interactions have been reported with the other $H_2$-receptor antagonists.

*Clinical use and dosage*

$H_2$-receptor antagonists can heal DUs and benign GUs. Patients with GU should have endoscopy and biopsy to exclude gastric carcinoma. Healing of GU should also be documented endoscopically. The $H_2$-receptor antagonists can be effective in some patients with gastro-oesophageal reflux disease (GORD), especially in milder grades of severity. For patients with erosive or ulcerative oesophagitis complicating GORD, the $H_2$-receptor antagonists are unlikely to be effective unless higher doses are given (see below).

---

**$H_2$-receptor antagonist doses**

Recommended doses for DU and GU are:
Ranitidine 150 mg twice daily or 300 mg in the evening
Cimetidine 400 mg twice daily or 800 mg in the evening
Nizatidine 300 mg in the evening
Famotidine 40 mg in the evening

---

Seventy-five to eighty per cent of DUs will heal within 4 weeks, increasing to around 90% by 8 weeks. GUs tend to be slower to heal, but over 80% should have healed by 8 weeks. If single evening doses are used, it is important that patients are advised to have nothing further by mouth after the dose. Eating food will stimulate gastric acid secretion through gastrin release and vagal activity and can reduce the pharmacological effect of the $H_2$-receptor antagonist.

Higher doses are recommended for GORD. Single evening dosage regimens are not appropriate. In GORD, $H_2$-receptor antagonists should be given at least twice daily. For ranitidine, the dose may go up to 300 mg four times daily.

$H_2$-receptor antagonists are of no proven value in the management of patients with upper gastrointestinal haemorrhage, whether from peptic ulceration or other sources. They may be used prophylactically in some critically ill patients in an effort to prevent stress-related gastric mucosal bleeding. However, this should not be a major problem in countries where high standards of intensive care are available.

*Comment.* Although $H_2$-receptor antagonists can heal peptic ulcers, relapse is common after stopping treatment. These drugs can be continued as long-term maintenance treatment, typically in half of their initial dose. However, the role of such treatment has become markedly reduced since the importance of eradication of *H. pylori* has been appreciated (see below).

$H_2$-receptor antagonists are of no proven value in non-ulcer dyspepsia. Their use in patients with undiagnosed upper abdominal pain is not recommended. Some of the $H_2$-receptor antagonists are now available in low doses 'over the counter'. They are likely to be used in this way by patients with mild GORD for relief of heartburn.

## Proton pump inhibitors: omeprazole, lansoprazole, pantoprazole, rabeprazole and esomeprazole

*Mechanism*
These drugs are irreversible inhibitors of the proton pump on the parietal cell membrane. The proton pump is an enzyme ($H^+/K^+$-ATPase) that actively secretes hydrogen ions into the gastric lumen. It is therefore responsible for the final step in the process of acid secretion. Blocking this enzyme causes a marked, but temporary, suppression of gastric acid secretion to any stimulus, including food.

*Pharmacokinetics*
The drugs are administered as delayed release preparations. The bioavailability of omeprazole after the first dose is limited, but increases with repeated once-daily dosing to reach a plateau by around the fifth day. These drugs have short elimination half-lives (1–2 h) but a prolonged pharmacological effect and are converted in the liver to inactive metabolites.

*Adverse effects*
These are mild and infrequent. Diarrhoea, skin rash and headache have all been reported. No serious life-threatening adverse effects have been encountered.

*Drug interactions*
Omeprazole reduces the clearance and prolongs the elimination of diazepam, phenytoin and the *R* enantiomer of warfarin through inhibition of their hepatic metabolism. No clinically important drug interactions have been reported with the other proton pump inhibitors.

*Clinical use and dosage*
Used in the treatment of severe, erosive oesophagitis; in the short-term management of DUs and GUs; in treatment and prophylaxis of NSAID-induced ulcers; in combination with antibiotics in the eradication of *H. pylori*; and in the treatment of Zollinger–Ellison syndrome. Intravenous preparations are also used, in combination with endoscopic treatment, for the treatment of bleeding peptic ulcers.

For DU, omeprazole 20 mg daily or lansoprazole 30 mg daily will heal around 90% of ulcers within 4 weeks. In patients with GU, the same doses are used, but treatment for 8 weeks is recommended.

## Synthetic prostaglandins: misoprostol
*Mechanism*
Prostaglandins are weak inhibitors of gastric acid secretion when given in pharmacological doses. Their mechanism of action is not fully understood.

In addition, prostaglandins have a series of properties loosely referred to as 'cytoprotection'. This means that they have been shown in animal studies to prevent or limit experimental damage to the gastric or duodenal mucosa from a variety of noxious stimuli. It is unclear whether or not this is an important property regarding their clinical use. Cytoprotection can be demonstrated at doses below those required for inhibition of gastric acid secretion.

*Pharmacokinetics*
Misoprostol has a short plasma half-life. It may act on the stomach both locally and systemically.

*Adverse effects*
There is diarrhoea in up to 40% of patients, but this is usually mild and self-limiting. Misoprostol and other prostaglandins are potentially abortifacient and so should not be given to women of child-bearing age.

*Clinical use and dose*
The main indication is to prevent gastric mucosal damage and GUs in patients on NSAIDs. Dose is 200 µg twice to four times daily.

   *Comment.* Misoprostol should be considered for those patients who genuinely require to take NSAIDs and who have a past history of peptic ulcer or upper gastrointestinal bleeding.

   For patients already on NSAIDs who are found to have a peptic ulcer, the NSAID should be stopped if possible. However, even if the NSAID has to be continued (in a patient with rheumatoid arthritis, for example) the ulcer can be healed with any type of anti-ulcer drug. There is no specific indication for misoprostol in this situation.

## Drugs that do not directly inhibit gastric acid secretion

### Chelated salts of bismuth: tripotassium dicitrato bismuthate
*Mechanism*
The means whereby bismuth salts heal ulcers are not fully understood. They do not directly inhibit acid secretion. However, they do suppress *H.*

*pylori* infection and thus reduce the hypersecretion of acid induced by the infection. In addition, they may form an insoluble protective layer over the ulcer base, preventing further damage by acid and pepsin. They may also stimulate local prostaglandin production.

*Pharmacokinetics*
A small quantity of bismuth is absorbed following oral administration. Urinary excretion of bismuth continues for over 2 weeks after stopping a course of treatment.

*Adverse effects*
The liquid preparation should be avoided because of an unpleasant smell and taste and the fact that it discolours the tongue. The liquid or tablet preparation may colour the faeces black. The long-term consequences of bismuth absorption are unknown, so this drug is not recommended for continuous or repeated administration.

   *Comment.* In the management of patients with peptic ulcer, the main use of a bismuth-containing compound is as part of a drug combination against *H. pylori*. This compound, when combined with metronidazole and another antibiotic, such as tetracycline, can eradicate the infection in 80–90% of patients within 2 weeks. However, frequent doses are necessary and compliance may be a problem.

### Sucralfate (sucrose aluminium octasulphate)
*Mechanism*
The exact mechanism of ulcer healing by sucralfate is unknown. It may act by coating ulcer bases or by stimulating local prostaglandin release. It does not directly affect acid secretion. However, like the bismuth salts it suppresses *H. pylori* infection and thus reduces the acid hypersecretion stimulated by the infection. It probably suppresses *H. pylori* by interfering with the ability of the organism to bind to the mucosal epithelial cells.

*Clinical use and dosage*
Sucralfate is indicated for the treatment of DU and benign GU. The usual dose is 1 g four times daily or 2 g twice daily. Healing rates are comparable to

those obtained with $H_2$-receptor antagonists. Sucralfate should not be used in patients with chronic renal failure because of the risk of aluminium absorption and toxicity.

*Pharmacokinetics*
Sucralfate acts locally; only small amounts of aluminium are absorbed.

*Adverse effects*
Constipation.

*Drug interactions*
Sucralfate can reduce the absorption of a number of different drugs, including phenytoin and tetracyclines.

## Drug combinations to eradicate *H. pylori*

Almost all patients with DU, and many patients with GU, are infected with *H. pylori*. Successful eradication of this bacterium is associated with prolonged remission from ulcer recurrence, and possibly with permanent cure of the ulcer diathesis. Re-infection with *H. pylori* after eradication appears to be rare, at least in developed countries.

Eradication of *H. pylori* usually requires both acid suppression and antibiotic treatment. The most widely used regimen combines a proton pump inhibitor with clarithromycin and amoxicillin for 1 week. Metronidazole can replace amoxicillin in allergic patients.

## Gastro-oesophageal reflux disease

### Aims

1 To relieve symptoms
2 To heal lesions of oesophagitis
3 To prevent complications.

### Relevant pathophysiology

Most patients have a functionally incompetent lower oesophageal sphincter that relaxes inappropriately, at times other than during swallowing. This allows excessive reflux of gastric contents,

containing acid and pepsin, into the oesophagus. Once refluxed into the oesophagus, acidic material remains in contact with the mucosa for prolonged periods as a result of impairment of physiological clearance mechanisms. This will be further exacerbated by the presence of a hiatus hernia. Gastric acid secretion is usually normal. Some patients have delayed gastric emptying.

## Drugs used in the treatment of gastro-oesophageal reflux disease

### Antacids and antacid/alginate preparations

Antacids are discussed above. In combination with an alginate, they are thought to provide a protective coating to the lower oesophagus, preventing some contact with refluxed gastric contents.

---

**Gastro-oesophageal reflux disease**

1 Antacids and antacid/alginate combinations
2 Drugs that inhibit gastric acid secretion:
   • $H_2$ receptor antagonists
   • Proton pump inhibitors: omeprazole, lansoprazole, esomeprazole, pantoprazole, rabeprazole
3 Drugs that act on oesophageal and/or gastric motility:
   • Metoclopramide, domperidone
   • Cisapride

---

## Drugs that inhibit gastric acid secretion

### $H_2$-receptor antagonists

These are discussed above. They have generally been less successful in the management of GORD than in peptic ulcer. To be effective in the treatment of GORD, they may have to be given in much higher doses than in peptic ulcer (e.g. ranitidine, 300 mg 6-hourly).

### Proton pump inhibitors

These drugs are discussed above. They are highly effective in treating all grades of GORD. They are superior to $H_2$-receptor antagonists in controlling the symptoms of the condition and in healing oesophagitis.

*Comment.* Based on the pathophysiology of the condition, it should be apparent that relapse will be rapid in most patients once treatment is withdrawn. Many patients, particularly those with severe grades of the condition, will require long-term treatment with a proton pump inhibitor. Patients with mild GORD may obtain sufficient symptom relief from an $H_2$-receptor antagonist taken as required.

## Drugs that act on oesophageal and/or gastric motility

### Metoclopramide, domperidone

These drugs are discussed in greater detail later in this chapter. They may be effective in patients with mild grades of GORD because of some of their actions on motility of the upper alimentary tract. They have a weak tonic effect on the lower oesophageal sphincter; they may improve oesophageal clearance and may also improve gastric emptying. They are seldom effective alone. They may be combined with another agent, such as an $H_2$-receptor antagonist, but this may not be cost-effective. Metoclopramide is not recommended for long-term use because of its adverse effects on the central nervous system (CNS) (see below).

## Diarrhoea and constipation

### Diarrhoea

In all patients presenting with diarrhoea it is important to identify and eliminate a cause where possible. If the cause is unclear, symptomatic relief may be helpful. The drugs used will depend upon the cause of the diarrhoea and are discussed below under the conditions that cause diarrhoea.

### Irritable bowel syndrome

This common condition is the most frequent cause of chronic, recurrent abdominal pain. It may also cause upset of bowel habit, with diarrhoea, constipation or both. The pathophysiology is poorly understood. There are abnormal motility patterns in the bowel, and patients may be unduly sensitive to distension or contraction of visceral smooth muscle. Some patients' diets are deficient in fibre. There is a relationship between psychological stress and symptoms in some patients.

Mebeverine is an antispasmodic agent which does not have significant anticholinergic effects. It is useful in relieving symptoms in some patients in a dose of 135 mg three times daily.

Enteric-coated capsules of peppermint oil are useful in relieving gut spasm in some patients. The capsules may cause heartburn if bitten into.

## Pancreatic insufficiency

A preparation of exogenous pancreatic enzymes containing trypsin, lipase and amylase is given for patients with chronic pancreatic exocrine insufficiency, as in chronic pancreatitis or cystic fibrosis. $H_2$-receptor antagonists may be given also in order to prevent denaturation of the pancreatic enzymes by gastric acid.

## Drugs used in non-specific diarrhoea

### Codeine phosphate

This is a useful agent for symptomatic control of diarrhoea. It raises intracolonic pressure and sphincter tone. It should not be given to patients with colonic diverticular disease and should be used only cautiously in patients with inflammatory bowel disease, and only under careful supervision.

### Morphine

Kaolin and morphine mixture British Pharmaceutical Codex (BPC) is a time-honoured remedy containing only small quantities of morphine. It is unpalatable and so is taken as a liquid.

### Diphenoxylate

This is an opiate derivative. It is combined with atropine in the preparation Lomotil. It is more expensive than codeine phosphate and probably no better.

### Loperamide

Loperamide is a synthetic opiate with some anticholinergic activity. It may cause dizziness or dryness of the mouth. The usual dose is 2 mg three or four times daily.

## Constipation

### Drugs used in non-specific constipation

**Drugs that increase faecal bulk**

These consist of non-absorbable polysaccharides as in bran, ispaghula or sterculia. They are generally effective in simple constipation, particularly where the intake of dietary fibre is poor. They are the agents of choice where treatment is likely to be prolonged.

**Stimulant laxatives**

These agents stimulate intestinal motility, probably through an effect on the myenteric nerve plexus. Examples are senna and bisacodyl. Prolonged use leads to hypotonicity of the bowel and thereby eventually exacerbates chronic constipation.

**Stool softeners**

The best known agent in this group is liquid paraffin. It acts by lubricating the faeces, which aids passage along the bowel. It may cause slight perianal irritation. Long-term use can lead to malabsorption of fat-soluble vitamins. It is not indicated for infants as inhalation of the liquid may produce a lipoid pneumonia.

**Osmotic laxatives**

These agents retain water in the bowel. They increase faecal bulk and moisten faeces. Examples are lactulose and salts of magnesium.

*Comment.* The commonest cause of constipation is lack of dietary fibre and most cases will respond to a high-fibre diet. Both the constipation and diarrhoea associated with diverticular disease may improve with a high-fibre diet.

## Nausea and vomiting

### Aims

1 To establish an underlying cause and give specific treatment if possible
2 To give symptomatic treatment.

### Relevant pathophysiology

Vomiting is controlled by two separate brainstem centres: the vomiting centre and the chemoreceptor trigger zone. The trigger zone may be activated endogenously or exogenously by toxins or drugs such as opiates. Activation of the trigger zone stimulates the vomiting centre. The act of vomiting is controlled by the vomiting centre, mainly through vagal action. The vomiting centre has afferent input from the gut, higher cortical centres and the vestibular apparatus. Muscarinic receptors and histamine $H_1$-receptors are highly concentrated around the area of the vomiting centre.

### Drugs used in treatment of vomiting

### Anticholinergic drugs: hyoscine

*Mechanism*
They compete with acetylcholine at muscarinic receptors in the gut and CNS and have antispasmodic action in the gut wall. They may be successful in motion sickness because of their central action.

*Adverse effects*
Adverse effects are drowsiness plus typical anticholinergic effects of dry mouth, blurred vision and difficulty in micturition.

**Clinical use**

A 0.3–0.6 mg dose of hyoscine is usually adequate prophylaxis for motion sickness.

## Antihistamines: promethazine

*Mechanism*

Antihistamines are competitive antagonists of histamine at $H_1$-receptors, acting mainly on the vomiting centre rather than on the chemoreceptor trigger zone. They have weak anticholinergic effects.

*Adverse effects*

Adverse effects are drowsiness, occasional insomnia and euphoria. Central effects are accentuated by alcohol.

*Clinical use*

Antihistamines are used in motion sickness or in vestibular disorders. They are widely used in the treatment of allergic rhinitis and other allergic reactions (see 'Immunopharmacology', Chapter 10).

Promethazine is given at a dose of 25 mg 8-hourly.

## Dopamine antagonists

### Phenothiazines: chlorpromazine, prochlorperazine

*Mechanism*

The general clinical pharmacology of phenothiazines is described in Chapter 16. These drugs act mainly on the chemoreceptor trigger zone. They have dopamine receptor antagonist properties as well as anticholinergic and other actions.

*Adverse effects*

Prolonged use may produce Parkinsonian-type tremor or other dyskinesias.

*Clinical use and dose*

Phenothiazines are effective in a variety of situations, including the vomiting of chronic renal failure and neoplastic disease, and drug-induced vomiting.

Recommended doses are:
Chlorpromazine 25–50 mg 8-hourly
Prochlorperazine 5–25 mg orally or 12.5 mg i.m. (tablets and suppositories, for buccal

and rectal administration respectively, are also available).

### Metoclopramide

*Mechanism*

Metoclopramide is a central dopamine receptor antagonist, effective at blocking stimuli to chemoreceptor trigger zone. It also has effects on upper gastrointestinal tract motility, as described above.

### Adverse effects

Metoclopramide may cause acute extrapyramidal reactions, such as opisthotonous, oculogyric crisis or other dystonias. These can be treated with an intravenous anticholinergic agent, such as benzotropine.

Metoclopramide raises serum prolactin levels and may cause gynaecomastia by virtue of its antidopaminergic effects.

*Drug interactions*

Metoclopramide potentiates the extrapyramidal side effects of phenothiazines.

### Clinical use and dose

Metoclopramide is effective in most causes of vomiting, apart from motion sickness. The usual dose is 10 mg 8-hourly, orally or parenterally.

### Domperidone

*Mechanism*

Domperidone is a dopamine antagonist, effective at the chemoreceptor trigger zone.

*Adverse effects*

Domperidone is less likely to cause extrapyramidal reactions than metoclopramide. It raises prolactin levels and may produce cardiac dysrhythmias following rapid intravenous injection.

*Clinical use and dose*

Domperidone is effective in most situations, especially nausea and vomiting related to cytotoxic drug therapy. The usual oral dose is 10–20 mg 4- to 8-hourly. It can also be administered rectally via suppository.

## Cannabinoids: nabilone

*Mechanism*

Tetrahydrocannabinol is one of the active constituents of marijuana. Nabilone is a synthetic cannabinoid used in the treatment of nausea and vomiting during cytotoxic therapy. Mode of action is unclear.

*Adverse effects*

Nabilone causes drowsiness, dizziness and dryness of the mouth. Euphoria and hallucinations are rare.

*Clinical use and dose*

Nabilone at a dose of 1–2 mg twice daily is of value in treating patients receiving cytotoxic agents. Prolonged use may produce toxic effects on CNS.

## Serotonin antagonists: ondansetron

*Mechanism*

Ondansetron is a selective antagonist of serotonin at 5-HT$_3$-receptors. Its exact mode of action in controlling nausea and vomiting is unclear but it has both CNS and peripheral actions.

*Adverse effects*

Ondansetron causes constipation and headache; flushing may occur.

*Clinical use and dose*

Ondansetron is indicated for the treatment of nausea and vomiting associated with cytotoxic therapy or radiotherapy. The dose and rate of administration depends on the severity of the problem and on the chemotherapy used.

## Inflammatory bowel disease

### Aims

1 To obtain remission in periods of relapse
2 To prolong periods of remission.

### Relevant pathophysiology

Ulcerative colitis and Crohn's disease are chronic inflammatory conditions of unknown aetiology but there is increasing appreciation of the importance of alterations in the mucosal immune response to resident luminal bacteria. Both are characterised by episodes of remission and relapse. Drug treatment is aimed at controlling inflammation and bringing about remission. Treatment of these conditions is not only pharmacological but also depends on psychological support, correction of nutritional deficiencies and possibly surgery.

## Drugs used in the treatment of inflammatory bowel disease

### Corticosteroids

These agents are discussed in detail in Chapter 11.

Steroids are of proven value in the treatment of acute relapses of ulcerative colitis and Crohn's disease. They may be given rectally, orally or intravenously depending on the extent and severity of the condition.

Budesonide is a synthetic corticosteroid with less systemic side effects as it undergoes extensive first-pass metabolism in the liver. An oral controlled release formulation of budesonide is used for the treatment of terminal Crohn's disease.

Steroids are of no value for ulcerative colitis in remission and should be withdrawn once clinical remission is achieved. There is no good evidence that long-term steroids help Crohn's disease.

### Aminosalicylates

Preparations are designed to deliver the drug to the distal gastrointestinal tract: Mesalazine (a controlled release preparation of 5-aminosalicylic acid (5-ASA)), olsalazine (two molecules of 5-ASA linked by an azo bond that is split by colonic bacteria to release 5-ASA within the colon) and balsalazide (a prodrug of 5-ASA). Sulphasalazine consists of 5-ASA linked to sulphapyridine by an azo bond that is split in the colon by bacterial azo-reductases.

*Mechanism*

It is thought that 5-ASA exerts a local anti-inflammatory effect.

*Adverse effects*
Blood dyscrasias, renal damage and (with olsalazine) watery diarrhoea.

*Clinical use*
These drugs are used in the management of mild–moderate ulcerative colitis and in the maintenance of remission.

## Azathioprine

*Mechanism*
This is an immunosuppressive agent which may be useful in improving control in patients with severe inflammatory bowel disease proving difficult to control on steroids and aminosalicylates.

*Side effects*
It may cause bone marrow suppression. It also reduces the immune response particularly to viral infection.

*Clinical use*
Patients on azathioprine should be told to report to their doctor immediately if they develop symptoms such as sore throat or a bleeding tendency. In addition, their blood count must be checked regularly.

## Other immunosuppressants

The use of these drugs is restricted to physicians with expertise in their use.

*Ciclosporin* is used in patients with severe ulcerative colitis that has not responded to parenteral corticosteroids (see also Chapter 5 (side effects)).

*Methotrexate* may induce remission in patients with Crohn's disease that have either not been able to tolerate or are unresponsive to azathioprine (see also Chapter 5 (side effects)).

*Infliximab* is a monoclonal antibody against tumour necrosis factor-$\alpha$. It has recently become available and is used for the treatment of severely active Crohn's disease that has not responded to corticosteroids, azathioprine or methotrexate (see also Chapter 5 (side effects)).

## Drugs adversely affecting gastrointestinal function

Virtually any drug may cause nausea, vomiting or diarrhoea and a detailed drug history is essential in patients with such complaints. Some specific drug-induced gastrointestinal problems are listed in Table 13.1.

**Table 13.1** Drugs that may adversely affect gastrointestinal function.

| Drug | Comment |
|---|---|
| Antacids containing aluminium sucralfate | Constipation |
| Antacids containing magnesium | Diarrhoea |
| Oral iron salts | Nausea; constipation or diarrhoea (only nausea is dose-related); darkens stools as does bismuth |
| Bisphosphonates | Severe oesophagitis, oesophageal ulcers and erosions |
| Antibiotics | Oral *and/or* oesophageal candidiasis; diarrhoea |
| Aspirin/NSAIDs* | Dyspepsia; gastric erosions (with or without significant bleeding); GUs; increased risk of perforation or bleeding of existing gastric or DU; NSAIDs may cause ulceration, stricture or perforation of small intestine; NSAIDs may promote relapse of inflammatory bowel disease |
| Oral potassium supplements | Ulceration or perforation at sites of stasis (e.g. oesophageal or intestinal stricture) |

* NSAIDs, non-steroidal anti-inflammatory drugs.

Diarrhoea is common in patients receiving antibiotics. This is usually attributed to an alteration in the intracolonic bacterial flora. In some patients a colitis may result from antibiotic therapy: antibiotic-associated colitis or pseudomembranous colitis. This is a result of the proliferation of *Clostridium difficile* in the bowel and the secretion of an endotoxin. Treatment of this condition depends on the prescription of an antibiotic, which is poorly absorbed when given orally. Two suitable agents are vancomycin and metronidazole.

# Chapter 14

# Drugs and the blood including anticoagulants and thrombolytic drugs

## Haemostasis

Vascular injury results firstly in vasoconstriction and formation of a platelet plug at the site of injury (primary haemostasis). The platelet plug is then stabilised by the formation of a fibrin meshwork, resulting from activation of the coagulation cascade. Eventually fibrin is cleared through digestion by fibrinolytic enzymes.

## Primary haemostasis

When endothelial integrity is breached, platelets adhere to exposed subendothelial collagen. The adherent platelets become activated resulting in:

1 Exposure of fibrinogen receptors, allowing fibrinogen to bind and cross-link adjacent platelets. This process is known as platelet aggregation. The platelet fibrinogen receptor consists of a complex of glycoproteins IIb and IIIa on the platelet membrane.

2 Release of contents of secretory granules including substances such as adenosine diphosphate (ADP) which promote further platelet activation.

3 Synthesis of thromboxane $A_2$ which also acts to promote further platelet activation and vasoconstriction.

## Activation of the coagulation cascade

As shown in Fig. 14.1, the coagulation cascade consists of a series of steps in which precursor proteins in plasma are converted to active enzymes in a sequential series of reactions. For convenience the coagulation cascade can be divided into three parts.

1 The *common* pathway consists of those reactions subsequent to the generation of factor $X_a$, culminating in the cleavage of fibrinogen by thrombin, with subsequent polymerisation of fibrin monomers into fibrin strands. Factor $X_a$ may be generated either by the extrinsic pathway or by the intrinsic pathway.

2 In the *extrinsic* pathway, tissue factor is expressed by cells or released following tissue injury. Binding of tissue factor to factor VII greatly accelerates the activation of factor VII and also the action of factor $VII_a$ in the activation of factor X.

3 The *intrinsic* pathway is initiated by the activation of factor XII by contact of blood with a 'foreign' surface. *In vivo*, this is usually the subendothelial tissues. A sequence of reactions as illustrated in Fig. 14.1 then result in the activation of factor X. Most coagulation factors are synthesised in the liver, and the synthesis of the procoagulant forms of factors II, VII, IX and X is dependent on the availability of vitamin K.

## Fibrinolysis

The fibrinolytic system, like the coagulation cascade, also consists of a series of enzymatic steps (see Fig. 14.2), this time resulting in the breakdown

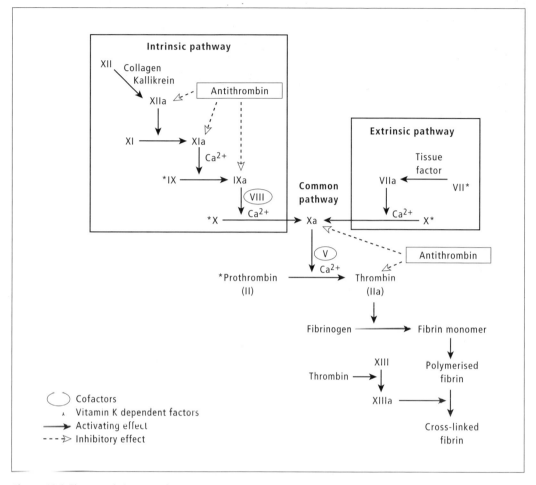

**Figure 14.1** The coagulation cascade.

of polymerised fibrin by plasmin into small degradation products (FDP). Plasmin is generated from the plasma protein plasminogen by the action of tissue plasminogen activator (tPA), which is most efficient in activation of plasminogen, when it is bound to fibrin. Furthermore, such localisation of fibrinolytic reactions protects plasmin from potent inhibitors present in plasma.

## Pathophysiology

Thrombosis is 'haemostasis in the wrong place'. When haemostasis proceeds unchecked within a large vessel, thrombosis occurs and vascular occlusion may result. Thrombi may also break up into small pieces and lodge at distant points within the circulatory system (embolism). The process of thrombosis in a blood vessel is promoted by one or more of three underlying pathological events: (i) abnormalities of the vessel wall; (ii) abnormalities of flow within a vessel; or (iii) abnormalities of blood constituents.

Thrombosis in arteries usually results from rupture of an atheromatous plaque, and arterial thrombi consist initially of platelets and subsequently of fibrin. Venous thrombosis often occurs in the context of stasis of blood flow, for example during periods of immobility or during pregnancy when pressure from the gravid uterus may impede venous return, and thrombi in veins are rich in

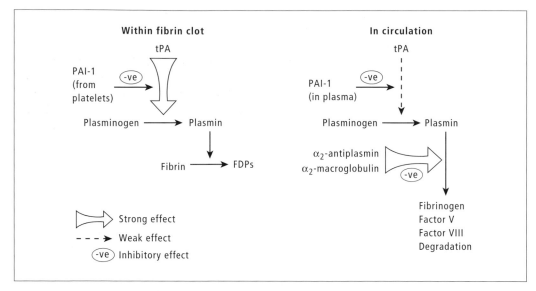

**Figure 14.2** The fibrinolytic system. Exogenous thrombolytic agents are plasminogen activators. FDPs, fibrin degradation products.

fibrin enmeshing all the cellular constituents of blood.

## Anticoagulant drugs

### Heparin

Anticoagulation can be achieved rapidly with heparin, and it is therefore the anticoagulant of choice in many acute thrombotic states such as treatment of deep vein thrombosis (DVT) or pulmonary embolism, and in severe unstable angina in which it has an additive effect to aspirin.

### Chemistry and pharmacology

Unfractionated heparin is a mixture of naturally occurring glycosaminoglycans with polysaccharide chains of varying length, and molecular weights ranging from 5000 to 30,000. Low molecular weight heparins are manufactured from unfractionated heparin to produce material with an average molecular weight of 4000–6500.

All heparins exert their anticoagulant activity by binding to and greatly accelerating the action of antithrombin as an inhibitor of thrombin (factor $II_a$), factor $X_a$ and other serine protease coagulation factors. Binding to antithrombin requires the presence of a specific pentasaccharide sequence on the heparin polysaccharide chain. A further requirement for heparin to enhance the anti-$II_a$ activity of antithrombin is the presence of a minimum chain length of 18 saccharides. As the proportion of chains of this length in low molecular weight heparins is less than in unfractionated heparin, it follows that low molecular weight heparins have a higher ratio of anti-$X_a$ to anti-$II_a$ activity. All heparins must be administered parenterally, either by the intravenous or by the subcutaneous route. For treatment of thrombosis, unfractionated heparin has traditionally been given by continuous intravenous infusion. The half-life of standard heparin following intravenous administration is 45–60 min, but heparins have complex kinetics, depending on dose, molecular weight and route of administration. Unfractionated heparin can also be given twice daily subcutaneously for treatment of DVT. Low molecular weight heparins demonstrate less binding to cells and to heparin-neutralising proteins than unfractionated heparin. This leads to improved bioavailability and to a longer half-life. These properties allow a more predictable anticoagulant response and once-daily subcutaneous administration, and there is no need to monitor therapeutic doses with coagulation time assays.

## Clinical use of unfractionated heparin

Heparin is used in the initial treatment of DVT and pulmonary embolism. In this situation, standard practice has been to administer 5000 IU unfractionated heparin intravenously as a loading dose, followed by a continuous infusion of 30,000–40,000 IU over 24 h, and to monitor the anticoagulant effect. Heparin is also used in unstable angina and in myocardial infarction to prevent coronary reocclusion following thrombolysis, and in the treatment and prevention of mural thrombus. It has a place as an adjunctive treatment to surgery or thrombolysis in the management of acute peripheral arterial occlusion. It is also used to prevent clotting in extracorporeal circulations such as renal dialysis circuits and cardiopulmonary bypass, and at low doses to flush indwelling vascular catheters.

Perioperative subcutaneous administration of low-dose heparin (usually 5000 IU b.d. unfractionated heparin) is effective in reducing the incidence of venous thrombosis and pulmonary embolism following general or orthopaedic surgery, and is also used for this purpose in acutely ill, immobile medical patients.

## Clinical use of low molecular weight heparin

Low molecular weight heparins have been evaluated extensively in the prevention of venous thrombosis in patients at risk, including those undergoing general or orthopaedic surgery and high-risk medical patients. They have been shown to be of similar efficacy to unfractionated heparin in all of these situations, and the convenience of once-daily administration makes their use attractive. They also cause less bleeding in medical patients. In orthopaedic surgery, particularly hip fractures, there is evidence that use of mechanical methods and aspirin is sufficient prophylaxis, and that heparins are not required.

Low molecular weight heparins administered once or twice daily subcutaneously with dose adjusted for body weight are as effective as unfractionated heparin administered intravenously in the treatment of DVT and pulmonary embolism. Once-daily administration allows outpatient treatment of DVT and minor pulmonary embolism in many patients, with savings on hospitalisation costs.

## Monitoring of heparin

Administration of therapeutic doses of unfractionated heparin must be monitored in the laboratory. A prolongation of the activated partial thromboplastin time (APTT) and the thrombin time is observed. The APTT, which tests the intrinsic and common pathways of coagulation, is the test usually chosen for therapeutic heparin monitoring. For the treatment of thrombosis, one should aim for an APTT 1.5–2.5 times the mid-point of the normal range, and it is important to achieve this in the first 24 h of treatment. An alternative is to measure plasma heparin levels that are based upon plasma anti-$X_a$ activity. It is not usually necessary to monitor heparin given in low doses for prophylaxis, and such regimens do not lead to prolongation of the APTT.

The APTT is insensitive to the effects of low molecular weight heparins. These may be measured by anti-$X_a$ assays (e.g. in renal failure) but monitoring is usually unnecessary because of the predictability of responses.

## Adverse effects

### Bleeding

Bleeding is a hazard, especially with full-dose heparin treatment. Bleeding complications are not entirely predictable by the APTT, and patient-related factors are also important. Hopes that low molecular weight heparins would have a substantially better safety profile compared with unfractionated heparin with respect to bleeding have not been confirmed for treatment, or for prophylaxis in surgical patients.

### Heparin induced thrombocytopenia

Significant thrombocytopenia occurs in approximately 3% of patients given full-dose unfractionated heparin. Mild early transient thrombocytopenia may be more common and is of no clinical significance. Thrombocytopenia occurring 4–14 days following heparin exposure is of greater significance, as potentially life-threatening thrombosis occurs in a small proportion of such patients. The thrombocytopenia is induced by a heparin-dependent antibody that causes platelet aggregation. Heparin-induced thrombocytopenia can occur with any dose or preparation of heparin, and although it appears to be much less common with low molecular weight heparin, antibody cross-reactivity has been documented. It is mandatory to monitor platelet counts during heparin therapy and prophylaxis from day 5 onwards: a baseline platelet count is useful. If heparin-induced thrombocytopenia is suspected, heparin should be withdrawn immediately and expert haematological advice sought.

### Osteoporosis

Reduction in bone density and bone fractures have been described following prolonged administration (usually greater than 20 weeks) and therefore have generally occurred in pregnant women. The mechanism is poorly understood. There appears to be a relationship with dose and duration of treatment, but individual susceptibility is also likely to be important. Monitoring of bone density may be considered in high-risk patients.

### Hypersensitivity

Local reactions at injection sites have been reported and, much more rarely, anaphylactoid reactions.

## Reversal of anticoagulation with heparin

Because of the short half-life of heparin, in the absence of clinical bleeding, it is reasonable simply to withhold therapy temporarily if over-anticoagulation has occurred. In the presence of haemorrhage, protamine should be administered intravenously. Protamine 1 mg neutralises the effects of 100 IU of unfractionated heparin. Protamine should never be given in doses of greater than 50 mg and should always be administered slowly to avoid hypotension and bradycardia.

## Contraindications to heparin

Active bleeding is an obvious contraindication. Others, including relative contraindications, are given below.

---

**Contraindications to heparin**

1 Uncorrected major bleeding
2 Uncorrected major bleeding disorder, e.g. thrombocytopenia, haemophilias
3 Active peptic ulcer, oesophageal varices, aneurysm, proliferative retinopathy or organ biopsy
4 Recent surgery, particularly neurosurgery or ophthalmic surgery
5 Severe renal or hepatic impairment (not including use for renal dialysis)
6 Recent stroke, intracranial or intraspinal bleed
7 Severe hypertension
8 Previous heparin-induced thrombocytopenia or thrombosis
9 Documented hypersensitivity

---

### Heparinoids and hirudins

These do not cross-react with heparin-dependent antibodies; hence, they can be used in heparin-induced thrombocytopenia. Danaparoid is a heparinoid; desirudin and lepirudin are recombinant hirudins, developed from hirudin, the natural anticoagulant of the medicinal leech.

### Fondaparinux

This is a pentasaccharide which selectively inhibits factor $X_a$. It is effective in prevention and treatment of DVT, but is more expensive than heparins.

## Warfarin

In practice, warfarin, a derivative of 4-hydroxycoumarin, is by far the most extensively used oral anticoagulant and is the drug of choice. Acenocoumarol (nicoumalone) and phenindione are also available but are rarely used. All of these drugs act as vitamin K antagonists. The remainder of this section on oral anticoagulants will refer only to warfarin, but similar principles apply to use of the other agents.

## Pharmacology

The coagulation factors II, VII, IX and X require gamma carboxylation on glutamic acid residues in order to bind calcium during coagulation reactions. Vitamin K is required for this carboxylation reaction, which is essential for procoagulant activity. Whilst acting as a cofactor, vitamin K is converted to vitamin K epoxide. The epoxide is then recycled via reductase reactions to active forms of vitamin K. Warfarin inhibits the reductase enzymes involved in the recycling of vitamin K, thus leading to a deficiency of procoagulant forms of factors II, VII, IX and X. Because some of these factors have prolonged half-lives, anticoagulation is not achieved for several days after initiating warfarin therapy, and loading doses are usually given in acute thrombosis. In acute situations, it is necessary to overlap heparin and warfarin therapy.

Warfarin is rapidly absorbed from the gut and is extensively bound to plasma albumin. Elimination of warfarin is by oxidative metabolism in the liver, with a half-life of 15–50 h.

## Monitoring of warfarin therapy

Warfarin therapy is monitored by the prothrombin time, which assesses the extrinsic and common pathways of coagulation. Standardisation is achieved by calibrating laboratory reagents used for measuring the prothrombin time against an international standard, and assigning an international sensitivity index (ISI) to each reagent. This allows the prothrombin time for the patient on treatment to be converted to an international normalised ratio (INR). The INR is the ratio of the patient's prothrombin time over the mean value in a normal reference population determined using the same batch of reagent and corrected for the ISI of the reagent. The development of the INR system of monitoring oral anticoagulation has allowed comparability of results between laboratories.
Clinical use of oral anticoagulants

---

**Clinical use of oral anticoagulants**

- Venous thromboembolism—prophylaxis and treatment
- Atrial fibrillation (high-risk patients)
- Valvular heart disease and prosthetic valve replacements, cardiomyopathy
- Mural thrombus

---

Warfarin is also used long-term if there is considered to be a significant risk of recurrent venous thrombosis. Table 14.1 shows recommended target INR ranges for some common indications for warfarin.

## Pregnancy

Warfarin crosses the placenta and is contraindicated in the first trimester of pregnancy because

**Table 14.1** Target INR ranges for oral anticoagulation.

| INR | Clinical condition |
| --- | --- |
| 2.0–2.5 | Prophylaxis of DVT and pulmonary embolism in high-risk patients (e.g. previous DVT, pulmonary embolism or thrombophilias) (for hip surgery 2.0–3.0) |
| 2.0–3.0 | Treatment of DVT and pulmonary embolism |
| | Prevention of systemic embolism in atrial fibrillation, mitral valve disease and other cardiac sources of embolism in the presence of previous systemic embolism |
| | Bioprosthetic heart valves with embolic risk factors |
| | Prevention of cardiac thromboembolism in high-risk patients following myocardial infarction |
| 3.0–4.5 | Mechanical prosthetic cardiac valves |
| | Recurrent thrombosis in patients with antiphospholipid syndrome |

of teratogenicity, and in the last few weeks of pregnancy because of fetal bleeding at delivery. Placental passage of warfarin leads to fetal anticoagulation at any stage in pregnancy, and so warfarin is not generally recommended in the management and prevention of venous thromboembolism during pregnancy. Because of the high risk and potentially catastrophic consequences of embolisation from artificial valves, warfarin is still the anticoagulant of choice from 12 to 36 weeks of pregnancy in patients with mechanical prosthetic valves.

## How to initiate anticoagulation with warfarin

Because of the kinetic considerations described above, anticoagulation with warfarin is not achieved for several days after initiating therapy, and in acute thrombosis loading doses are given at the start of treatment. A baseline coagulation screen should be checked prior to initiating treatment. Common practice for loading would be to administer 5–10 mg warfarin on two consecutive days and to check the INR on the third day. Lower doses are used in congestive cardiac failure, in the presence of abnormalities of liver function or a prolongation of baseline prothrombin time, and in the elderly. It is also necessary to avoid loading doses in patients known to be suffering from familial protein C or protein S deficiency (see below).

Maintenance doses usually lie between 3 and 9 mg warfarin. Daily or alternate-day monitoring of the INR should be carried out until stable values are achieved within the target range. In many instances, patients being induced with warfarin will also be receiving heparin for treatment or prevention of thrombosis. It is important to continue heparin until a therapeutic INR is achieved with warfarin.

Once stabilised, all patients, before discharge from hospital, should be enrolled in their local anticoagulant service and should receive education (e.g. by a pharmacist), using a national anticoagulant book where warfarin dosage and INR results are documented. The book should also contain important information for the patient (or carers) regarding therapy, including side effects and information about drug interactions. The following information should always be supplied to the supervising anticoagulant clinic: full personal patient details, indication for anticoagulation, proposed duration of treatment, desired target INR, and full details of all of the patient's medication. The patient should be advised to show the book to all doctors whom they attend, as well as the dentist.

## Drug interactions

Drug interactions are the most common reason for loss of anticoagulant control, bleeding and thrombosis in patients previously stabilised on warfarin. Great care should be taken in prescribing any additional medication to patients on oral anticoagulants. Drugs may potentiate the effects of warfarin by inhibiting liver enzymes involved in warfarin metabolism, by competing for protein binding, by reducing vitamin K availability or by affecting other aspects of haemostasis. Note that alcohol dose-dependently potentiates the effects of warfarin, and patients on oral anticoagulants should keep their alcohol consumption stable and less than 2 units/day. Drugs usually antagonise the effects of warfarin by inducing liver enzymes but in one case (colestyramine) the underlying mechanism is interference with warfarin absorption. Common drug interactions are illustrated in Table 14.2, but this list is by no means exhaustive: consult the *British National Formulary* before any change of drugs!

## Adverse effects

*Bleeding* is the most common adverse event encountered in patients on oral anticoagulants. Bleeding is usually related to prolongation of the INR above the therapeutic range, and underlying causes should be sought if bleeding occurs at

**Table 14.2** Important drug interactions with warfarin.

| Potentiation | Antagonism |
| --- | --- |
| *Analgesics* | |
| NSAIDs—azapropazone, phenylbutazone | |
| Aspirin | |
| Co-proxamol | |
| Ketorolac (postoperative) | |
| *Antibiotics* | |
| Co-trimoxazole | Rifampicin |
| Metronidazole | Griseofulvin |
| Ampicillin | |
| Cephalosporins | |
| Erythromycin | |
| Aminoglycosides | |
| Tetracycline | |
| Miconazole | |
| *Cardiovascular drugs* | |
| Amiodarone | Spironolactone |
| Fibrates | Colestyramine (cholestyramine) |
| *Endocrine agents* | |
| *Corticosteroids* | |
| Thyroxine | |
| Tamoxifen | |
| Anabolic steroids | |
| Glucagon | |
| *Gastrointestinal drugs* | |
| Cimetidine | |
| Omeprazole | |
| *Others* | |
| Allopurinol | Vitamin K |
| Alcohol | Phenytoin |
| Chlorpromazine | Carbamazepine |
| *Tricyclic antidepressants* | Barbiturates |
| | Antihistamines |

coagulation inhibitors by warfarin, which occurs quickly compared with the suppression of the procoagulant factors. Adequate heparinisation and the avoidance of loading doses of warfarin should help to prevent this complication in patients at risk. Such patients should be managed by haematologists.

## Treatment of haemorrhage and reversal of oral anticoagulation

For elective situations such as surgery including tooth extractions, warfarin should be stopped at least 48 h in advance of the procedure and the INR monitored, with the option of substituting heparin if there is high risk of thrombosis (e.g. mechanical heart valves).

When haemorrhage occurs in patients on oral anticoagulants, there are well-defined guidelines for management. These are shown in Table 14.3. The advice of a haematologist should always be sought. Several general points are important regarding the use of vitamin K. Note that vitamin K takes 6 h to have any effect, and in an emergency fresh frozen plasma or coagulation factor concentrates must be administered to provide an immediate source of vitamin K dependent factors. Small doses of vitamin K (0.5–2 mg) are sufficient for reversal of warfarin effects in all but the most extreme cases. Furthermore, caution should be exerted in the administration of vitamin K to patients with prosthetic cardiac valves. The administration of large doses of vitamin K, e.g. 10 mg, makes further use of oral anticoagulants impossible for several weeks.

therapeutic levels (e.g. endoscopy for gastrointestinal bleeding or haematuria).

Other adverse effects are rare and include alopecia and skin rashes. There was a high incidence of hypersensitivity reactions with phenindione, and so it is now rarely used.

Patients with protein C or protein S deficiency are susceptible to skin necrosis during induction phases of oral anticoagulation. This is a result of the suppression of these vitamin K dependent

## Contraindications to oral anticoagulants

These are similar to the previously listed contraindications to heparin, except for the following:
1 Lack of patient co-operation for any reason (e.g. mental impairment, alcoholism) or continued intravenous drug use constitutes a contraindication to oral anticoagulants.
2 Oral anticoagulants are teratogenic and are contraindicated in the first trimester of pregnancy except in certain rare circumstances.

**Table 14.3** Reversal of oral anticoagulation.

| Condition | Action |
| --- | --- |
| *Major bleeding* | Stop warfarin; give phytomenadione (vitamin $K_1$) 5 mg by slow intravenous injection; give prothrombin complex concentrate (factors II, VII, IX and X) 30–50 units/kg or (if no concentrate available) fresh frozen plasma 15 ml/kg |
| *INR > 8.0, no bleeding or minor bleeding* | Stop warfarin, restart when INR < 5.0; if there are other risk factors for bleeding give phytomenadione (vitamin $K_1$) 500 μg by slow intravenous injection or 5 mg by mouth (for partial reversal of anticoagulation give smaller oral doses of phytomenadione e.g. 0.5–2.5 mg using the intravenous preparation orally); repeat dose of phytomenadione if INR still too high after 24 h |
| *INR 6.0–8.0, no bleeding or minor bleeding* | Stop warfarin, restart when INR < 5.0 |
| *INR < 6.0 but more than 0.5 units above target value* | Reduce dose or stop warfarin, restart when INR < 5.0 |
| *Unexpected bleeding at therapeutic levels* | Always investigate possibility of underlying cause, e.g. unsuspected renal or gastrointestinal tract pathology |

**3** Heparin-induced thrombocytopenia is *not* a contraindication to oral anticoagulants, which may be used as antithrombotic agents when the platelet count increases.

## Thrombolytic agents

### Clinical use of thrombolytic agents

Thrombolytic agents have gained an established role in the treatment of acute myocardial infarction with ST segment elevation (STEMI) or left bundle branch block. Their early administration leads to angiographically demonstrable coronary artery patency, limitation of infarct size, improved left ventricular function and, most importantly, reduced mortality (for streptokinase and alteplase).

Thrombolysis is also used in selected cases of acute peripheral arterial occlusion (usually by local arterial infusion) and in massive ileofemoral vein thrombosis or massive pulmonary embolism. The role of thrombolysis in peripheral arterial or venous thromboembolism is less widely accepted.

The role of thrombolysis with alteplase (less than 3 h after onset of symptoms) in acute ischaemic stroke has recently been established, under strictly controlled circumstances in acute stroke units. In particular, haemorrhage or established infarction must be excluded by brain imaging with computerised tomography (CT) or magnetic resonance (MR). Whether or not delayed thrombolysis is beneficial is currently being studied in large randomised trials.

### General aspects of thrombolysis

All thrombolytic agents act by activating plasminogen to plasmin, leading to degradation of fibrin, not only in thrombi but also in haemostatic fibrin plugs, which frequently causes major bleeding (there is a 1% risk of intracranial bleeding which is often fatal or disabling).

## Streptokinase

This is a protein produced by group A $\beta$-haemolytic streptococci. Streptokinase requires a complex to be formed with plasminogen before it can cleave other plasminogen molecules to form plasmin. As it is a foreign protein, streptokinase may cause allergic reactions. Many patients already have antibodies to streptokinase because of previous streptococcal infection, but streptokinase administration also frequently leads to antibody formation. Use of an alternative agent such as tPA is recommended if a patient who has previously received streptokinase requires thrombolysis (such patients should carry a card indicating this).

## Alteplase (tPA)

Recombinant tPA (alteplase) is developed from an endogenous fibrinolytic enzyme, release of which initiates physiological fibrinolysis. It lyses thrombi more rapidly, but carries a higher risk of intracranial haemorrhage than streptokinase and is more expensive; hence, its main indication in STEMI is previous streptokinase therapy. It is the thrombolytic agent of choice in selected cases of acute ischaemic stroke (less than 3 h from onset) in acute stroke units.

## Other thrombolytic agents

Reteplase and tenectaplase are also licensed for treatment of acute myocardial infarction. They are given by intravenous injection (tenecteplase by a bolus injection).

## Anaemia and haematinics

### Aims

1 To relieve symptoms
2 To correct the underlying disorder
3 To replace any deficiencies: iron, vitamin $B_{12}$, folic acid.

## Relevant pathophysiology

The cellular constituents of the blood—the red cells, white cells and platelets—exist as a result of the balance between production and destruction. Anaemia occurs when the concentration of haemoglobin in the blood falls below normal for the age and sex of the patient. The lower limits of normal are:

1 For adult males: 13.0 g/dl
2 For adult females: 11.5 g/dl.

The balance between production and destruction may be disturbed by:

1 Blood loss
2 Impaired red cell formation: haematinic deficiency or bone marrow depression
3 Increased red cell destruction: haemolysis.

Iron, vitamin $B_{12}$ and folic acid are essential for normal marrow function. Deficiency of any or all of these results in defective red cell synthesis and eventual anaemia. As each of the agents plays a different part in cellular production in the marrow, individual deficiencies are manifested in different ways. Accurate diagnosis is therefore essential before any specific agent is given. Lack of iron causes a hypochromic, microcytic anaemia with low serum ferritin. Lack of vitamin $B_{12}$ or folic acid causes a macrocytic anaemia with a megaloblastic bone marrow. If the marrow is deprived of either or both vitamin $B_{12}$ and folic acid, the blood picture and the marrow look the same, but it is essential to determine which substance is missing. If folic acid is given to a patient who has vitamin $B_{12}$ deficiency, neurological damage (subacute combined degeneration of the cord) may be provoked or aggravated.

## Iron deficiency anaemia

### Iron

As iron is usually absorbed from the gut, a satisfactory response is achieved in most patients when iron salts are given orally. Several ferrous salts are available. There is little to choose between them although they vary greatly in cost. The cheaper salts such as ferrous sulphate should be used unless gastrointestinal adverse effects are severe. Slow-release preparations should be avoided because of unreliable absorption. The duration of treatment, and its success, depends on the underlying cause of the anaemia. Haemoglobin should rise by approximately 1g/dl/week. The achievement of normal haemoglobin levels should then be followed by further treatment for 6 months in an attempt to replenish iron stores throughout the body.

### Adverse effects

Some people cannot tolerate oral iron preparations. The main complaints are nausea, epigastric discomfort, constipation and diarrhoea. A change in the ferrous salt form may help but improvement may be related to a lower content of iron in the alternative preparation.

### Dose

Ferrous sulphate is given at a dose of 200 mg three times daily until anaemia is corrected and iron stores are replenished.

## Parenteral iron

Oral iron therapy occasionally fails to achieve its objective because of lack of patient cooperation, severe adverse effects or gastrointestinal malabsorption. The total dose of parenteral iron required is calculated for each patient on the basis of body weight and haemoglobin level. Iron sucrose is given by slow intravenous injection of infusion only. Iron dextran is given either by deep intramuscular injection into the gluteal muscle or by slow intravenous injection or infusion. Anaphylactic reactions can occur with parenteral iron, and patients should be given a test dose initially, and carefully monitored.

## Megaloblastic anaemia

### Vitamin B$_{12}$

Vitamin B$_{12}$ deficiency demands that vitamin B$_{12}$ should be injected in adequate doses for life. Usually the underlying disease, such as pernicious

anaemia, cannot be corrected and a route that bypasses the defective absorption mechanism in the gut therefore must supply the vitamin. Treatment should correct the anaemia and then maintain a normal blood picture. It should arrest, reverse or prevent lesions of the nervous system and replenish depleted stores.

A dramatic response often follows within 2–3 days of the start of vitamin B$_{12}$ therapy. Symptoms improve and the haemoglobin concentration rises progressively to normal. An early index of success is a rise in the reticulocyte count, which reaches a peak after about 1 week and then gradually declines to normal in the next 2 weeks.

Marrow changes reverse rapidly.

### Adverse effects

These are rare and probably related to contamination or impurities in the injected solution.

### Dose

Hydroxocobalamin is given at a dose of 1 mg on alternate days by intramuscular injection for 1 week, then at 2- to 3-monthly intervals for life.

## Folic acid

Folic acid deficiency in Western countries is frequently the result of low dietary intake. Less commonly it is the consequence of malabsorption. Pregnancy makes such demands on iron and folic acid stores in the mother that it has been routine for iron and folic acid to be prescribed throughout pregnancy. Recent evidence that periconceptional maternal folic acid deficiency is associated with the birth of infants with neural tube defects has led to the recommendation of the use of supplements of small doses of folic acid by women who are planning pregnancy until at least 12 weeks gestation. Folic acid should never be given alone for vitamin B$_{12}$ deficiency, as it may precipitate subacute combined deficiency of the spinal cord.

### Dose

An oral dose of 5 mg daily is given for 4 months. When combined with iron for prophylactic use in pregnancy, 200–500 µg is given daily. A dose of 400 µg daily is recommended for routine periconceptional prophylaxis, but 5 mg daily (until week 12 of pregnancy) is recommended for women who have already given birth to an infant with a neural tube defect.

## Haemopoietic growth factors

These naturally occurring glycoproteins have a physiological role in the regulation of haemopoiesis. Most are synthesised by bone marrow stromal cells. Some act on pluripotent stem cells, whilst others are lineage-specific and act only on committed progenitors. Molecular biological techniques have made possible the production of recombinant forms of some of the haemopoetic growth factors, and these are now in clinical use for a number of specialised indications. All these agents are given parenterally, usually by subcutaneous or sometimes by intravenous injection.

## Recombinant erythropoietin (epoetin, darbepoetin alfa)

Physiologically, erythropoietin is synthesised in the kidney, and its synthesis is regulated by the oxygen tension in renal tissues. It acts on committed erythroid precursors to increase erythropoiesis. In severe renal failure erythropoietin production is defective and this contributes to the anaemia of renal disease. Recombinant human erythropoietin was the first of the growth factors to come into therapeutic use and is indicated for the treatment of anaemia associated with severe renal failure. Patients on dialysis and those not yet being dialysed are suitable. Haematinic deficiency, infections and aluminium accumulation should be ruled out as major contributory causes of anaemia before prescribing erythropoietin to renal patients. Potential adverse effects of erythropoietin include hypertension, clotting of vascular access sites, flu-like symptoms and seizures. It follows that erythropoietin is contraindicated in patients with uncontrolled hypertension.

## Recombinant human granulocyte-colony stimulating factor (filgrastim, lenogastim, perfilgrastim)

Granulocyte-colony stimulating factor (G-CSF) is a growth factor that acts at relatively late stages of myelopoiesis in a lineage-specific manner to enhance the production and function of neutrophils. Recombinant human G-CSF (rhG-CSF) has been available for therapeutic use in recent years. It is effective in shortening the duration of neutropenias, e.g., following myelosuppressive chemotherapy, including bone marrow transplantation. Its use should be confined to specialised haematology or oncology units.

## Drug-induced blood conditions

### Drug-induced blood loss

Drugs used to relieve pain and inflammation in rheumatoid and osteoarthritis are often associated with chronic, occult blood loss from the gastrointestinal tract. Aspirin ingestion is a well-recognised cause of this type of anaemia and all other non-steroidal anti-inflammatory drugs, e.g. indomethacin, ibuprofen and COX-2 inhibitors, carry this risk (see 'Symptom modifying antirheumatic therapies', Chapter 9). Oral anticoagulants carry a similar risk.

### Drug-induced megaloblastic anaemia

Two important mechanisms result in drug-induced megaloblastic anaemia:
1 Interference with cellular DNA synthesis by cytotoxic drugs such as cytosine arabinoside, 5-fluorouracil or 6-mercaptopurine
2 Interference with folate absorption or use of anticonvulsants such as phenytoin and phenobarbital or the cytotoxic drug methotrexate, which inhibits dihydrofolate reductase.

### Drug-induced sideroblastic anaemia

Some drugs and chemicals are involved in the aetiology of sideroblastic anaemia (a type of refractory anaemia) in a small proportion of patients. This can occur following administration of the antituberculous drug isoniazid, or following excessive alcohol consumption or exposure to lead.

## Drug-induced marrow depression: aplastic anaemia

This occurs when cellular activity in the bone marrow is suppressed and is usually associated with the suppression of white cell and platelet formation (pancytopenia). Rarely, pure red cell aplasia may occur. Cytotoxic drugs are the commonest cause.

Drugs causing aplastic anaemia usually incorporate a benzene ring with closely attached amino groups. The outcome depends on the dose and the length of exposure, and to less well-defined factors such as the degree of susceptibility, idiosyncracy or hypersensitivity exhibited by an individual.

Certain drugs have a high risk of causing aplastic anaemia. These include gold salts. In other cases this is a rare idiosyncratic adverse effect, e.g. with antimicrobials such as chloramphenicol and the sulphonylureas.

Some drugs have a tendency to suppress white cells, e.g. phenylbutazone, meprobamate and chlorpromazine, while others inhibit platelet production, e.g. gold salts.

Unless the risk is acceptable, as in the treatment of some forms of malignant diseases, aplastic anaemia should be prevented at all costs. The risks can be minimised by avoiding known marrow depressants, especially in patients with a history of allergy or idiosyncracy. If the risk is accepted, then every effort should be made to detect early signs and symptoms of bone marrow depression. The patient should be advised that sore throat, fever, malaise and bruising may be an indication. Regular peripheral blood examination should be performed. In many circumstances, where the degree of exposure to the causative agent has not been excessive, withdrawal of the agent leads to recovery within 2–3 weeks. Otherwise, intensive therapy is required, including reverse barrier nursing antibiotics, transfusion of blood products, administration of androgens or rhG-CSF and, in extreme cases, bone marrow transplantation.

## Drug-induced haemolytic anaemia

A haemolytic anaemia occurs when the rate of red cell destruction is increased and red cells survive for a shorter time than the normal 100–200 days. Many drugs can reduce red cell survival:
1 Those that inevitably cause haemolytic anaemia (direct toxins)
2 Those that cause haemolysis because of hereditary defects in red cell metabolism
3 Drugs that cause haemolysis because of the development of abnormal immune mechanisms.

### Direct toxins

Drugs and chemicals that have powerful oxidant properties are likely to cause haemolysis. Damage by these agents results in fragmentation and irregular contraction of red cells, spherocytosis, basophilic stippling, Heinz bodies, methaemoglobinaemia and sulphaemoglobinaemia. In addition to many domestic and industrial agents, haemolytic anaemia may follow the use of sulphones in the treatment of leprosy and sulphonamides, including sulphasalazine and dapsone.

### Interaction with hereditary defects in red cells

Glucose-6-phosphate dehydrogenase deficiency in Negroid and Mediterranean races may give some protection against falciparum malaria, but the red cells in these individuals are abnormally sensitive to oxidising agents, resulting in haemolysis.

A large number of compounds may cause this haemolytic reaction, notably:
1 Antimalarial drugs, e.g. primaquine and pamaquin
2 The sulphones used in leprosy, e.g. dapsone
3 Some sulphonamides including co-trimoxazole
4 Quinolone antibiotics including ciprofloxacin and nalidixic acid
5 Water-soluble vitamin K analogues.

### Immune mechanisms

Drugs can be associated with two immune haemolytic mechanisms.

## Immune haemolytic anaemia

Antibodies may be formed against the drug or its metabolites. Antibodies can only be demonstrated *in vitro* in the presence of the drug. They may be stimulated by the drug binding directly to red cells forming a drug–red cell complex (the hapten cell mechanism, e.g. penicillin and cephalothin) or by the drug itself with subsequent adsorption on to the red cell surface. Activation of complement then causes lysis (immune complex mechanism, e.g. quinidine, *p*-aminosalicylic acid and rifampicin).

## Autoimmune haemolytic anaemia

Antibodies are formed against the red cells. They can be demonstrated *in vitro* in the absence of the drug. This not uncommon form of haemolytic anaemia has been associated most often with the antihypertensive drug methyldopa. While at least 15% of patients on methyldopa develop a positive direct antiglobulin test, less than 0.1% develop overt haemolytic anaemia. If the drug is withdrawn, the haemoglobin level recovers but it may take many months for the antiglobulin test to become negative. Other drugs occasionally causing this kind of haemolytic anaemia are levodopa and mefenamic acid.

## Drug-induced neutropenia

---
**Drugs and neutropenia**

1 Antibiotics: chloramphenicol, co-trimoxazole
2 Anti-inflammatory drugs: phenylbutazone
3 Oral hypoglycaemics
4 Psychotropic drugs including phenothiazines and the antipsychotic agent clozapine which may cause agranulocytosis in 1 in 300 patients and which requires patient registration for use
5 Anticonvulsants: carbamazepine
6 Antithyroid drugs

---

The most common adverse effect of drugs on the white cell system is a reduction in the number of neutrophils below the lower limit of normal (neutropenia).

Drugs causing this do so either as part of aplastic anaemia (pancytopenia) or as a selective neutropenia that does not involve the red cells or platelets. Drugs causing pancytopenia have been discussed in relation to aplastic anaemia.

Drugs may also cause selective neutropenia. This may occur either because of selective myeloid suppression, or because of an immune mechanism that may affect mature neutrophils only, or may also involve late myeloid precursors in the bone marrow (agranulocytosis). A large number of agents have been documented as causes of neutropenia, and a careful drug history should be taken in patients presenting with neutropenia. In most cases individual patient susceptibility to a particular drug underlies the problem. The following have a particular association with neutropenia:

Treatment of drug-induced neutropenia calls for:
1 Withdrawal of the drug
2 Haematological advice and bone marrow examination
3 In severe cases expert supportive care for the prevention and treatment of infection
4 In selected cases treatment with myeloid growth factors, e.g. rhG CSF.

## Drug-induced thrombocytopenia

Platelets may be reduced in number (thrombocytopenia) or function by drugs and chemicals. This may be part of aplastic anaemia or selective thrombocytopenia. The latter is a rare effect of various drugs, including heparins, thiazides, sulphonamides and sulphonylureas, and sodium valproate.

Drug-induced thrombocytopenia may occur as a result of suppression of platelet production or may involve an immune mechanism, akin to drug-induced immune haemolysis. A further mechanism is drug-induced platelet aggregation, for example, heparin-induced thrombocytopenia which is a consequence of antibody-dependent platelet aggregation. Rarely, drugs may be involved in the aetiology of microangiopathic syndromes associated with thrombocytopenia (thrombotic thrombocytopenic purpura and haemolytic uraemic syndrome). Oral contraceptive agents and ciclosporin have occasionally been implicated in such cases.

Drug-induced thrombocytopenia should be treated according to haematological advice. The offending agent should be withdrawn and a bone marrow examination is usually indicated. If an immune mechanism is implicated, intravenous immunoglobulin treatment may be helpful. In others, particularly if platelet production is suppressed and the thrombocytopenia is severe or the patient is haemorrhagic, platelet transfusion may be indicated. Platelet transfusion should *not* be given in suspected cases of heparin-induced thrombocytopenia. Heparin should be stopped and advice regarding alternative anticoagulation sought from a haematologist. Platelet transfusions are also contraindicated in microangiopathic syndromes.

*Comment*. Whenever a disorder of blood cell formation is observed and an adverse drug effect suspected, take a careful drug history and consult reference books describing adverse effects.

# Chapter 15

# Anaesthesia and the relief of pain

## Relevant pathophysiology

Sensory receptors for pain are found in all tissues of the body. A variety of noxious stimuli (thermal, chemical, mechanical or electrical) cause them to respond and lead to the subjective experience of pain.

1 The first-order afferent neurones transmitting pain impulses are of two types:
- The rapidly conducting (12–30 m/s) small-diameter myelinated fibres of the A group (delta)
- The slow (0.5–2 m/s) non-myelinated C fibres.

Both the rapidly and slow-conducting fibres terminate in the dorsal horns of the spinal cord.

2 Second-order neurones carry the pain stimuli to the thalamus in the lateral spinothalamic tracts. Branches from both A and C fibres form synapses with cells in the dorsal horns of the spinal cord. A network of cells in this area, which includes the substantia gelatinosa, regulates transmission between the nociceptive neurones and those in the spinothalamic tract. Descending fibres from higher centres act to inhibit transmission.

3 From the thalamus, third-order neurones convey pain impulses to the post-central gyri of the cerebral cortex. The thalamus is the main region responsible for the integration of pain input but the cortical area is concerned with the exact and meaningful subjective interpretation of pain.

The transducing qualities of free nerve endings are affected by chemical changes in the immediate vicinity, e.g. changes in the concentrations of hydrogen ions, substance P, 5-hydroxytryptamine (5-HT), histamine, bradykinin and eicosanoids. Bradykinin and related substances are formed in extracellular fluid whenever there is tissue damage and account for the vascular and exudative changes of inflammation. Bradykinin sensitises and stimulates nerve endings and causes pain. The analgesic effects of aspirin and other non-steroidal anti-inflammatory drugs result from the impaired release of mediator by mechanisms including inhibition of prostaglandin synthesis (Chapter 9).

Within the central nervous system (CNS), opioid receptors are localised in the spinal cord dorsal horn, and in the brain stem, thalamus and cortex, in what constitutes the ascending pain transmission system, as well as structures that comprise a descending inhibitory system that modulates pain at the level of the spinal cord. There are four distinct opioid receptor types and each of these has an endogenous ligand. Mu and kappa receptors, stimulated naturally by $\beta$-endorphins and dynorphins respectively, are responsible not only for analgesia but also for many of the adverse effects of morphine including respiratory depression and miosis. The consequences of stimulating the delta receptor, whose endogenous ligand is the enkephalins, with morphine in humans are unclear. The recently identified opioid receptor-like (ORL1) receptor is stimulated naturally by nociceptin/orphanin FQ (N/OFQ). Although the ORL1-N/OFQ system clearly belongs to the opioid receptor family and has a role in a variety of processes such as pain modulation and anxiety, it does not bind classical opiates and has distinct pharmacological actions. It is no longer believed that there is a sigma opioid receptor.

In addition to the endogenous ligands of the opioid receptor family, many other substances influence the pain pathways of the CNS including nitric oxide, cholecystokinin, substance P, biogenic amines like 5-HT and excitatory amino acids such as glutamate.

## Principles of drug treatment

From a practical point of view, there are two types of pain:

1 Visceral pain, which is a dull, poorly localised pain, e.g. peritoneal pain

2 Somatic pain, which is sharply defined, e.g. pain of a fractured femur.

Pain is a valuable symptom of underlying pathology and may be vital in the diagnosis of disease, e.g. in management of the acute abdomen. However, inadequate administration of relief to a patient in distress while steps are taken to confirm the diagnosis should be avoided.

There is a pronounced placebo effect in the treatment of pain. Thirty per cent of patients in pain experience some relief from a doctor taking an interest in their pain and prescribing any drug.

## Opioid analgesics

Opiates are drugs derived from opium, a term for the juice of the poppy plant. Opioid is a more inclusive term, applying to all agonists or antagonists with morphine-like activity. The term narcotic is no longer used pharmacologically because of its pejorative legal meaning.

## Morphine

### Mechanism of action

Morphine produces a range of depressant effects by a central action on mu opioid receptors within the CNS and in peripheral tissues.

The CNS effects include analgesia, euphoria and sedation; depression of respiration; depression of the vasomotor centre resulting in hypotension; cough suppression; release of antidiuretic hormone; miosis; and nausea and vomiting. Peripheral effects include smooth muscle contraction with reduced motility of the gastrointestinal tract; reduced secretion of gastrointestinal tract; biliary spasm; urinary retention; constriction of bronchi partly as a result of histamine release; vasodilatation; and itching.

### Pharmacokinetics

Morphine is unreliably absorbed after oral administration and subject to high first-pass metabolism in the gut wall and the liver; the oral bioavailability of morphine is typically 20%. However, there is a slow-release oral preparation that results in delayed but sustained therapeutic plasma morphine concentrations. The drug can be given intravenously, intramuscularly or subcutaneously. After intramuscular injection, peak brain concentrations occur between 30 and 45 min but relatively little of the administered drug crosses the blood–brain barrier. Morphine can also be injected into the subarachnoid and epidural spaces although its high water solubility makes it a less attractive drug for this purpose than diamorphine or fentanyl (because of the risk of secondary respiratory depression) and its side-effect profile is relatively poor when administered via these routes.

The major route of elimination is conjugation with glucuronic acid to form morphine-3-monoglucuronide, which is excreted in the urine. Only a very small amount of free morphine appears in the urine, bile or faeces. About 90% of the administered dose is eliminated within the first 24 h.

## Adverse effects

Many of the adverse effects of morphine represent an extension of its pharmacological effects as a result of relative overdosage (see below).

---

### Adverse effects of morphine

**1** Respiratory depression, periodic breathing or apnoea
**2** Hypotension
**3** Nausea and vomiting
**4** Constipation
**5** Tremor
**6** Urticaria and itching
**7** Tolerance and addiction to the drug. These are rare when morphine is given during anaesthesia or for the relief of pain after surgery

---

## Drug interactions

Morphine delays the absorption of other drugs when they are given orally. In addition, other drugs such as phenothiazines and tricyclic antidepressants potentiate its depressant effects. Morphine will, in turn, potentiate the effect of most hypnotics and all volatile anacsthetic agents.

## Clinical use and dose

**1** The relief of visceral and somatic pain
**2** The relief of anxiety and pain after myocardial infarction
**3** In acute left ventricular failure (pulmonary oedema) to reduce preload by venodilation (Chapter 6)
**4** Before, during and after anaesthesia, as part of a balanced anaesthetic technique
The usual intramuscular or subcutaneous dose for relief of severe pain is 0.1–0.2 mg/kg but this dose may need to be adjusted to take into account factors such as age and co-morbidity that may alter an individual's response. For post-operative pain, morphine is often given intravenously using syringe drivers activated by the patient (patient-controlled analgesia)
**5** Opioids, particularly codeine derivatives, are used as antitussives (Chapter 8) and antidiarrhoeal agents (Chapter 13).

## Other opioid analgesics

Many opioid drugs are available and the properties of some are summarised in Table 15.1. Others

**Table 15.1** Comparison of opioid analgesic drugs.

| | Dose (mg) | Route | Duration of action (h) | Notes |
|---|---|---|---|---|
| *Natural opiates* | | | | |
| Morphine | 10–15 | i.m., s.c. | 4 | |
| | 10–30 | oral as sustained | 8 | Slow onset, needs regular dosage |
| | | release | 8 | to be useful |
| *Semi-synthetic* | | | | |
| Diamorphine | 5 | i.m., s.c. | 4 | |
| Oxycodone | 10 | i.m. | 4–6 | Used in chronic pain |
| | 30 | Rectal | 4–8 | |
| Dihydrocodeine | 50 | i.m., s.c. | 4 | |
| | 30–60 | Oral | 4 | |
| *Synthetic* | | | | |
| Pethidine | 100–150 | i.m., s.c. | 2–3 | |
| Buprenorphine | 0.3 | i.m., s.c. | 8 | Partial agonist |
| | 0.3 | Sublingual | 8 | Slow onset |
| Methadone | 5–10 | Oral/i.m. | 5–6 | Used in chronic pain |
| Tramadol | 50–100 | Oral | 5–6 | Used in chronic pain |
| | 100 | i.m. | 5–6 | Used in post-operative pain |

such as papaveretum, pentazocine, butorphanol, dextromoramide, levorphanol and dipipanone have very limited use.

## Diamorphine or heroin

This is more potent and more lipid-soluble than morphine. It is metabolised to monoacetylmorphine and then morphine. It is claimed to be less emetic than morphine but there is little evidence for this. When patients receiving palliative care require large doses of morphine for pain relief, diamorphine can be administered by continuous subcutaneous infusion in a smaller volume of solution than the equivalent dose of morphine. This is an important consideration in patients with cachexia.

## Codeine or methylmorphine

The actions of codeine are similar to those of morphine but codeine is a less potent analgesic. A number of fixed dose preparations containing paracetamol, ibuprofen or aspirin in combination with codeine phosphate are available for the treatment of pain of mild to moderate severity. Codeine is also used as a cough suppressant and to control diarrhoea. Ten per cent of the dose is demethylated in the liver to form morphine.

## Pethidine

This is a synthetic analgesic that has a more rapid onset than morphine and a shorter duration of action. Smooth muscle contraction is less prominent and therefore pethidine is used in biliary and ureteric colic. Constipation does not occur to the same extent. One of its metabolites, norpethidine, is active and may accumulate and cause convulsions in patients with hepatic or renal impairment. The risk of toxicity may be increased in patients taking other drugs that induce hepatic enzymes. Pethidine effectively inhibits post-anaesthetic shivering.

## Fentanyl

This is the most potent analgesic used in the United Kingdom. When given in small intravenous doses, it has a rapid onset and a short duration of action (about 30 min), whereas large doses may be effective for several hours. Cardiovascular stability is present even when the drug is administered in large doses and the role of fentanyl in cardiovascular anaesthesia is well established. Because fentanyl is highly lipid-soluble, it may be absorbed transdermally and this property is exploited in palliative care.

## Alfentanil

This is given solely by the intravenous route. When compared to fentanyl, alfentanil has a slightly faster onset of action but, following a bolus dose, its effects last only 5–10 min. The pharmacokinetics of alfentanil is consistent with administration by a continuous intravenous infusion and it can be included in the sedation regimes of intensive care units. The clearance of alfentanil is unaffected by renal disease.

## Remifentanil

This is given solely by the intravenous route. It has a rapid onset of action (similar to alfentanil) and an ultra-short duration of action. The context-sensitive half-time of a drug is a pharmacokinetic measure of the time required for the drug's plasma concentration to decrease by 50% after cessation of an infusion; the "context" is the duration of the infusion. By virtue of its relatively small volume of distribution and widespread metabolism by non-specific esterases, the context-sensitive half-time of remifentanil remains consistently short (3.2 min) even following an infusion of long duration (>8 h). This clinically important feature distinguishes remifentanil from other opioids, the context-sensitive half-times of which are highly dependent upon the duration of the infusion, and is largely independent of the degree of hepatic and renal function.

## Tramadol

Tramadol is a non-selective agonist at mu, kappa and delta opioid receptors. It also inhibits neuronal reuptake of 5-HT and noradrenaline, and enhances 5-HT release. It is used in the management of moderate to severe acute pain, in chronic pain and in palliative care. Advantages include a low incidence of respiratory depression and a low potential for abuse. The main disadvantages are nausea, sedation and diaphoresis.

## Partial agonists and opiate antagonists

### Buprenorphine

This is a partial agonist at mu opiate receptors. It is a potent long-lasting analgesic drug that can be absorbed sublingually. Dependence or addiction potential is claimed to be low. Respiratory depression is not reversed by the opiate antagonist naloxone except in very high doses (15 mg or more). Hallucinations can occur. Note that it is not advisable to give buprenorphine to augment inadequate analgesia from morphine and more potent agents.

### Nalbuphine and meptazinol

These are synthetic opioids used parenterally in the treatment of surgical and chronic pain.

### Naloxone

This is a specific opioid antagonist without agonist activity. It is used to antagonise all of the actions of opioid analgesic drugs. It precipitates withdrawal symptoms if given to addicts or the neonate born to a mother addicted to opioids. Naloxone may be given intravenously or intramuscularly in a dose of 0.4–1.2 mg. When given intravenously, the onset of action occurs within 1–2 min and it lasts 20–30 min. Thus, if it is used to reverse an opioid that has a longer duration of action it may have to be given repeatedly, preferably by intravenous infusion.

## Local (regional) anaesthesia

Transmission of impulses in peripheral nerves is associated with depolarisation of the nerve cell membrane, which is the result of increased membrane permeability to sodium ions. Local anaesthetic agents produce a localised, reversible block to nerve conduction by reducing the permeability of the membrane to sodium. Most of the clinically useful local anaesthetic agents act by reversibly blocking the sodium channel through a direct interaction between the anaesthetic molecule and a few amino acids of the receptor protein. These agents may exist in the charged and uncharged form in solution. The uncharged form diffuses more readily through the neural sheath while the charged form attaches to the receptor. The relative proportion of the charged and uncharged form depends upon the $pK_a$ of the drug, the pH of the solution and the pH at the injection site. The smaller the nerve fibre, the more sensitive it is to local anaesthetic block. Thus it is possible, but practically difficult, to block pain and autonomic fibres and leave proprioception, i.e. touch and movement, intact.

Local anaesthetics are administered locally and do not rely on the circulation to take them to their site of action. However, uptake into the systemic circulation terminates their effects. The rate of systemic absorption is determined by the factors listed below.

| Systemic absorption of local anaesthetics |
| --- |
| **1** Pharmacokinetic properties of the drug |
| **2** Vascularity of the injection site |
| **3** Concentration of the solution used |
| **4** Rate of injection |

A vasoconstrictor, such as adrenaline, may be used in solution with the local anaesthetic to delay systemic absorption, prolong the local block and limit toxicity.

Local anaesthetics are weak bases with $pK_a$ values between 7.5 (mepivacaine) and 8.9 (procaine). Marked changes in the ratio of ionised to non-ionised drug occur with changes in acid–base balance. They are extensively bound to plasma proteins. Differences in binding between agents may influence the intensity and duration of effect and placental transfer.

Table 15.2 Comparison of local anaesthetic drugs.

| Agent | Relative dosage | $pK_a$ | $t_{1/2}$ (h) | Onset | Duration |
|---|---|---|---|---|---|
| *Amides* | | | | | |
| Lidocaine | 1.0 | 7.9 | 1.6 | Rapid | Medium |
| Bupivacaine | 0.25 | 8.1 | 2.7 | Slow | Long |
| Prilocaine | 1.0 | 7.9 | — | Slow | Medium |
| Ropivacaine | 0.33 | 8.1 | 3.3 | Slow | Long |
| *Esters* | | | | | |
| Cocaine | 1.0 | — | * | Slow | Medium |
| Procaine | 2.0 | 8.9 | * | Slow | Short |
| Tetracaine (Amethocaine) | 0.25 | 8.5 | * | Slow | Long |
| Chloroprocaine | 3.0 | 8.7 | * | — | — |

* $t_{1/2}$ is very short owing to hydrolysis in plasma.

Local anaesthetic drugs are of two types:

1 *Esters*, e.g. procaine, which are metabolised in the plasma by esterases

2 *Amides*, e.g. lidocaine (lignocaine), which are extensively metabolised in the liver, the clearance being dependent on liver blood flow. In the liver, *N*-dealkylation of the tertiary amine produces a more soluble secondary amine that may be active and is in turn dealkylated. Very little of an injected dose of local anaesthetic is excreted unchanged in the urine.

The physicochemical and pharmacokinetic properties of several local anaesthetics are shown in Table 15.2.

## Lidocaine

Lidocaine (lignocaine) has both local and systemic effects. Local effects include loss of pain and other sensations, vasodilatation and loss of motor power. Various preparations of lidocaine are used for topical, infiltration, conduction and epidural anaesthesia. One or two per cent solutions, containing 10 or 20 mg/ml of lidocaine respectively, are popular and the first effects are noted 5–10 min after administration with the duration of action being around 2–3 h. Systemic effects follow absorption from the site of local administration or systemic administration and result from generalised membrane stabilisation. Myocardial excitability is depressed and lidocaine may be used in the treatment of ventricular tachyarrhythmias (Chapter 6) because it possesses class I anti-arrhythmic activity.

Adverse effects include anxiety and excitement progressing to sedation, disorientation, lingular and circumoral anaesthesia, restlessness, twitching, tremors, convulsions and unconsciousness. Coma may be accompanied by apnoea and cardiovascular collapse. The maximum 'safe' dose of lidocaine is 3 mg/kg without adrenaline and 7 mg/kg with adrenaline. However, factors that influence toxicity include peak plasma level and rate of rise of plasma level. Adverse effects can therefore occur not only after an overdose, but also following a rapid injection into a highly vascular area; recommended maximum doses are a guide only.

## Other local anaesthetics

### Bupivacaine

This is an amide that is four times as potent as lidocaine. It is available in 0.25, 0.5 or 0.75% solutions, containing 2.5, 5 or 7.5 mg/ml of bupivacaine respectively, and these are used for infiltration, conduction, spinal and epidural anaesthesia. The maximum 'safe' dose is 2 mg/kg (with or without adrenaline) and, in comparison with lidocaine, its action has a slower onset but a longer duration.

## Levobupivacaine

Bupivacaine exists as a racemic mixture of two enantiomers—levobupivacaine and dextrobupivacaine. Levobupivacaine has a similar efficacy but an enhanced safety profile when compared to bupivacaine and, as a result of progress in chiral synthetic technology, is now available in 0.25, 0.5 or 0.75% solutions.

## Prilocaine

This is equipotent with lidocaine and can be used for all types of local analgesia. It is less toxic than lidocaine because of its greater degree of tissue uptake. Large doses may produce methaemoglobinaemia, which is caused by a metabolite, $O$-toluidine. The maximum dose is 6 mg/kg (8 mg/kg with felypressin). The drug is widely used for intravenous regional anaesthesia. Reformulated in a mixture of prilocaine and lidocaine crystals (eutectic mixture of local anaesthetic—EMLA), it is absorbed transdermally and gives good surface analgesia for procedures such as venepuncture in children.

## Ropivacaine

Although structurally similar to bupivacaine, ropivacaine may cause less motor block and cardiotoxicity. However, this may simply relate to reduced potency.

## Cocaine

This is an ester and is unique in that, in addition to its local anaesthetic properties, it may act as a CNS stimulant. It has been used clinically for topical anaesthesia and for its central euphoriant effects in the management of terminal malignant disease.

## General anaesthesia

General anaesthesia is characterised by a balanced technique in which drugs are used specifically to produce loss of consciousness, analgesia and muscle relaxation. Nowadays, a single drug is rarely used to produce all the components of general anaesthesia.

## Intravenous anaesthetic agents

These drugs are used to produce a rapid and pleasant induction of sleep. In most cases, other agents will maintain anaesthesia and thus it is rapidity of onset and not brevity of action that is the most desirable property. The mechanism of action of these agents remains unclear. They are all highly lipid-soluble agents and cross the blood–brain barrier rapidly. Their rapid onset of action is a result of this rapid transfer into the brain and high cerebral blood flow. Action is terminated by distribution of the drugs away from the brain to less well-perfused tissues.

## Non-barbiturate anaesthetics

### Propofol

Propofol is the most widely used intravenous anaesthetic. It is a phenol derivative that is available as a white oil-in-water emulsion containing 1 or 2% propofol in soybean oil, glycerol and purified egg phosphatide. After administration of 1.5–2.5 mg/kg, sleep occurs in one arm–brain circulation time (10–20 s) but this may be delayed in patients with cardiac disease or shock. Loss of consciousness is pleasant and lasts for 2–5 min. Recovery is rapid following redistribution of propofol from the brain to other tissues. Elimination is faster than with other intravenous anaesthetics because of glucuronide conjugation in the liver. There is thus no pronounced after-effect. Similarly, infusion of the drug does not produce significant cumulation, making it suitable for total intravenous anaesthesia. Advantages include depression of upper airway reflexes and an anti-emetic effect; disadvantages are hypotension, respiratory depression and pain on injection.

### Etomidate

This is an imidazole derivative with a very short duration of action owing to rapid redistribution. It has minimal effect on the cardiovascular system and traditionally it has been the induction agent of choice in very sick patients. It is metabolised in the liver and has a half-life of 4.6 h. Injection may be painful and causes muscle twitching with involuntary movements. Post-operative nausea and vomiting are also associated with etomidate. The drug blocks 11-$\beta$-hydroxylation in the adrenal cortex, inhibiting cortisol synthesis for up to 24 h after a bolus dose. The clinical implications of this finding are unclear but the use of etomidate infusions for sedation in the intensive care unit is associated with an increased mortality.

### Ketamine

This is a derivative of phencyclidine. It may be administered intravenously, intramuscularly or into the epidural space. It is now used infrequently in the United Kingdom but is given extensively in developing countries. It is almost devoid of hypnotic properties and produces a state of dissociative anaesthesia characterised by anterograde amnesia and profound analgesia. In contrast to other intravenous anaesthetic agents, ketamine stimulates respiration and increases blood pressure. Adverse effects include emergence delirium, unpleasant dreams and hallucinations. Post-operative nausea and vomiting are common.

## Barbiturates

### Thiopental (thiopentone)

Thiopental, the sulphur analogue of pentobarbitone, was once the most widely used intravenous anaesthetic. After administration, the initial decay of plasma concentration is very rapid and the half-life of the initial distribution phase is 2.5 min. Elimination is by hepatic metabolism and the terminal half-life is 6.2 h (Table 15.3).

The adverse effects of thiopental include respiratory depression, myocardial depression and vasodilatation. Laryngeal reflexes are not depressed and laryngospasm may occur. The drug has no analgesic properties. Thiopental, like all barbiturates, may exacerbate porphyria.

## Inhalation anaesthetic agents

These agents, usually with others, such as intravenous analgesics, are used to maintain a state of general anaesthesia after induction. The depth of anaesthesia produced is related to the tension of the agent in the blood. Because the alveolar epithelium of the lung presents virtually no barrier to diffusion, the partial pressure of the agent in the alveoli determines the depth of anaesthesia. This alveolar partial pressure is influenced by several factors including inspired concentration, pulmonary ventilation and cardiac output. However, the rate of onset of anaesthetic action is mainly determined by the agent's solubility in blood; as a general rule, drugs with low blood–gas solubility, such as sevoflurane, act rapidly and drugs with high blood–gas solubility, such as ether, act slowly.

> **Factors affecting alveolar concentration of anaesthetics**
>
> 1 The concentration of the drug in the inspired gas
> 2 Alveolar ventilation
> 3 Cardiac output
> 4 The solubility of the drug in the blood

The potency of these agents is related to, but is not dependent on, fat solubility. The minimum alveolar concentration (MAC) is the alveolar

**Table 15.3** Comparison of intravenous anaesthetic induction agents.

| Drug | Distribution volume (l/kg) | Clearance (ml/min) | Plasma half-life $t_{1/2}$ (h) |
|---|---|---|---|
| Propofol | 5.0 | 1500 | 2.0 |
| Etomidate | 4.5 | 740 | 4.6 |
| Ketamine | 3.3 | 1296 | 3.4 |
| Thiopental | 1.6 | 144 | 6.2 |

concentration that produces a state of surgical anaesthesia in 50% of patients. Put another way, it is the dose that abolishes movement in response to incision in 50% of patients. MAC is a population median that varies with age and other factors.

In practice, clinical signs are used to monitor depth of anaesthesia. Inspired and end-tidal concentrations of inhalational agent are routinely measured but depth of anaesthesia monitors have not gained widespread acceptance in the United Kingdom.

## Nitrous oxide

This is a vapour at room temperature. Although it cannot produce surgical anaesthesia when administered alone (i.e. its MAC is over 100%), a concentration of 70% in oxygen is conventionally used as an adjunct to more potent inhalational agents. An equal mixture of nitrous oxide and oxygen is used to produce analgesia during labour and other painful procedures. Adverse effects include postoperative nausea and vomiting, and prolonged exposure to nitrous oxide may result in bone marrow depression.

## Isoflurane

This is a halogenated ether that is a liquid at room temperature and must be vaporised before use. Over 99% of an administered dose is excreted unchanged by the lungs and the remainder is metabolised in the liver. In common with other volatile anaesthetics, it depresses the respiratory and cardiovascular systems but causes less myocardial depression and arrhythmias than other agents.

## Desflurane

This differs from isoflurane by the substitution of a fluorine for a chlorine atom. It boils at around room temperature and requires a heated, pressurised vaporiser. Its solubility in blood is similar to that of nitrous oxide allowing rapid uptake and, more importantly, rapid elimination of the drug. Its properties are otherwise similar to those of isoflurane.

## Sevoflurane

Like desflurane this is an ether halogenated solely with fluorine atoms. Its low solubility in blood allows rapid emergence from anaesthesia and its low level of airway irritation makes it suited for inhalational induction of anaesthesia.

## Halothane

This is a halogenated hydrocarbon. The liver metabolises 20%; hepatic damage very rarely occurs 7–10 days after halothane anaesthesia, especially following repeated exposures, because of an immunological response to one of its metabolites. This has virtually abolished the use of halothane in adults. Arrhythmias, bradycardia and myocardial depression are more troublesome than with other volatile agents.

## Enflurane

A halogenated ether, its properties are similar to those of halothane. As the liver metabolises much less enflurane than halothane, the risk of hepatitis is reduced.

## **Neuromuscular blocking drugs**

When an electrical impulse in a motor nerve reaches the nerve ending it releases acetylcholine at the neuromuscular junction. Acetylcholine acts on nicotinic cholinergic receptors on the muscle membrane, resulting in a wave of depolarisation. The acetylcholine is then destroyed rapidly by a specific cholinesterase.

Neuromuscular blocking drugs may interfere with neurotransmission in one of two ways:
1 Prolongation of the normal depolarisation, e.g. suxamethonium
2 Competitive inhibition of acetylcholine at the receptors, e.g. vecuronium, atracurium.

These drugs are used during general anaesthesia to:
1 facilitate tracheal intubation and controlled ventilation

2 facilitate surgery, e.g. abdominal surgery, if muscle relaxation is deemed advantageous.

After administration, the anaesthetist must always ventilate the patient's lungs because paralysis includes all voluntary muscles, notably the respiratory muscles. The use of these drugs is an integral part of a balanced anaesthetic technique, but great care must be taken to ensure that the patient is unconscious.

Factors that influence the action of neuromuscular blocking drugs are listed below.

---

**Factors affecting neuromuscular blockade**

**1** Muscle blood flow (the most important factor). Muscles with high blood flow have the earliest onset and shortest duration of action
**2** Changes in temperature
**3** pH
**4** Potassium concentrations influence the degree of paralysis
**5** Aminoglycoside antibiotics prolong competitive blockade by reducing acetylcholine release
**6** Drugs that produce central muscle relaxation, e.g. benzodiazepines or isoflurane, prolong the muscle paralysis
**7** Renal disease, as most competitive blockers are excreted unchanged in the kidney to a greater or lesser extent. Atracurium is, however, metabolised in the blood
**8** Hereditary atypical cholinesterase markedly prolongs the effect of suxamethonium

---

## Suxamethonium

This is a very short-acting depolarising neuromuscular blocking drug. A dose of 1 mg/kg produces muscle fasciculations within 30 s followed by complete paralysis for 3–5 min.

Respiration must be maintained artificially. The drug is broken down very rapidly by plasma cholinesterase. In patients with a genetically determined abnormality in this enzyme's activity, paralysis is prolonged. Adverse effects of suxamethonium include bradycardia, muscle pains and raised intraocular pressure.

## Non-depolarising muscle relaxants

### Vecuronium

This is an aminosteroid that produces competitive neuromuscular paralysis. It has replaced the traditional relaxants tubocurarine, a benzylisoquinolinium compound, and pancuronium, also an aminosteroid. Its advantages are its lack of effects on the heart and an intermediate duration of action (20–40 min). Rocuronium is structurally similar. Duration of action is similar to that of vecuronium but its onset is more rapid.

Neuromuscular blockade may be reversed at the end of surgery by administering an anticholinesterase such as neostigmine. This drug is always given with atropine or glycopyrrolate, which prevent the muscarinic effects of acetylcholine and allow the nicotinic effects to be manifest.

### Atracurium

This is a benzylisoquinolinium compound with few cardiovascular side effects. It has an intermediate duration of action because of rapid non-enzymatic degradation in plasma and is particularly favoured in patients with renal or hepatic disease. The principal disadvantage is histamine release. This can be avoided by using cisatracurium, an isomer of atracurium, which does not provoke histamine release.

### Mivacurium

Mivacurium is also a benzylisoquinolinium compound. It is hydrolysed rapidly by plasma cholinesterase and has a shorter duration of action than atracurium or vecuronium, making it suitable for shorter procedures.

# Chapter 16

# Drugs and psychiatry

The last 50 years have seen major changes in psychiatric practice, with the advent of effective psychotropic drugs and the trend away from custodial to community care. The introduction of the phenothiazines in the 1950s transformed the lives of many patients with schizophrenia by abolishing troublesome symptoms and permitting a return to more normal behaviour. Next came the antidepressants, a welcome alternative to the effective but to some, controversial, electroconvulsive therapy. Since the 1960s lithium has been used effectively in acute mania, as prophylaxis in bipolar affective illness and more recently as adjunctive therapy for refractory depression. The 1960s also saw the introduction of chlordiazepoxide, the first clinical use of benzodiazepines. These sedative and anxiolytic agents were a welcome improvement upon the more dangerous barbiturates they replaced but their widespread use has led to concerns over dependency. A relatively quiescent couple of decades then gave way to an explosion of new pharmacotherapies. Antidepressant treatments expanded, first with the introduction of selective serotonin reuptake inhibitors (SSRIs) followed by a range of other novel agents. Lithium now shares a stage with several anticonvulsant drugs shown to be effective as mood stabilisers. The management of schizophrenia and related psychoses has benefited from a new generation of antipsychotics with improved side-effect profile and, particularly in the case of clozapine, evidence of improved efficacy.

Most recently, pharmacotherapy for substance use disorders and dementia has also been the focus of renewed interest.

The classification of psychiatric disorders remains heavily dependent upon the identification of clusters of symptoms, and as a result diagnostic categories have a disconcerting tendency to merge. In general, where a particular illness does not fall clearly into a diagnostic category, treatment is best directed at relief of the predominating symptoms. Table 16.1 presents a working outline of the major categories in which drug treatment is likely to be required.

*Comment.* Elucidation of the cause of psychiatric symptoms is frequently difficult. It is important to try to characterise the principal underlying abnormality, as specific drug treatment is available for most of these categories. Misdiagnosis may exacerbate psychiatric symptoms; for example, sedative benzodiazepines given to a depressed patient may lead to further impairment of function and even increased risk of suicide. Tricyclic antidepressants may precipitate or aggravate psychotic symptoms in a patient with schizophrenia.

## Antipsychotic drugs

### Aims

The main aims are to inhibit the most florid subjective and behavioural disturbances of psychosis,

**Table 16.1** Psychiatric disorders in which drug treatments are commonly used.

Acute and chronic organic brain syndromes (including delirium, dementia and drug-related psychoses)
Bipolar affective (manic-depressive) disorder
Unipolar depression (psychotic and non-psychotic)
Schizophrenia and delusional disorders (paranoid psychoses)
Generalised anxiety and panic disorders
Phobias
Obsessive compulsive disorder
Less commonly, complications of drug dependence, alcohol misuse and personality disorder may require
    drug treatment

and to restore the patient to as near normal a life in society as possible. Some atypical antipsychotics also aim to diminish 'negative symptoms' of schizophrenia such as amotivation, flattened affect and social withdrawal.

## Relevant pathophysiology

The antipsychotics are used in acute schizophrenia to diminish disturbance as a consequence of delusional thinking, hallucinations, inappropriate behaviour and anxiety. In chronic schizophrenia maintenance antipsychotic therapy reduces risk of relapse. Atypical agents may also reduce negative symptoms more resistant to conventional antipsychotics. In affective disorders antipsychotics are used to control manic symptoms, and in depression where delusions, or anxiety and agitation are prominent. They are also used to treat drug-related psychoses.

The pathophysiology of the psychoses is still unclear and the mechanisms by which drugs exert their effect are still largely hypothetical. The 'dopamine hypothesis', which proposes an over-activity of the brain dopamine system in schizophrenia, is the most favoured explanation for the antipsychotic effects of these drugs. The finding of increased dopamine concentrations in the brains of both treated and untreated patients with schizophrenia, together with the dopamine receptor antagonistic effects of antipsychotics, is in keeping with this hypothesis. On the other hand, 'atypical' antipsychotics such as clozapine, which have additional pharmacological properties, may be effective where typical antipsychotics

have failed. Furthermore, traditional antipsychotic agents have little effect upon the 'negative' symptoms of schizophrenia. Thus it is important to recognise that although the 'dopamine hypothesis' might help to explain some of the therapeutic effects of antipsychotics, it does not in itself explain the pathophysiology of schizophrenia.

## Conventional antipsychotics

### Mechanism

Conventional antipsychotics act as competitive antagonists of dopamine (particularly $D_2$) receptors in the central nervous system and compete for dopamine binding sites *in vitro*. Although all have similar efficacy, they show a range of other pharmacological properties that might contribute to their therapeutic effects and which are also of importance in determining the profile of adverse effects for any individual drug.

1 Muscarinic blockade causing anticholinergic activity is considerable with thioridazine and much less with fluphenazine and haloperidol.

2 $\alpha_1$-Adrenoceptor blockade is prominent with chlorpromazine and thioridazine and less so with fluphenazine.

3 Histaminergic ($H_1$) blockade results in sedation most commonly with chlorpromazine and thioridazine.

4 Dopaminergic blockade is greater with 'high-potency' drugs such as haloperidol. This is also closely linked to propensity for adverse extrapyramidal (Parkinsonian) side effects (EPS).

EPS may need to be controlled by reduction in the dose of antipsychotic or temporary co-administration of anticholinergic drugs such as procylidine, trihexyphenidyl (benzhexol), orphenadrine or benzatropine (benztropine) (see 'Movement disorders', Chapter 17).

## Pharmacokinetics

Chlorpromazine, the prototype antipsychotic, is absorbed orally and metabolised by the liver to many active and inactive metabolites. It has a plasma half-life of over 16 h that, together with the long-lived active metabolites, makes once-daily dosing practical although rarely used. No clearcut therapeutic range can be defined because of the presence of unmeasured active metabolites and a wide range of individual responses in patients. Plasma or urine drug levels are only of help in assessing compliance. First-pass metabolism is immense, of the order of 80%, making intramuscular administration considerably more potent than the oral alternative.

## Adverse reactions

Dose-related adverse reactions from known pharmacological properties include those listed below.

## Clinical use and dose

Chlorpromazine: orally 75–300 mg daily, increasing up to 1 g gradually if required. Chlorpromazine: intramuscular injection, 25–50 mg 6- to 8-hourly as required to control acute symptoms. Haloperidol: orally 1.5–3 mg, 2–3 times daily with doses of up to 120 mg daily in treatment resistant cases.

Antipsychotics administered in lower doses are used in nausea and vomiting (see 'Nausea and vomiting', Chapter 13), hiccough, vertigo and labyrinthine disturbances, and during drug withdrawal reactions. They are also widely used as pre-medication in anaesthesia (see 'General anaesthesia', Chapter 15). Other psychiatric indications are mentioned above.

## Atypical antipsychotics

These include clozapine, risperidone, olanzapine, quetiapine, zotepine and amisulpride. They differ from conventional antipsychotics (and from each other) in their pattern of receptor binding, e.g. clozapine has affinity for 5-hydroxytryptamine (5-HT) and $D_4$ receptors in addition to the more conventional sites listed above. All atypicals share

---

**Adverse effects of conventional antipsychotics**

Dose-related adverse reactions from known pharmacological properties
**1** Extrapyramidal side effects, caused by dopamine receptor blockade, including: (i) acute dystonia; (ii) parkinsonism; (iii) akathisia; and (iv) tardive dyskinesia—involuntary choreoathetoid movements which, unlike other EPS, may persist even after withdrawal of the antipsychotic drug. Tardive dyskinesia may be aggravated by anticholinergic drugs and treatment is generally unsatisfactory. Benzodiazepines, diazepam and clonazepam may be helpful
**2** Increased prolactin (also resulting from dopaminergic blockade), e.g. galactorrhoea, infertility and impotence
**3** Anticholinergic effects, e.g. blurred vision, constipation, urinary hesitancy, dry mouth, tachycardia or arrhythmias
**4** $\alpha_1$–Adrenoceptor blockade, e.g. postural hypotension
**5** Histamine$_1$–receptor blockade, e.g. sedation
**6** Antipsychotic malignant syndrome (potentially fatal hyperthermia, muscle rigidity and autonomic dysfunction)
**7** Hypothermia in the elderly
**8** Other adverse effects such as confusion, nightmares and insomnia and weight gain

Hypersensitivity reactions not related to dose
**1** Cholestatic jaundice with portal infiltration occurs in 2–4% of patients, usually early in treatment. It presents the biochemical features of cholestasis and resolves slowly on drug withdrawal
**2** Agranulocytosis (rare)
**3** Skin rashes, including photosensitivity dermatitis and urticaria may occur

a reduced propensity to cause EPS (most importantly tardive dyskinesia). Claims have been made for their effectiveness in treating negative symptoms but only clozapine has been demonstrated clearly to be superior to conventional antipsychotics in treatment-resistant patients.

Other adverse effects of atypicals include weight gain (most commonly with clozapine, olanzapine and quetiapine) and sedation. Clozapine may cause agranulocytosis and prescription is restricted initially to hospital patients who can be provided with weekly blood monitoring.

## Depot antipsychotics

Long-acting depot antipsychotic preparations play an important part in the community maintenance of more disabled and therefore poorly compliant psychiatric patients. A number of different antipsychotics are used in this way. Commonly used examples are fluphenazine and flupentixol (flupenthixol). Fluphenazine is a phenothiazine derivative. As the decanoate or enanthate ester it can be given as a depot by intramuscular injection at intervals of 14–40 days. Adverse effects of fluphenazine are similar to those of chlorpromazine but sedation and anticholinergic adverse effects are less common. EPS are correspondingly more common, particularly dystonia and akathisia or restlessness. Liver and bone marrow toxicity and skin rashes have been reported, as with most other phenothiazines. Flupentixol is a thioxanthine, and as such is somewhat less sedating than other classes of antipsychotic. It is more likely to cause EPS.

### Dose

Fluphenazine decanoate: 25–100 mg by injection into the gluteal muscles every 15–40 days, determined by response and side effects. A test dose (12.5 mg) should be given when treatment is begun, to assess possible extrapyramidal reactions.

Flupentixol decanoate: 40–400 mg (test dose 20 mg) similarly administered.

*Comment.* Antipsychotic drugs play a central role in the initial treatment and long-term management of psychoses. The dose should be determined individually from response and adverse effects. Novel drugs (with the exception of clozapine) are increasingly prescribed now as first-choice interventions. Ineffectiveness after a minimum of 6 weeks treatment on any one drug should result in a trial of a second drug of a different class. Clozapine should be considered if there is lack of response to two antipsychotics. Depot intramuscular preparations are useful for long-term outpatient management. Adverse effects are common and may be disabling or even dangerous. Patients on long-term antipsychotic medication should remain under close medical supervision.

Antipsychotics should not be used in the management of simple anxiety as an alternative to anxiolytics, minor tranquillisers or other forms of treatment.

## Antidepressants

### Aims

The main aims are to relieve symptoms of depression, restore normal social behaviour and prevent further episodes.

### Relevant pathophysiology

Depression is common in all populations. Its prevalence is increasing worldwide and it is anticipated to become the second commonest cause of global morbidity (after ischaemic heart disease) by 2020. Pathological feelings of sadness and despair may be associated with physical and emotional withdrawal. Depressive illnesses are a common factor in suicide.

Major depression is characterised by low mood and anhedonia (loss of pleasure). Other key symptoms include psychomotor changes, cognitive impairment and changes in sleep, appetite and weight. Psychotic symptoms, such as delusions of unworthiness, may also occur. Episodes may be recurrent (unipolar depression) or alternate with mania (bipolar affective disorder).

A range of drugs, including sedatives, steroids, opiates and the antihypertensive methyldopa may cause depressive symptoms. The causative drug should be withdrawn if possible.

The neurobiological basis of depression is thought to involve underactivity of central neuronal pathways where noradrenaline or serotonin act as transmitters. This amine hypothesis is supported by biochemical measurement of these transmitters and their metabolites *in vivo* in cerebrospinal fluid and in brain tissue at post-mortem, and from neuroendocrine evidence of abnormal aminergic neurotransmission in depressed patients. There is further support from the therapeutic actions of drugs that modify amine turnover. It is currently thought that mona-aminergic change is the beginning of a molecular cascade in depression. Most modern antidepressants are concerned with aminergic reuptake inhibition. As a result of this there is associated pre-synaptic autoregulatory desensitisation, up- and down-regulation of post-synaptic receptor sites, receptor-mediated second messenger and neurotrophic intracellular signalling effects.

Monoamine oxidase inhibitors (MAOIs) block the intrasynaptic breakdown of noradrenaline and serotonin and thus increase transmitter activity.

Tricyclic antidepressants block neuronal reuptake (uptake 1) of noradrenaline and/or serotonin into noradrenergic/serotonergic neurones, altering transmitter levels in the synaptic cleft.

The SSRIs selectively inhibit the reuptake of serotonin.

Other 'atypical' antidepressants influence noradrenergic and/or serotonergic neurotransmission in a variety of other ways.

*Comment.* The diagnosis of depression is complicated by frequent non-specific somatic symptoms of anorexia, malaise, weight loss and constipation. Conversely, the symptoms of depression often accompany non-psychiatric physical illness and understandably depressing adjustments such as bereavement. Nevertheless, pathological depression is common, responsive to drug treatment and therefore important to identify and treat appropriately. Suicide is a serious and well-recognised complication of depression.

## Tricyclic antidepressants

### Mechanism

This group of drugs includes the closely related agents amitriptyline, nortriptyline, imipramine and clomipramine. They competitively block neuronal uptake of noradrenaline and serotonin into nerve endings and in the short term increase transmitter levels in the synaptic cleft. In the long term these agents lead to down-regulation of pre- and post-synaptic adrenoceptors and serotonin receptors in the brain.

All tricyclics have a range of other pharmacological properties that may contribute to their therapeutic actions and adverse effects:
1 $\alpha_1$–Adrenoceptor blockade
2 Anticholinergic effects
3 Antihistaminergic effects
4 Other non-specific sedative actions.

The therapeutic response to tricyclics develops over 3–4 weeks. Suicide by overdose of antidepressant is a risk during this lag period during treatment. There is some evidence that long-term tricyclic treatment is superior to placebo in reducing the frequency of recurrent depressive symptoms. Amitriptyline, which has more sedative properties, may be useful in agitated depression or where insomnia is troublesome. Imipramine, with less sedative properties, is indicated in those who have marked motor retardation.

### Pharmacokinetics

Tricyclics are extensively metabolised by the liver. The half-life of amitriptyline is >24 h and the formation of metabolites with antidepressant activity further extends the duration of drug activity. Once-daily dosing, ideally at night, is indicated for most tricyclics.

Hepatic metabolism of tricyclics is determined by genetic and environmental factors. There are wide differences in plasma level when the same dose is given to a group of individuals. Thus the dose of tricyclic should be titrated individually, with therapeutic response or adverse effects as end points.

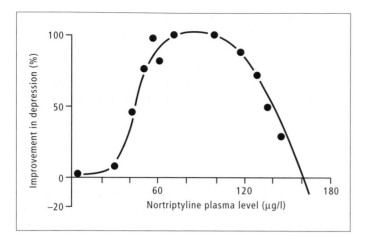

**Figure 16.1** Relationship between drug plasma level and effect with nortriptyline.

Studies with nortriptyline have shown an unusual relationship between drug plasma level and effect (Fig. 16.1). At low drug levels and also at high drug levels there is little effect, while optimal effect is seen within a very narrow concentration range (50–150 µg/l) or therapeutic window. This has led some to propose drug level monitoring as a guide to antidepressant therapy, but this is not routine clinical practice.

## Adverse effects (box below)

## Clinical use and dose

As the many side effects can limit compliance, it is often prudent to begin with a relatively low dose and titrate upwards to a therapeutic dose over a period of 1–2 weeks: 25–75 mg orally, titrated to 100–200 mg daily. Imipramine may also be useful in nocturnal enuresis and hyperactivity syndrome in childhood. Amitriptyline is also used in some forms of neurogenic pain.

## Other related antidepressants

Monocyclic, bicyclic and tetracyclic drugs have been developed with similar therapeutic properties to the tricyclics

## SSRIs

Drugs in this group include fluoxetine, fluvoxamine, paroxetine, sertraline and citalopram

## Mechanism

These drugs inhibit the reuptake of serotinin 5-HT into neurones in the central nervous system.

## Pharmacokinetics

SSRIs have good oral bioavailability and are eliminated by liver metabolism. They have long half-lives (e.g. fluoxetine 2 days) and can be given once daily.

## Adverse effects

SSRIs have the same *incidence* of adverse effects as the tricyclics but the nature of these effects is

---

**Adverse effects of tricyclics**

**1** Sedation and confusional states, especially with amitriptyline
**2** Anticholinergic effects, e.g. dry mouth, constipation, urinary symptoms, sexual dysfunction and precipitation of glaucoma
**3** Postural hypotension, especially in the very young and old
**4** Cardiac tachyarrhythmias (seen in overdose) and conduction defects that are quinidine/procainamide-like. May occur more frequently in patients treated with long-term tricyclics
**5** Self-poisoning by tricyclic overdose is common and its management is discussed further in Chapter 20 (see 'The management of specific complications')
**6** Fits may occur on withdrawal of tricyclics

different: nausea, diarrhoea, headache, insomnia and agitation are the main problems. They are less sedative than tricyclics and safer in overdose. Those with shorter half-lives should be withdrawn slowly—a discontinuance syndrome is recognised. SSRIs increase the levels of carbamazepine, phenytoin, MAOIs (2 weeks should elapse between treatments and 5 weeks in the case of fluoxetine), benzodiazepines, lithium and possibly warfarin.

*Comment.* Tricyclic antidepressants and SSRIs have similar efficacy but a different range of side effects. The main significance of SSRIs is that they have much reduced toxicity in overdose.

## Monoamine oxidase inhibitors

### Mechanism

Phenelzine, tranylcypromine and iproniazid are non-competitive irreversible antagonists of monoamine oxidase (MAO). They block MAO type A, in contrast to selegiline, which is described in Chapter 17. The enzyme is blocked not only in brain monoamine neurones but also in peripheral neurones, enterocytes in the gut wall and platelets. Inhibition of MAO leads to increases in serotonin, noradrenaline and dopamine in the brain.

The problems with MAOIs result from widespread enzyme inhibition, and as a result other drug treatments for depression have been favoured. There are now reversible MAOIs, such as moclobemide, which promise a safer alternative. Apart from therapeutic failure with other antidepressants, indication for the use of MAOIs include phobic states and 'agitated' depression.

When used, the response may be delayed for 2–3 weeks. After the use of irreversible MAOIs the enzyme recovers slowly (2–3 weeks) after the drug is stopped, as it requires re-synthesis. This problem does not accompany the use of reversible MAOIs.

### Adverse effects

1 Postural hypotension
2 Headache

3 Anticholinergic side effects
4 Drug-induced liver damage (phenelzine and isocarboxazid)
5 Hypertensive crisis.

The most important adverse effect is hypertensive crisis following amine-containing foods, beverages or drugs. Inhibition of MAO in the gut wall allows absorption of tyramine and other sympathomimetic substances in food or drink. MAO usually metabolises these to inactive products during absorption. The amines are taken up from the circulation by peripheral sympathetic nerve endings. They displace endogenous noradrenaline from storage sites (indirect sympathomimetic action) leading to hypertension, tachycardia and headache.

Severe paroxysmal hypertension may cause a cerebrovascular accident. Foods rich in tyramine, particularly cheese, meat, yeast extract and red wine, should be avoided.

*Comment.* The dangers of hypertension, the limitations on food intake and the availability of alternatives have greatly reduced the role of MAOIs in depression. They are rarely used as first line agents.

## Other antidepressants

### Mianserin

A tetracyclic compound with sedative properties and low cardiotoxicity. Blood dyscrasias can occur in patients (particularly the elderly) treated with this drug. A 30–60 mg daily dose is given at bedtime, increasing if necessary and if tolerated to 200 mg daily.

### Nefazodone

Causes 5-HT reuptake inhibition and 5-HT$_2$ blockade. The commonest side effects of nausea and restlessness can be minimised by building up the dose gradually to an optimal range of 300–600 mg daily. There is a beneficial effect on sleep.

### Venlafaxine

A combined serotonin and noradrenaline reuptake inhibitor (SNRI) but without the anticholinergic and sedative effects commonly seen with the tricyclics. Dosage should be 75 mg daily or greater and a once-daily slow-release form is available. The most frequent side effect is nausea, usually resolving after a week, but blood-pressure elevation may occur at higher doses.

## Mirtazepine

Termed a 'noradrenergic and specific serotonergic antidepressant' this drug has a novel action in enhancing noradrenaline and (indirectly) serotonin transmission by blocking pre-synaptic $\alpha_2$-adrenergic receptors. It also causes $5-HT_2$- and $5-HT_3$-receptor blockade, minimising serotonergic side effects. Dose range is 15–45 mg, with sedation more prominent at lower doses.

## Reboxetine

Specifically causing noradrenaline reuptake inhibition, reboxetine is administered in a dose range of 4–12 mg daily. Claims have been made for its greater effect on social functioning. Dry mouth is the commonest side effect.

## Mood stabilising agents

### Relevant pathophysiology

Mania and hypomania are characterised by a pathologically elevated mood and disinhibited behaviour. They usually occur as part of a bipolar affective (manic depressive) disorder. Mania is characterised by elated mood and irritability with motor over-activity, non-stop talk, flight of ideas, grandiosity and a progressive lack of contact with reality.

Treatment of an acute manic episode includes sedation with haloperidol or other major tranquillisers, together with general supportive measures. Specific therapy with lithium salts is used both in the acute attack (the main disadvantage to its use as sole agent being its delayed onset of effect) and for prophylaxis between attacks. Lithium is also now recognised to have a place in the prophylaxis against recurring depressive disorder and as

adjunctive therapy in antidepressant-resistant depression. The anticonvulsants carbamazepine and sodium valproate are also used as prophylactic agents in bipolar disorder.

## Lithium carbonate

### Mechanism

The monovalent lithium cation, given as the carbonate salt, modifies the effect in mania. The mechanism of action of lithium is not clear. It appears to substitute for sodium and potassium cations in cellular transport processes. It has effects on the release of monoamine neurotransmitters and alters intracellular and extracellular ion concentrations, fluxes across excitable membranes and the concentrations of 'second messengers' such as inositol phosphate. Lithium may take several days to achieve its effect.

### Pharmacokinetics

Lithium is rapidly and completely absorbed after oral dosing. It is not metabolised and is excreted unchanged by the kidney with a half-life of 12 h. Lithium is distributed in total body water, and it slowly enters cells and reaches steady-state levels after dosing for 5 days. There is a narrow therapeutic range for lithium (0.5–1.0 mmol/l, with higher levels sometimes used in acute mania), with severe adverse effects occurring at higher levels. Monitoring of drug levels in plasma is essential for optimal control of therapy (Chapter 2, p. 18). Change in renal function is the most important factor modifying elimination and thus plasma levels. Lithium clearance is 0.2 times the creatinine clearance, and the dose must be modified in the presence of renal impairment and in the elderly. The sodium and potassium status of the patient also influences lithium levels and response. Thus dehydration, salt depletion or diuretic therapy all tend to increase the plasma drug concentration.

> **Adverse effects of lithium carbonate**
>
> **1** Nausea and vomiting
> **2** Drowsiness, confusion and fits
> **3** Ataxia, nystagmus and dysarthria
> **4** Hypothyroidism by interference with iodination; rarely hyperthyroidism
> **5** Oedema and weight gain
> **6** Nephrogenic diabetes insipidus

## Adverse effects (see above)

These are more common and severe when the plasma lithium level exceeds 1.2 mmol/l or in the presence of salt depletion or diuretic therapy.

## Drug interactions

Lithium levels rise following the introduction of diuretics. Other drugs altering sodium balance (e.g. steroids, ACE inhibitors) may have the same effect. Lithium potentiates the neurotoxicity of haloperidol and flupentixol. Owing to the wide range of further possible interactions, always check carefully before administering another drug with lithium.

## Dose

Lithium carbonate: 0.4–2.0 g daily in divided doses, depending on renal function and drug plasma levels achieved.

## Other mood stabilisers

### Carbamazepine

This commonly used anticonvulsant is an effective treatment both for acute mania and as prophylaxis in bipolar disorder. Trials suggest that its prophylactic effect is less marked than lithium and so should be reserved for those where lithium is contraindicated or has proven ineffective. There is an uncertain relationship between blood levels and treatment response. A dose of 600–800 mg should be aimed for, depending on response and side effects.

### Sodium valproate

While there is not as much evidence available for valproate, what there is suggests effectiveness in treatment of acute mania and prophylaxis of bipolar disorder. Blood levels above 45 mg/l are associated with response but side effects are prominent at levels above 100 mg/l.

## Antipsychotic drugs

Haloperidol and other antipsychotic major tranquillisers have long been used in the management of acute mania. Symptoms are controlled, but it is not clear whether the duration of the manic episode is reduced. These drugs are useful in the treatment of acute attacks.

Haloperidol or chlorpromazine have been used successfully and may be used either alone or in combination with lithium carbonate so long as the dose of haloperidol does not exceed 15 mg/day and the plasma lithium concentration does not exceed 0.8 mmol/l. For adverse effects, see 'Epilepsy' in Chapter 17.

*Comment.* Lithium carbonate is used for long-term prophylaxis in bipolar affective disorder and recurring depressive illness, and it is used together with phenothiazines for control of symptoms in acute attacks. The daily dose of lithium depends on renal function and should be determined individually. Monitoring of lithium plasma levels is essential for optimal treatment without unacceptable adverse effects.

Carbamazepine and valproate may be more effective in lithium-resistant cases (e.g. rapid-cycling affective disorder, mania with depressive symptoms) and combinations of any two of the three mood stabilisers may be more effective than monotherapy.

## Anxiolytics

### Aim

The aim is to control symptoms of anxiety without interfering with normal physical or mental function.

## Relevant pathophysiology

The experience of anxiety, with physical and psychological symptoms, is a universal phenomenon. Furthermore, better defined and clearly morbid anxiety disorders such as agoraphobia are amongst mankind's commonest seriously disabling conditions. As a result there has always been widespread and excessive use of whatever anxiolytic agents are available. Since the introduction of chlordiazepoxide in 1960, the anxiolytic benzodiazepines have become the most widely prescribed group of drugs in the United Kingdom and in the United States (15–20% of the population at any one time). Medical practitioners, conditioned to 'treat', often find it extremely difficult to resist demands for a pill to relieve anxiety even though such problems invariably require other forms of intervention.

The principal groups of drugs used in the management of anxiety are the benzodiazepines, the β-receptor blockers and recently developed agents affecting 5-HT systems. There is also growing interest in the use of imipramine and SSRIs in the treatment of patients with panic attacks, the use of serotonergic agents in the treatment of patients with obsessional or compulsive disorders and the use of MAOIs in the treatment of certain phobic conditions.

*Comment.* Anxiety in appropriate circumstances is a normal response. If anxiety symptoms are frequent or persist in a severe form, they may interfere with normal function. Such pathological anxiety is an indication for assessment and appropriate treatment, which might include a pharmacological agent.

## Benzodiazepines

### Mechanism

Benzodiazepines have a relatively selective action on the limbic system, cerebral cortex and the ascending amine systems that govern arousal. They potentiate gamma-aminobutyric acid (GABA) transmission. The identification of specific binding sites for benzodiazepines has led to speculation that these 'receptors' are normally present to be activated by an, as yet, unidentified 'endogenous benzodiazepine', deficient in anxiety states. Clear proof of this has yet to emerge.

The amnesic action of benzodiazepines is useful in addition to sedation for use as pre-medication for minor investigative procedures like gastroscopy and bronchoscopy.

The benzodiazepines currently available range from very short-acting drugs such as flurazepam or temazepam, which are used as hypnotics, to longer-acting agents such as diazepam, chlordiazepoxide and oxazepam, which are most useful as anxiolytics. Variations in pharmacokinetics and metabolism are responsible for these differences.

## Pharmacokinetics

Diazepam is rapidly absorbed from the gastrointestinal tract and extensively metabolised by oxidation in the liver. It forms several active metabolites, including oxazepam, which is used therapeutically in its own right. The plasma half-life is long (24 h) and its duration of effect even longer, as the active metabolites have half-lives of several days. The half-life may be increased in the elderly, who may also be more sensitive to the drug.

Oxazepam is an active metabolite of diazepam. It is cleared by conjugation in the liver and has a half-life of 10–20 h.

Chlordiazepoxide was one of the earlier benzodiazepines. It is still used as an anxiolytic, and is the drug of choice in serious alcohol withdrawal states.

## Adverse effects

Benzodiazepines are drugs of dependence. The risk of physical dependence is apparently greater with short-acting agents. Prescriptions should be limited to short-term use (no longer than 6 weeks) and in the case of anxiety only if the condition is severely disabling.

Other adverse effects are listed below.

## Adverse effects of benzodiazepines

**1** Drowsiness, agitation, ataxia and lightheadedness, especially in the elderly
**2** Incontinence, nightmares and confusion
**3** Excessive salivation
**4** Changes in libido
**5** Respiratory depression, hypotension
**6** Impaired alertness with motor and intellectual dysfunction, e.g. driving, operating machinery
**7** Paradoxical stimulant effects in some violent patients
**8** Disinhibition can lead to suicidal behaviour
**9** Withdrawal can be associated with rebound increased agitation, hallucinations and epileptic seizures
**10** Thrombophlebitis may follow intravenous diazepam
**11** Psychological adjustment to bereavement may be inhibited by benzodiazepines

**Table 16.2** Anxiolytic drugs and dose range used.

| Drug | Group | Dose (mg) |
|---|---|---|
| Chlordiazepoxide | | 75–100 |
| Diazepam | | 4–30 |
| Lorazepam | Benzodiazepines | 1–10 |
| Medazepam | | 10–30 |
| Oxazepam | | 30–120 |
| Propranolol | Beta-blocker | 40 (when need anticipated) |
| Buspirone | $5\text{-}HT_{1a}$-receptor agonist | 15–30 |

## Drug interactions

Benzodiazepines have additive or synergistic effects with other centrally acting drugs—antihistamines, alcohol, barbiturates. This may increase the impairment of motor or intellectual function or worsen respiratory depression.

Diazepam and chlordiazepoxide do not interfere with the metabolism of other drugs and do not interact with warfarin.

## Clinical use and dose

Benzodiazepines are appropriate in the short-term management (2–4 weeks) of severe disabling anxiety. Chlordiazepoxide is the treatment of choice in severe alcohol withdrawal states including delirium tremens.

Diazepam: orally, 4–30 mg daily in divided doses titrated to control symptoms and continued only as long as is necessary; intramuscularly or slow intravenous injection, 10 mg repeated after 4–6 h if required. Diazepam is used as a sedative in acutely agitated hospitalised patients or as pre-medication before minor procedures.

Comparable doses of the benzodiazepines are shown in Table 16.2.

*Comment.* Use the lowest possible dose.

The use of benzodiazepines to treat mild anxiety is unjustifiable. Long-term use is to be avoided. If a patient has taken a benzodiazepine for a long time, the drug should be withdrawn slowly, at a rate determined by the severity of the withdrawal syndrome.

## Other drug treatment of anxiety

### β-Receptor blockers

β-Receptor blockers reduce cardiovascular and other β-receptor mediated effects of increased sympathetic activity. Most experience has been acquired with propranolol, a non-selective beta-blocker. Their value in the treatment of morbid anxiety is limited but occasional use in patients disabled by performance anxiety can be of value. The clinical pharmacology and adverse effects of beta-blockers are discussed in Chapter 6. Beta-blockers should be used with caution in patients with a past history of asthma, peripheral vascular disease, cardiac failure or bradyarrhythmias.

### Dose

Propranolol: 40 mg before a predictably anxiety-provoking situation.

### Serotonergic agents

Buspirone is a $5\text{-}HT_{1a}$ receptor agonist for which reasonable evidence of clinical efficacy exists. It does not appear to interact with the same receptors as the benzodiazepines, but early claims of freedom from physical dependence should be treated with caution.

## Clomethiazole

Clomethiazole has few advantages over benzo-diazepines, and prolonged use may lead to dependence and severe respiratory depression can occur.

## Tricyclic antidepressants, SSRIs and MAOIs

Imipramine and SSRIs have a part to play in the treatment of patients disabled by recurrent panic attacks. SSRIs and clomipramine are used in the treatment of obsessive-compulsive disorder, and MAOIs used in the treatment of certain phobic disorders. Their effects are probably a result of long-term changes in central noradrenergic and/or serotonergic activity. Optimal treatment of such patients also involves an appropriate psychological intervention. Use of these agents depends upon careful assessment of the clinical problem and requires specialised advice.

*Comment.* Anxiety symptoms should only be treated with drugs if they are severe and interfere with the patient's lifestyle or if alternative social or psychotherapy is not possible or appropriate. Treatment should be regularly revised and stopped as soon as possible. Benzodiazepines are effective but beta-blockers may be an alternative, with fewer dependence problems and less abuse potential. The treatment of more severely disabled patients with anxiety disorder may benefit from one of the various noradrenergic or serotonergic agents traditionally used in the treatment of depression, but such use should be restricted to specialised services.

## Hypnotic drugs and the treatment of insomnia

### Aim

By short-term use the aim is to restore normal restful sleep without a residual hangover the next day and to aid a return to normal sleep without drugs.

## Relevant pathophysiology

Insomnia is an interference with the quality or quantity of sleep and is a very common complaint. Insomnia is a subjective symptom and reflects what the patient considers to be the 'normal' length and quality of sleep. Individuals vary in their expectation of sleep. Requirements for sleep may vary and diminish with advancing age. A reduced duration of total sleep is common in the elderly and may not be pathological.

The treatment of sleep disorders requires:
1 Assessment of the type of sleep disorder
2 Assessment of accompanying symptoms of anxiety or depression and their treatment
3 Diagnosis and treatment of other physical symptoms interfering with sleep, e.g. pain, nocturnal dyspnoea or urinary frequency
4 Consideration of non-pharmacological strategies, including changes in lifestyle. Simple measures like bathing, exercising or enriched milk drinks at bedtime may help.

Drug treatment should be offered only when the alternatives given above have been excluded, and where there is evidence of frequent and marked sleep impairment. Hypnotics should ideally be used for short periods of days or weeks when required, and not given for regular long-term use.
*Comment.* A successful hypnotic should act rapidly, allow the subject to wake if necessary without severe sedation and be free from residual hangover effects in the morning. Unfortunately, few of the available agents meet these criteria.

## Benzodiazepines

### Mechanism

Benzodiazepines exert hypnotic effects by similar mechanisms to their anxiolytic actions but at higher doses. At the peak of drug action, in

**Table 16.3** Benzodiazepine hypnotic drugs.

| Drug | Plasma half-life (h) | Active metabolite |
|------|----------------------|-------------------|
| Nitrazepam | 20+ | None |
| Flurazepam | 2–4 | Yes, with long half-life |
| Temazepam | 5–6 | None |

addition to the anxiolytic effect, the drugs affect brain arousal systems by potentiating the inhibitory effects of GABA.

Nitrazepam, flurazepam and temazepam are widely used (Table 16.3). They induce sleep within 20–40 min of dosing and produce sleep with a reduction in deep sleep (stage 4) and a reduction in rapid eye movement (REM) sleep.

Residual hangover effects with cumulative adverse reactions in chronic dosing may occur with nitrazepam and flurazepam, which have a long half-life and an active metabolite, respectively.

Temazepam appears to have the advantage of a short half-life and no active metabolites. Residual impairment is less with temazepam than with other benzodiazepines.

### Adverse effects

Benzodiazepines are drugs of dependence. Particular problems relevant to their use as hypnotics include oversedation (especially in the elderly), 'hangover' effect, paradoxical agitation, and withdrawal phenomena including rebound insomnia, vivid dreams and fits.

### Clinical use and dose

Benzodiazepines are indicated in the short-term management of severe, disabling insomnia.
Temazepam: 10–30 mg 30 min
Nitrazepam: 5–10 mg before going to bed
Flurazepam: 15–30 mg at bedtime
*Comment.* Hypnotic drugs should only be used for short periods of time. They should certainly not be prescribed without very careful thought. Other

physical, psychiatric and social factors may well require attention.

## Drug-induced psychiatric disorder

Central nervous system adverse effects of drugs are common, especially in the case of lipid-soluble drugs with specific effects on:
1 Receptors
2 Transmitter synthesis
3 Degradation of transmitters
4 Electrophysiological effects on excitable membranes.

A careful history of recent drug ingestion is an essential feature of the evaluation of a patient with psychiatric illness and, where possible, the first step in the management of drug-induced psychiatric symptoms should be withdrawal of the offending drug.

There are many well-documented examples of drugs causing behavioural adverse effects, and these are summarised in Table 16.4.

## Abuse of psychoactive drugs

Abuse of drugs and related agents is a major social problem amongst young people, especially in urban communities. Therapeutic drug use may also lead to dependence, e.g. benzodiazepines used for anxiety or insomnia, or opiate analgesic abuse in patients first treated for chronic severe pain. However, the concept of drug misuse or abuse must be judged in a cultural and historical context. Attitudes to the non-therapeutic use of cannabis and even opiates differ greatly throughout the world.

The problems of drug abuse are:
1 The direct specific toxic effects, e.g. respiratory depression with opiates
2 Generalised actions on mood, disinhibition of social behaviour and impaired level of consciousness
3 Short-term consequences of drug withdrawal, e.g. psychological and physical symptoms of dependence
4 Long-term medical complications of the contemporary drug 'subculture', e.g. hepatitis,

**Table 16.4** Drug-induced psychiatric disorder.

<table>
<tr><td colspan="3" align="center">Depression</td></tr>
<tr><td>Antihypertensives</td><td>Steroids</td><td></td></tr>
<tr><td>Methyldopa</td><td>Corticosteroids</td><td></td></tr>
<tr><td>Clonidine</td><td>Oral contraceptive pill</td><td></td></tr>
<tr><td>Reserpine</td><td></td><td></td></tr>
<tr><td>Propranolol</td><td>Analgesics</td><td></td></tr>
<tr><td>Guanethidine</td><td>Opiates</td><td></td></tr>
<tr><td>Non-steroidal anti-inflammatory drugs</td><td></td><td></td></tr>
<tr><td>Sedatives</td><td></td><td></td></tr>
<tr><td>Benzodiazepines</td><td>Others</td><td></td></tr>
<tr><td>Alcohol</td><td>Levodopa</td><td>Cimetidine</td></tr>
<tr><td>Barbiturates</td><td>Tetrabenazine</td><td>Triamcinolone</td></tr>
<tr><td></td><td>Methysergide</td><td>Mefloquine</td></tr>
<tr><td>Antipsychotics</td><td></td><td></td></tr>
<tr><td>Phenothiazines and other antipsychotics</td><td></td><td></td></tr>
<tr><td colspan="3" align="center">Psychotic states</td></tr>
<tr><td colspan="3">Sympathomimetics (amfetamine (amphetamine))<br>and the amfetamine-derived 'designer' drug Ecstasy<br>Anticholinergic drugs (atropine, trihexyphenidyl (benzhexol))<br>Levodopa and dopamine agonists (bromocriptine, apomorphine)<br>Steroids (prednisolone, dexamethasone)<br>Phencyclidine (PCP: 'angel dust')<br>Cannabis</td></tr>
<tr><td colspan="3" align="center">Anxiety and anxiety symptoms</td></tr>
<tr><td colspan="3">Sympathomimetics (amfetamine, ephedrine, phenylpropanolamine, etc.)<br>$\beta_2$-Adrenoceptor agonists (isoprenaline, salbutamol, terbutaline)</td></tr>
<tr><td colspan="3" align="center">Drug-withdrawal states</td></tr>
<tr><td colspan="3">Benzodiazepines, clonidine, barbiturates, opiates and alcohol</td></tr>
</table>

septicaemia, acquired immunodeficiency syndrome (AIDS) and bacterial endocarditis.

Psychoactive drugs, like analgesics or sedatives, have a high potential for abuse because of:

1 *Central effects*. They modify mood or behaviour, leading to either pleasurable experiences, depersonalisation or intoxication and amnesia.

2 *Tolerance*. If there is tolerance to the effect with regular use, and thus a need to increase the dose to get the same effect, then not only is the drug-taking habit reinforced but there is a greater risk of chemical toxicity or adverse effects at the higher doses.

3 *Withdrawal symptoms*. Symptoms on withdrawal of the abused drug further reinforce the need for continued drug use (or abuse). While these withdrawal symptoms may often be psychological, in the case of benzodiazepines, opiates and barbiturates, physical symptoms on withdrawal create further dependence or 'addiction'.

Drugs with a high abuse potential can be divided into:

1 Therapeutic agents:
- Benzodiazepines
- Barbiturates
- Other hypnotics and sedatives
- Opiate analgesics and analogues, including dextropropoxyphene.

2 Non-therapeutic agents ('street' drugs):
- Cannabis
- Cocaine

- Opiates
- Amfetamines (amphetamines); their therapeutic use now is very limited
- LSD, psylocybin, phencyclidine and other hallucinogens
- Solvents
- Alcohol.

The following agents are used in the management of psychoactive substance misuse.

## Benzodiazepines

Their primary use is in the management of severe alcohol withdrawal states, which may present with autonomic overarousal and fits, and delirium tremens. Long-acting compounds such as chlordiazepoxide are preferred and prescribed on a reducing dose regime over 5–7 days. Initial doses are judged on symptom severity and may range from 60 to 160 mg/day. Vitamin supplementation (B$_1$) ought to also be given to minimise risk of amnesic (Wernicke–Korsakoff) syndrome. Vitamin deficiency and malabsorption require high doses to be used.

## Disulfiram

The metabolism of ethanol is blocked by disulfiram, which causes inhibition of ALDH leading to accumulation of acetaldehyde. Symptoms of the alcohol–disulfiram reaction include flushing, tachycardia, headache, nausea, vomiting and hypotension. Rarely, significant medical complications can arise. The practice of patients receiving a test challenge has now been abandoned and disulfiram therefore acts as a deterrent to drinking in patients who are motivated toward abstinence. Enzyme inhibition (and thus potential for reaction) lasts up to 7 days and patients must be warned of potential interactions with alcohol in foods and over-the-counter medications.

## Acamprosate

Acamprosate enhances GABA inhibitory neurotransmission and antagonises glutamate excitation. This is thought to be the mechanism by which it reduces craving for alcohol. It is prescribed in a usual dose of 666 mg three times daily. It should be commenced while abstinent but can be maintained during brief relapses.

## Opiate dependence

May be treated by use of substitute prescribing (methadone) or by drugs that abolish the euphoric effects of opiates (naltrexone). Drugs such as lofexidine are used to minimise symptoms of opiate withdrawal.

*Comment.* The management of drug abuse is not easy and involves:

1 Management of acute pharmacological toxicity
2 Treatment of any acute medical complications, e.g. septicaemia, endocarditis
3 Psychiatric assessment and treatment of any underlying psychopathology, e.g. depression
4 Controlled planned withdrawal of the drug, if necessary, with temporary substitution, e.g. methadone for heroin
5 Long-term measures such as family or community support (Alcoholics Anonymous), psychotherapy or drug therapy (disulfiram for alcoholics).

## Treatment of dementia

### Aim

Traditionally, drugs have been used to minimise behavioural disturbance in dementia. New agents, such as donepezil, stabilise or reverse cognitive decline, albeit temporarily.

### Relevant pathophysiology

Dementia is a chronic, progressive organic brain disorder resulting in memory decline and eventual loss of all aspects of cognitive functioning. A small number of cases are reversible where certain specific aetiologies can be found (e.g. vitamin B$_{12}$ deficiency, normal pressure hydrocephalus, hypothyroidism). The majority, however, are irreversible, the commonest being Alzheimer's disease (and its variant, Lewy Body dementia) and multi-infarct dementia.

Alzheimer's disease is characterised by post-mortem findings of senile plaques, neurofibrillary tangles and reduced neurotransmitter levels, particularly of acetylcholine, the severity of which correlates with neuronal loss. Acetylcholinesterase inhibitors have recently been introduced in the management of mild to moderate Alzheimer's disease. Compounds currently available include donepezil and rivastigmine. They may slow the rate of cognitive and non-cognitive decline in 40% of patients.

## Donepezil

This is prescribed in an initial dose of 5 mg daily, rising to 10 mg/day after 1 month. Side effects, which include nausea, vomiting and diarrhoea, are minimised by careful dose titration.

## Rivastigmine

Similar side effects to donepezil are seen. Rivastigmine is prescribed twice daily in doses of 6–12 mg/day, titrated weekly to maximum tolerated dose.

*Comment.* While drugs may slow cognitive decline, they do not alter ultimate disease progression and, on withdrawal, rapid deterioration may occur, even when no clear response has been seen. This should be explained to patients and their relatives. Baseline assessment of cognitive functioning should precede treatment and patients should be reassessed again at 3 months. If no clear improvement has occurred the drug should be stopped. Other drugs, including antidepressants and antipsychotics are often used to control behavioural disturbance. However, antipsychotics should be avoided if at all possible in patients with Lewy Body dementia, where they may cause severe EPS.

# Chapter 17

# Drugs and neurological disease

## Epilepsy

### Pathophysiology

Epilepsy is recurrent unprovoked seizures. A seizure is a paroxysmal event resulting from abnormal, hypersynchronous discharges of cortical neurones. Convulsions refer to a seizure where motor manifestations predominate. Two major categories of seizures are recognised: generalised seizures and partial seizures. Generalised seizures lead to loss of consciousness and are bilaterally symmetric. In a partial seizure, symptoms begin locally and may progress to a secondary generalised seizure. Common types of primary generalised seizures are grand mal (tonic–clonic), tonic, myoclonic, petit mal (absence) and atonic (akinetic). There are two main types of partial seizures: simple, with no impairment of consciousness, and complex, where consciousness may be altered and patients may have automatism (lip-smacking or aimless walking). An aura is the subjective onset of a minor partial seizure and may appear as olfactory, visual or psychic symptoms. Seizures that occur as the consequence of an identifiable brain pathology (trauma, tumour or infarction) are called secondary or symptomatic epilepsy; all other types of epilepsy are primary. *Generalised status epilepticus* is a medical emergency in which epileptic activity persists for 30 min or more. Other types of *status epilepticus* (including simple partial, complex

partial and absence status epilepticus) are often associated with delayed diagnosis and treatment, but have a much lower risk of morbidity.

### Aim and principles of therapy

In treating epilepsy, the drug chosen needs to be matched to the individual patient and the type of epileptic seizures. A wide range of treatments is currently available and 70–80% of epileptic patients will become seizure-free with appropriate drug therapy.

Sodium valproate is the first choice for generalised seizures; lamotrigine is an alternative. Valproate is also the treatment of choice for juvenile myoclonic epilepsy. For partial seizures, carbamazepine is the first choice; lamotrigine, oxcarbazepine and valproate are alternatives. Ethosuximide is the only available alternative to valproate for petit mal (absence seizures); phenytoin or carbamazepine is ineffective. Clonazepam is usually an adjunct to valproate for treating myoclonic seizures and clobazam is particularly useful for seizures occurring in clusters (e.g. during menstrual periods). Phenobarbital is a cheap and effective treatment for generalised seizures but is currently used only when other treatments fail. Phenobarbital is also the active ingredient in primidone, effective in all types of epilepsy except absence seizures. It is rarely used now.

The therapeutic goal in epilepsy treatment is complete remission of seizures without side effects, using a single drug (monotherapy). Table 17.1 is a list of anti-epileptic drugs with their doses, common side effects and interactions. Most anticonvulsants have important interactions with other drugs, especially those that are highly protein bound or are metabolised by the liver, including other anticonvulsants and oral contraceptives. Interactions between anti-epileptic drugs are complex and may enhance toxicity without a corresponding increase in the anti-epileptic effect. There is good correlation between therapeutic effect and drug level only with phenytoin and to some extent with phenobarbital and carbamazepine; valproate and newer anti-epileptic drugs do not require monitoring of plasma levels. If ineffective, medications should be increased to the maximum tolerated dose on clinical grounds rather than serum levels. Approximately one third of patients will require polytherapy with two or more drugs.

## Newer anti-epileptic drugs

These are expensive. Lamotrigine has entered common usage, especially in adolescents, young women and the elderly, because it is well tolerated, has a favourable cognitive and behavioural profile, does not induce the metabolism of lipid-soluble drugs (such as the oral contraceptive pill) and does not lead to weight gain. Oxcarbazepine is also well tolerated and licensed as monotherapy. Levetiracetam is currently licensed as adjunctive therapy in partial epilepsy with or without secondary generalisation, but is effective as monotherapy and in idiopathic generalised epilepsies, and has the advantage of having no significant drug interactions with other anti-epileptics. Vigabatrin, gabapentin and tiagabine are primarily indicated as add-on therapy for seizures poorly controlled with optimal doses of the conventional first-line therapy. Vigabatrin has been recommended as monotherapy only for infantile spasms (West's syndrome). Experience with felbamate, zonisamide and flunarizine has been largely restricted to trials.

Patients with certain epilepsy syndromes (e.g. temporal lobe epilepsy) refractory to medical therapy will benefit from surgical excision of the seizure focus and could achieve significant reduction or permanent discontinuation of their anti-epileptic drug therapy.

## Anti-epileptic drugs in common use

### Carbamazepine

A tricyclic derivative, it is likely that carbamazepine acts by blocking the neuronal calcium and sodium channels. It is also effective in neuralgia and certain forms of dystonia. It is metabolised in the liver and is a powerful enzyme inducer, inducing its own metabolism so that its elimination half-life falls from an initial 24–48 h following a single dose to 8–12 h on chronic therapy. For this reason, carbamazepine must be started at a low dose (e.g. 100–200 mg once daily in an adult) and then the dose is gradually titrated upwards over several weeks. It is contraindicated in patients with cardiac conduction defects, a history of bone marrow depression and porphyria, and in combination with monoamine oxidase (MAO) inhibitors. A measles-like skin rash is the commonest side effect (5–15%) that may occasionally proceed to erythema multiforme. Patients must be cautioned about the rare idiosyncratic risk of bone marrow suppression (leucopenia and thrombocytopenia) and liver disorders. Other side effects include vestibulo-cerebellar symptoms as a manifestation of acute toxicity, hyponatremia as a consequence of the syndrome of inappropriate antidiuretic hormone (ADH) secretion and a 1% risk of spina bifida in babies exposed in utero. Cognitive and behavioural effects are also recognised. Paradoxic seizures may occur with carbamazepine toxicity. Carbamazepine is available as a suppository for use in small children.

### Valproate

Sodium valproate acts by increasing the level of the inhibitory neurotransmitter gamma-aminobutyric acid (GABA) by a combination of mechanisms that

Table **17.1** Anti-epileptic drugs.

| Generic name | Principal uses | Typical dosage and dosing intervals | Half-life | Therapeutic range | Adverse effects | | Drug interactions |
| --- | --- | --- | --- | --- | --- | --- | --- |
| | | | | | Neurologic | Systemic | |
| Valproic acid | Tonic–clonic absence, atypical absence, myoclonic focal-onset | 750–2000 mg/day (920–60 mg/kg) b.i.d.-q.i.d. | 9–20 h | 50–150 mg/l (400–700 μmol/l) | Ataxia, sedation, tremor | Hepatotoxicity, thrombocytopenia, gastrointestinal irritation, weight gain, transient alopecia, hyperammonaemia | Level decreased by carbamazepine, phenobarbital (phenobarbitone), phenytoin |
| Carbamazepine | Tonic–clonic focal onset | 600–1800 mg/day (15–35 mg/kg, child) b.i.d.-q.i.d. | 12–17 h | 4–12 mg/l (17–42 μmol/l) | Ataxia, dizziness, diplopia, vertigo | Aplastic anaemia, leukopenia, gastrointestinal irritation, hepatotoxicity | Level decreased by erythromycin, propoxyphene isoniazid, cimetidine |
| Phenytoin (diphenylhydantoin) | Tonic–clonic (grand mal), focal-onset | 300–400 mg/day (3–6 mg/kg, adult; 4–8 mg/kg, child) q.i.d.-b.i.d. | 22 h (wide variation. dose-dependent) | 10–20 mg/l (40–80 μmol/l) | Ataxia, incoordination, confusion, cerebellar | Gum, hyperplasia, lymphadenopathy, hirsutism, osteomalacia, facial coarsening, skin rash | Level increased by isoniazid, sulphonamides; level decreased by carbamazepine, phenobarbital; altered folate metabolism *(Continued)* |

**Table 17.1** (*Continued*)

| Generic name | Principal uses | Typical dosage and dosing intervals | Half-life | Therapeutic range | Adverse effects | | Drug interactions |
|---|---|---|---|---|---|---|---|
| | | | | | Neurologic | Systemic | |
| Topiramate | Monotherapy and adjunctive treatment of partial seizures and primary and secondarily generalised tonic–clonic seizures. Adjunctive therapy for Lennox–Gastaut syndrome | 50 mg daily initially (25 mg in children), then slowly increased to 200–400 mg/day b.i.d. | 18–30 h | Not established | Impaired memory and concentration, impaired speech, mood disorder and depression; paresthesia, dizziness, ataxia | Renal calculi, leukopenia, taste disturbance, weight loss, fatigue, asthenia | Accelerated metabolism of contraceptives |
| Phenobarbital | Tonic–clonic focal-onset | 60–180 mg/day (1–4 mg/kg, adult; 3–6 mg/kg, child) q.i.d. | 90 h (70 h in children) | 10–40 mg/l (50–170 μmol/l) | Sedation, ataxia, confusion, dizziness, decreased libido, depression | Skin rash | Level increased by valproic acid, phenytoin. Enhances metabolism of other drugs via liver enzyme induction |
| Primidone | Tonic–clonic focal onset | 750–1000 mg/day (10–25 mg/kg) b.i.d.–t.i.d. | Primidone 8–15 h, phenobarbital, 90 h | Primidone 4–12 mg/l phenobarbital 10–40 mg/l | Same as phenobarbital | Same as phenobarbital | Same as phenobarbital |
| Ethosuximide | Absence (petit mal) | 750–1250 mg/day (20–40 mg/kg) q.d.–b.i.d. | 60 h, adult; 30 h, child | 40–100 mg/l (283–708 μmol/l) | Ataxia, lethargy, headache | Gastrointestinal irritation, skin rash, bone marrow suppression | No known significant interactions |

| Drug | Indications | Dose | Half-life | Therapeutic level | Side effects | | Interactions |
|---|---|---|---|---|---|---|---|
| Gabapentin | Focal-onset | 900–2400 mg/day t.i.d.–q.i.d. | 5–9 h | Not established | Sedation, dizziness, ataxia, fatigue | Gastrointestinal irritation | No known significant interactions |
| Clonazepam | Absence, atypical absence, Myoclonic | 1–12 mg/day (0.1–0.2 mg/kg) q.i.d.–t.i.d. | 18–48 h | 10–70 pg/l | Ataxia, sedation, lethargy | Anorexia | Increased sedation with hypnotics |
| Lamotrigine | Monotherapy and adjunctive treatment of partial seizures and primary and secondarily generalised tonic–clonic seizures, Lennox–Gastaut syndrome | 150–500 mg/day b.i.d. (with enzyme-inducers); 59 h (with valproic acid) | 25 h, 15 h | Not established | Dizziness, diplopia, sedation, ataxia, headache | Skin rash, Stevens–Johnson syndrome | Level decreased by carbamazepine, phenobarbital, phenytoin; level increased by valproic acid |
| Vigabatrin | Monotherapy for infantile spasms (West's syndrome); add-on for focal and secondary generalised seizures | 0.5 g (40 mg/kg in child) starting dose; increased to 2–4 g (100 mg/kg in children and up to 150 mg/kg in West's syndrome) b.i.d. | 12–18 h | Not established | Visual field defects, nystagmus, ataxia, irritability, depression, memory loss, psychoses; excitation in children; rarely photophobia and retinal disorders | Weight gain, oedema, alopecia, gastrointestinal irritation | Level decreased by carbamazepine, phenobarbital |

*(Continued)*

**Table 17.1** (Continued)

| Generic name | Principal uses | Typical dosage and dosing intervals | Half-life | Therapeutic range | Adverse effects | | Drug interactions |
|---|---|---|---|---|---|---|---|
| | | | | | Neurologic | Systemic | |
| Tiagabine | Add-on for focal-onset seizures with or without generalisation | 5 mg initially, increased to 30–45 mg/day, NOT in children | 7–9 h | Not established | Dizziness, tremor, depression, drowsiness, speech and memory problems | Fatigue, leukopenia | No significant interaction |
| Oxcarbazepine | Monotherapy and adjunctive treatment of partial seizures with or without secondarily generalised tonic clonic seizures | 0.6 to 2.4 g daily in divided dosages | 8–10 h | Not established | Diplopia, vertigo, dizziness, ataxia | Leucopenia, Stevens–Johnson Syndrome, hyponatraemia | Sometimes lowers carbamazepine; sometimes increases phenytoin, often increases phenobarbital; accelerates metabolism of oestrogens |
| Levetiracetam | Adjunctive treatment of partial seizures | 1–3 g in divided doses | 6–8 h | Not established | Drowsiness, dizziness, ataxia, depression, tremor | Leucopenia, rash | None |

may involve its accelerated synthesis (induction of glutamic acid decarboxylase) and reduced breakdown (inhibition of GABA-transaminase). It can be used in all forms of epilepsy and also for migraine prophylaxis, neuralgia, chorea and cerebellar tremors. It is well absorbed, extensively protein bound and metabolised in the liver, and thus contraindicated in active liver disease and porphyria. Fatal hepatic failure has occurred especially in children under 3 years of age and those with metabolic or degenerative disorder and those on multiple anti-epileptic drugs for severe seizure disorder, usually in the first 6 months of therapy. Monitoring of liver function tests is recommended before and during the first 6 months of therapy, especially in patients most at risk. Common adverse effects include weight gain, gastric irritation, ataxia, tremors, polycystic ovary-like symptoms in women, rarely pancreatitis, leukopenia and bone marrow depression. An interesting side effect is loss of hair followed by regrowth of curly hair. The risk of spina bifida in babies exposed *in utero* is 2–3%. A parenteral therapy is available for continuation or initiation of valproate treatment when oral therapy is not possible. Some physicians use this preparation in *status epilepticus*.

## Phenytoin

It acts by neuronal membrane stabilisation and blockade of sodium channels. Despite its proven efficacy in tonic–clonic and partial seizures, phenytoin is no longer a first-line therapy because of its narrow therapeutic window and long-term side effects. The relationship between dose and plasma concentration is non-linear; small dosage increases in some patients may produce large rises in plasma concentration at saturation (zero-order) kinetics. Monitoring of plasma concentration is extremely useful with phenytoin. It is also an enzyme inducer and is commonly implicated in drug interaction. Phenytoin is also effective in neuralgia and myotonia. It is unsuitable in adolescent patients as a result of its cosmetic side effects (coarse facies, acne, hirsutism and gingival hyperplasia). It is to be avoided in porphyria and in second degree or complete heart block. Phenytoin is the cause

of a common drug-induced systemic lupus erythematosus (SLE). Concentration-dependent side effects include anorexia, insomnia, nausea, cerebellar symptoms (nystagmus and ataxia), peripheral neuropathy, chorea, obtundation and seizures. Long-term use can cause osteomalacia (vitamin D malabsorbtion), megaloblastic anaemia (folate malabsorbtion), Dupuytren's contracture and generalised lymphadenopathy that may appear indistinguishable from Hodgkin's lymphoma on histology. Rarely, blood dyscrasias (agranulocytosis), hepatitis, skin rash and erythema multiforme are reported.

The parenteral preparation of phenytoin is the first-line therapy in patients with status epilepticus. The injection must only be given intravenously. The injection solution is strongly alkaline and if extravasated, it can cause intense irritation of tissues and in the hands, swelling and discoloration ('purple glove' syndrome). Because of its alkaline pH, phenytoin should not be mixed with solutions with acidic pH, e.g. 5% dextrose in water, which will precipitate the salt (dihydantoin sodium). Rapid intravenous injections may also cause cardiovascular and central nervous system (CNS) depression, heart block, hypotension and respiratory arrest; patients over the age of 50 years are more susceptible. The rate of infusion should not exceed 50 mg/min; resuscitation facilities and a cardiac rhythm monitor must be available.

## Fosphenytoin

Fosphenytoin is a new, water-soluble prodrug of phenytoin that is suitable for intramuscular or intravenous injections. It is more neutral in solution and is better tolerated at infusion sites. It is converted to phenytoin (half-life: 15 min) by nonspecific phosphatases. Doses of fosphenytoin are expressed as phenytoin equivalents (PE), which are the amount of phenytoin released by the prodrug in the presence of phosphatases. Unlike parenteral phenytoin, fosphenytoin is not formulated with propylene glycol that has been implicated in the cardiovascular side effects of intravenous phenytoin. It can be also administered more rapidly at PE doses up to 150 mg/min. Although cardiovascular complications are less likely, cardiac monitoring is still recommended during intravenous infusion.

## Lamotrigine

It acts by blocking the neuronal sodium channels and is effective as monotherapy in partial and generalised seizures. It is well absorbed, fully bioavailable and is metabolised largely as a glucuronide conjugate in the liver. It is contraindicated in hepatic impairment. Elimination half-life of lamotrigine is reduced to around 15 h by the enzyme-inducing anti-epileptic drugs (carbamazepine and phenytoin), whereas sodium valproate inhibits its metabolism and doubles the half-life to nearly 60 h. It must be given at a very low dose (12.5 mg daily or 25 mg every alternate day) with slow weekly dose increment in patients on concomitant valproate therapy. A pharmacodynamic interaction is common when lamotrigine is co-prescribed in patients taking carbamazepine and the symptoms of neurotoxicity (headache, nausea, dizziness, diplopia and ataxia) can be avoided or ameliorated by reducing the carbamazepine dose. The commonest side effect of lamotrigine is skin rash (3–5%) and there is good evidence that starting with a high dose increases the risk of rash with lamotrigine. Other side effects that are concentration dependent include dizziness, nausea, diplopia and ataxia. Increased toxicity and paradoxic deterioration of seizure control may occur when lamotrigine is used in combination with other anti-epileptic drugs.

## Anti-epileptic drug therapy in pregnancy

There is an increased risk of teratogenicity associated with the use of anti-epileptic drugs in pregnancy that may be less with monotherapy. In view of the increased risk of neural tube and other defects associated, in particular, with valproate, carbamazepine and phenytoin ('foetal hydantoin' syndrome), women taking anti-epileptic drugs who may become pregnant should be informed of the risks and must be screened antenatally ($\alpha$-fetoprotein measurement and a second

trimester ultrasound scan) if they become pregnant. All women on anti-epileptic drug therapy should take folic acid before and during pregnancy; a dose of 5 mg daily is appropriate for women receiving established anti-epileptic drugs. In view of the increased bleeding associated with carbamazepine, phenobarbital and phenytoin, prophylactic Vitamin $K_1$ should be given to the mother on any of these drugs before delivery. Breast feeding is acceptable with most anti-epileptic drugs with the exception of barbiturates, ethosuximide and some of the more recently introduced drugs.

## Status epilepticus

The treatment protocol for convulsive (tonic–clonic) status epilepticus is outlined in Table 17.2.

## Migraine, other headaches and neuralgic pain

### Pathophysiology

Migraine (corrupted from hemicrania) may be classical (headache with aura) or common (headache without aura). Family history is often positive and migraine is more common in women. The triad of a classical migraine is visual scotomata or scintillations, unilateral throbbing headache and nausea or vomiting. Headache may be bilateral or generalised in common migraine with a more gradual onset. An attack usually lasts for 2–6 h and may be provoked by wine, cheese, chocolate, contraceptives, stress, exercise or travel. Cluster headache is characterised by recurrent, unilateral throbbing headache that is typically nocturnal, commoner in males, provoked by alcohol and accompanied by retro-orbital searing pain, conjunctival and nasal congestion. Headache as a result of temporal arteritis affects elderly people (two-thirds are women) and may lead to blindness if untreated.

### Aim and principles of treatment

The principles of treatment in migraine consist of three steps: (i) elimination of known precipitant or trigger; (ii) pharmacological treatment of acute attacks and (iii) prophylaxis.

**Table 17.2** Anti-epileptic drug therapy for convulsive status epilepticus.

| Time frame (min) | Intervention |
| --- | --- |
| (continuing seizures) | |
| 0–5 | *In all*: monitor vital signs, administer $O_2$, establish i.v. access, collect blood for biochemistry, blood gases and toxic screen; drug levels (phenytoin, carbamazepine) if on treatment. Put patient in recovery position. 50 ml of 50% dextrose i.v. (+100 mg thiamine i.m./i.v. if known alcoholic) |
| | *Lorazepam* 0.1 mg/kg i.v. at 2 mg/min (maximum dose: children 2 mg and adults 8 mg) |
| 5–25 | *Phenytoin* 15–20 mg/kg i.v. at 50 mg/min (typically 1 g in an adult) |
| | *or* |
| | *Fosphenytoin* 15–20 mg/kg PE i.v. at 150 mg/min. If on oral phenytoin, use 50% of calculated dose. *If seizures persist, then* |
| 25–30 | Additional phenytoin (5–10 mg/kg) or fosphenytoin (5–10 mg/kg PE) i.v. |
| >30 | Patient must be admitted to an ICU; EEG monitoring if possible |
| 30–50 | *Phenobarbital* (phenobarbitone) 10–15 mg/kg at 50 mg/min i.v. |
| 50–60 | Additional phenobarbital 5–10 mg/kg (not exceeding a cumulative total dose of 20 mg/kg or 1 g) *Alternatively Paraldehyde* by deep intramuscular injections (5 ml in each buttock, maximum 10 ml using all glass equipment with a steel needle |
| If seizure activity persists beyond 60 min | *Use one of the following infusions:* |
| | *Midazolam* (loading dose 0.1–0.2 mg/kg slow i.v., then maintained at a dose of 0.75–10 μg/kg/min) |
| | *Clomethiazole* (chlormethiazole) as an 0.8% solution intravenously 40–120 mg/min up to a maximum of 800 mg (80 μg/kg in children), then maintained at a rate of 4–8 mg/min |
| | *Propofol* (loading dose 1–2 mg/kg i.v., followed by 2–10 mg/kg/h) |
| | *If this fails, only then use* |
| | *Thiopental* (thiopentone) (2.5% solution), given i.v. 100–150 mg in adults over 10–15 s (2–7 mg/kg in children), then maintained at 0.5–1 mg/kg/h If EEG facilities are available, then the dose may be adjusted on the basis of EEG monitoring, the end point is suppression of spikes. If blood pressure is stable, secondary end point is burst-suppression pattern in the EEG with intervals of <1 s between bursts |

*Notes*: (1) Maintenance doses of phenytoin (5–6 mg/kg) and phenobarbital (3–5 mg/kg) must be continued; measure plasma concentrations for optimal doses. (2) Taper infusions of midazolam, clomethiazole or thiopentone after 12 h; if seizures recur, reinstate infusion for at least 12 h. (3) There is a risk of convulsions with propofol. (4) EEG monitoring, though not mandatory, may be useful when available; an ictal EEG also helps to exclude pseudo-status epilepticus. (5) Use i.v. fluids and low-dose dopamine ± dobutamine to treat hypotension.

## Treatment of acute attack

This should begin at the very onset of headache. Any standard non-steroidal anti-inflammatory drug (NSAID), e.g. aspirin, paracetamol, naproxen or ibuprofen, often with an anti-emetic in combination (metoclopramide, domperidone or a phenothiazine), is the first choice. Tolfenamic acid is a new NSAID that has been indicated specifically for migraine attacks. Because serotonin (5-hydroxy tryptamine or 5-HT), plays a key role in the neurovascular inflammation that is characteristic of migraine, $5\text{-HT}_1$ agonists ('triptans') are of considerable value in the treatment of an acute attack, especially in those who fail to respond to simple analgesics. The first-generation triptans consist of sumatriptan, naratriptan and zolmitriptan. The second-generation triptans (rizatriptan and eletriptan) cross the blood–brain barrier and have better bioavailability on oral administration. It should be noted that triptans do not abolish nausea or vomiting and require the additional use of an anti-emetic. Unremitting attacks of severe migraine lasting for days ('status migrainosus') require the short-term use of corticosteroids in an anti-inflammatory dose, although this diagnosis should always be made with caution and after exclusion of all other possibilities even in a patient known to be a migraine sufferer. Corticosteroids are also indicated as first-line therapy in the treatment of the headache of temporal arteritis and in severe cluster headache.

Great care should be exercised when prescribing analgesics to patients with headache, because with frequent use, a large proportion will develop chronic daily headaches resulting from the drugs ('analgesic headache') in addition to their primary headache type. Opioid-containing preparations are particularly likely to produce this effect but it does occur with simple analgesics and NSAIDs. Prolonged use of triptans can also give rise to 'rebound headache'.

## Treatment for migraine prophylaxis

In patients with two or more attacks in a month, use of prophylactic agents for prevention of migraine is justified. Amitriptyline and propranolol are the two main prophylactic agents that are often used in combination. Other beta-blockers (e.g. atenolol) are also effective. Other prophylactic agents that may be used in migraine are pizotifen, valproate, topiramate, carbamazepine, methysergide or selected calcium channel blockers (verapamil). Verapamil (160–240 mg/day) is used for prophylaxis in cluster headache.

## Antimigraine drugs in common use

### Sumatriptan

A $5\text{-HT}_{1D}$ agonist, sumatriptan is used for acute attacks of migraine (oral preparation, intranasal spray or subcutaneous injections) and cluster headache (subcutaneous injections only). It should not be taken until 24 h after stopping any preparation containing ergotamine. It has poor bioavailability and less than half of the orally administered dose is absorbed. Further reduction may occur in patients with migraine-induced gastroparesis and vomiting. The dose by mouth is 50 mg (some patients may require 100 mg) and patients not responding should not take a second dose for the same attack. In responders, the dose may be repeated if migraine recurs (maximum 300 mg in 24 h). It is available as an intranasal spray and subcutaneous injection for prompt relief. The dose by subcutaneous injection using an auto-injector is 6 mg (maximum 24 mg in 24 h) and 1 spray (20 mg) intranasally (maximum 40 mg in 24 h). Sumatriptan is also effective in cluster headache. None of the 5-HT agonists should be used for prophylaxis and all are contraindicated in ischaemic heart disease, previous myocardial infarction, coronary vasospasm, uncontrolled hypertension and in attacks of migraine with brain stem dysfunction ('basilar migraine'). Side effects of triptans include sensations of tingling, heat, heaviness, pressure or tightness in the chest, flushing, dizziness, weakness, vomiting and fatigue.

### Ergotamine

It is used in rare cases of acute attacks of migraine and cluster headache. Ergotamine has a high affinity for 5-HT$_1$ receptors, which probably explains its mode of action in this condition. Ergot alkaloids are $\alpha$-receptor blockers and also have a direct vascular effect causing vasoconstriction. This may lead to peripheral vasoconstriction with Raynaud's phenomenon, ischaemia and digital gangrene ('ergotism') in patients with co-existing vascular disease and in chronic users who take it habitually to counteract the symptoms of headache caused by vasodilation when the drug is withdrawn. It is contraindicated in patients with known coronary artery disease. The dose of ergotamine (as tartarate) is 1–2 mg sublingually to a total dose of 6–8 mg per attack or maximum 12 mg/week; rectally the dose is 2 mg repeated after 1 h to the same total dose; and by aerosol, 360 μg inhalation repeated up to six inhalations daily or 15 per week.

## Beta-blockers

Propranolol, a non-selective beta-blocker, is effective in reducing the frequency of migraine attacks in daily doses of 40–120 mg (this may be increased up to 480 mg according to effectiveness) given orally. Other cardioselective beta-blockers (bisoprolol or atenolol) are better tolerated and probably equally effective. Their mechanism of action in migraine prophylaxis is unknown.

## Amitriptyline

A tricyclic antidepressant, its antimigraine effect is not a result of its antidepressant property and small doses are often effective (20–50 mg/day). Sedation and dry mouth are two common side effects. The detailed pharmacology of amitriptyline is given elsewhere in this book.

## Pizotifen

It is an antihistamine and serotonin antagonist structurally related to the tricyclic antidepressants. It affords good prophylaxis for migraine but may cause weight gain and drowsiness. The treatment may be started at 500 μg at night; maximum dose is 3 mg/day.

## Methysergide

A 5-HT$_2$ antagonist, methysergide is a very effective drug for prophylaxis of migraine and cluster headache but carries serious long-term side effects (retroperitoneal, pleural and cardiac valvar fibrosis, arterial and coronary vasospasm) that widely limit its use now. These risks can be minimised by taking periodic 'drug holidays' (5 months on the drug and 1 month off in a 6-month cycle). The usual dose is 1–2 mg 2–3 times daily. Methysergide is also used in 'serotonin syndrome' and to treat diarrhoea caused by carcinoid tumour in higher doses.

## Facial pain and neuralgias

The most common cause of facial pain is dental, triggered by hot, cold or sweet foods. Facial neuralgias (trigeminal and glossopharyngeal) consist of paroxysmal, fleeting pain akin to electric shock. Most cases are idiopathic although structural diseases (e.g. multiple sclerosis) are likely in younger patients. Carbamazepine (400–1200 mg/day) is usually effective; gabapentin, phenytoin, valproate and baclofen are other options.

## Cerebrovascular disease

### Pathophysiology

A stroke is the sudden onset of neurological deficit from a vascular mechanism. Eighty per cent of strokes are a consequence of ischaemia; a transient ischaemic attack (TIA) is an ischaemic neurodeficit that rapidly resolves. The accepted boundary between a TIA and a completed stroke is 24 h. The remaining 20% of strokes are primary haemorrhages, including subarachnoid, lobar and hypertensive deep cerebral haemorrhages. Multiple factors, both non-modifiable (age and sex) and modifiable (e.g. hypertension and diabetes), influence the risk of cerebrovascular disease. Prolonged hypertension and diabetes are specific risk factors for small vessel cerebral stroke (lacunar infarcts); smoking is a risk factor for all vascular mechanisms causing stroke.

Cerebral venous thrombosis may be spontaneous (as seen during pregnancy) or may be secondary to a hypercoagulable state, focal intracranial or ear infections.

## Aim and principles of treatment

### Intracranial haemorrhage

The specific treatment is often surgical and pharmacological interventions are directed to the reduction of raised intracranial pressure (ICP). Nimodipine, a calcium channel blocker that crosses the blood–brain barrier, may be effective in minimising symptomatic vasospasm following subarachnoid haemorrhage if begun early (by day 4). Cerebral vasospasm after aneurysm surgery is best treated by improving cerebral perfusion with vasopressor agents.

### Acute treatment of ischaemic stroke

Patients with TIA or an established ischaemic stroke should receive aspirin (75–300 mg/day) as soon as the diagnosis is confirmed. If fever and/or hyperglycemia are present, these should be treated promptly. Anticoagulation is strictly reserved for patients with high risk of venous thromboembolism, cerebral venous thrombosis without major haemorrhage, recurrent thromboembolic arterial stroke from a known source (e.g. cardiogenic emboli with atrial fibrillation) and progressive stroke in the basilar artery territory (stroke-in-evolution). Systemic or selective intra-arterial thrombolytic therapy with recombinant tissue plasminogen activator (rtPA) may be offered in centres with expertise in patients seen within the first 3 h of the ischaemic event in the absence of any major ischaemia or haemorrhage on the computerised tomography (CT) scan. Despite a higher risk of cerebral haemorrhage as a consequence of thrombolytic therapy in ischaemic stroke, both short-term outcome and long-term disabilities significantly improve in thrombolysed patients.

## Secondary prevention of stroke

Lifestyle and risk factor modifications will remain the cornerstone of secondary stroke prevention. All patients with ischaemic stroke or TIA should receive life-long aspirin (75–300 mg daily). Higher doses of aspirin have little advantage and only worsen gastrotoxicity. Identical doses of aspirin are given to patients after carotid endarterectomy. Clopidogrel (75 mg/day) is an alternative for patients intolerant of aspirin. Addition of dipyridamole (200 mg twice daily) to aspirin is recommended for patients with recurrent ischaemic events despite aspirin. Warfarin is indicated for patients with atrial fibrillation or cardioembolic stroke. The combination of aspirin and warfarin carries a high risk of cerebral haemorrrhage, especially in the elderly.

Blood pressure reduction should be considered in all patients with cerebrovascular disease. Existing data favours the use of a diuretic/ACE inhibitor combination, introduced a few weeks after the onset of the symptoms. Strategies to lower blood pressure may need to be modified in the context of significant carotid stenosis: aggressive blood pressure reduction in such patients may aggravate cerebral ischaemia.

There is some evidence that statin therapy reduces risk of further vascular events in patients with ischaemic stroke. Further trials of lipid lowering in stroke patients are underway. For a more detailed discussion of vascular risk modification see Chapter 5.

## Drugs used in cerebrovascular diseases

(For aspirin and warfarin, see Chapter 14.)

## Raised intracranial pressure (ICP)

Acute rises in ICP can occur as a result of intracerebral or subarachnoid haemorrhage, cerebral infarction, tumours, Reye's syndrome and after head injury. The aim of medical therapy is to maintain cerebral perfusion and prevent global cerebral ischaemia. General treatment of acutely raised

ICP (best carried out in an intensive care unit) involves: (i) head elevation to 45 degrees; (ii) restriction of free water by the use of intravenous normal (0.9%) saline to 1000 ml/day; (iii) aggressive treatment of fever; (iv) careful intubation (without causing gagging or coughing) in comatose patients; (v) avoiding a drop in systemic blood pressure and (vi) stool softeners to prevent straining. Specific treatment depends on the cause of raised ICP. Mannitol, an osmolar diuretic, lowers ICP by decreasing interstitial brain fluid and is given as intravenous boluses of 0.5–1 g/kg every 4–6 h, maintaining plasma osmolality above 295 mOsm/kg. Furosemide (frusemide) is less effective. Longer periods of treatment with mannitol may not be effective. Dexamethasone is the treatment of choice for raised ICP resulting from vasogenic oedema, as in cerebral tumours or metastases. It is given as an initial dose of 8–12 mg intravenously, followed by 4–6 mg every 6 h. Mechanical hyperventilation in intubated patients to reduce arterial $P_{co2}$ to 3.5 kPa is sometimes helpful.

Cases of chronically raised ICP without any focal cerebral pathology (idiopathic intracranial hypertension) are treated with oral acetazolamide (750–1000 mg/day).

Acetazolamide is an inhibitor of the carbonic anhydrase enzyme that is present in the choroid plexus where cerebrospinal fluid (CSF) is formed. It probably reduces the synthesis of CSF and is the most effective treatment for idiopathic intracranial hypertension (and open-angle glaucoma). It is also used in neurology with remarkable success to prevent attacks of periodic paralysis and episodic ataxia and it is occasionally helpful as an adjuvant therapy in atypical absence, atonic and tonic seizures especially in children. Its use to reduce hydrocephalus caused by choroid plexus papilloma is only of historical interest. The main side effects are nausea, taste disturbance, loss of appetite, paraesthesia, fatigue, metabolic acidosis and electrolyte disturbances; rarely renal calculi, abnormal liver function, blood disorders including agranulocytosis and thrombocytopenia and erythema multiforme are reported.

## Infections of the nervous system

Infections of the CNS may be acute or chronic. The pathogens involved may be bacterial, viral, protozoal or parasitic. Brain abscess and subdural empyema are focal suppurative infections of the brain and require surgical drainage in addition to antibiotics. Treatment for acute bacterial meningitis and herpes simplex encephalitis must begin as soon as possible on clinical suspicion alone, with intravenous benzylpenicillin and aciclovir, respectively. In tropical countries, cerebral malaria (caused by choloroquine-resistant forms of *Plasmodium falciparum*) and tuberculous meningitis are important causes of mortality and morbidity. HIV infections can involve any part of the nervous system and should be treated with standard antiretroviral combination therapy. Leprosy is the commonest infection of the peripheral nerves in the world. The pharmacology of antimicrobial chemotherapy is given elsewhere in this book (Chapter 19).

## Disorders of sleep

Excessive daytime sleepiness (EDS) causes impaired alertness leading to accidents and is associated with increased cardiovascular morbidity and mortality. Many disorders of EDS are consequences of neurological diseases, e.g. narcolepsy and periodic limb movements during sleep (PLMS). EDS in narcolepsy is often associated with cataplexy (sudden loss of muscle tone, provoked by an emotional stimulus like laughter). Narcoleptic EDS is usually treated with stimulants (methylphenidate, pemoline, dextroamfetamine, methamfetamine, mazindol), all of which carry the risk of dependence with long-term use. Modafinil is a recent addition to this list that has been claimed to act differently with less risk of dependence. Cataplexy and other sleep-related phenomena in narcolepsy frequently respond to tricyclic or SSRI antidepressants. The most effective treatments for the restless leg syndrome and PLMS are dopaminergic agents (levodopa, bromocriptine and pergolide) taken before retiring to bed. Tricyclic antidepressants paradoxically aggravate these movements.

## Neuroimmunology

### Pathophysiology

Immunological mechanisms are recognised to play an important role in a number of diseases affecting different parts of the nervous system (Table 17.3). One of three treatments may be selected to treat an acute attack following neuroimmunological injury: (i) high doses of corticosteroids (e.g. intravenous methylprednisolone); (ii) human immunoglobulin (IVIg) or (iii) plasma exchange (plasmapheresis). However, one particular treatment may be more specific for one disease than the other. In diseases with an established autoimmune mechanism (e.g. myasthenia gravis or vasculitic neuropathy), long-term immunosuppression is required as well. Azathioprine is the most commonly used immunosuppressive drug in neurology, but methotrexate, cyclosporine and cyclophosphamide are used in specific situations when more aggressive immunosuppression is required.

### Methylprednisolone

Methylprednisolone is usually used for rapid suppression of inflammatory and allergic disorders; its side effect profile is similar to prednisolone except that rapid intravenous administration of large doses has been associated with cardiovascular collapse. Patients often experience a metallic taste at the time of infusion, and psychosis and restlessness are reported occasionally. It is usually given in short courses (1 g daily for 3 days or 500 mg daily for 5 days) When oral prednisolone is used for long-term immunosuppression, care must be taken to avoid long-term complications like osteopenia and prophylactic use of bisphosphonates may be desirable in high-risk cases (e.g. post-menopausal women). For the pharmacokinetics and adverse effects of corticosteroids

Table 17.3 Neurological disorders with a proven or presumed immunological mechanism.

| | |
|---|---|
| *Central nervous system (CNS)* | |
| Acute | Disseminated encephalomyelitis |
| | Haemorrhagic leukoencephalitis |
| | Demyelinating optic neuritis |
| | Transverse myelitis |
| | CNS vasculitis (isolated angiitis of CNS) |
| Subacute | Neuro-systemic lupus erythematosus (SLE) |
| | Subacute cerebellar degeneration and limbic encephalitis (usually paraneoplastic) |
| Chronic | Multiple sclerosis (MS) |
| | Stiff-person syndrome |
| *Peripheral nervous system* | |
| Acute | AIDP (Guillain–Barré syndrome) |
| | Vasculitis of peripheral nerves |
| Chronic | CIDP, MMN (multi-focal motor neuropathy) |
| | Acquired neuromyotonia |
| *Neuromuscular junction* | |
| | Myasthenia gravis |
| | LEMS |
| *Skeletal muscles* | |
| | Polymyositis and dermatomyositis |

and immunosuppressive drugs, please refer to the relevant sections in this book.

## Interferons

Interferons are naturally occurring recombinant proteins with complex effects on immunity and cell function. Three classes of interferons are available for treatment: alpha, beta and gamma. Interferon-$\alpha$ is used in selected cancer treatment and chronic viral hepatitis (B and C); interferon $\gamma$-1b is indicated in chronic granulomatous disease to reduce the frequency of infections; only interferon-$\beta$ is effective in reducing relapse frequency and severity in patients with relapsing multiple sclerosis. Effects on disease progression are unclear.

## Human immunoglobulin (IVIg)

The mechanism of action of IVIg in acute and chronic inflammatory demyelinating polyneuropathies (AIDP and CIDP) and in other neuroimmunological disorders is unclear; exogenous IVIg may neutralise putative autoantibodies as a result of the presence of anti-idiotype antibodies in the healthy donor pool contributing the human IVIg. Another explanation is that administered IVIg increases the catabolism of endogenous IVIg that may carry the circulating autoantibody fraction. The usual dose is 2 g/kg given i.v. over 3–5 days; a dose of 1 g/kg may be adequate for maintenance. IVIg is also used for replacement therapy in patients with congenital a$\gamma$ or hypo-$\gamma$ globulinemia, for the treatment of idiopathic thrombocytopenic purpura, Kawasaki syndrome and for the prophylaxis of infection following bone marrow transplantation. Common side effects are allergic reaction, urticaria, hypotension, venous thrombosis and increased blood viscosity. In patients who are IgA-deficient, oliguric renal failure may occur.

## Specific diseases

### Multiple sclerosis

In multiple sclerosis (MS), there is destruction of myelin in the CNS. An acute attack causes oedema around the area of demyelination, called a plaque. Recurrent attacks cause destruction of axons that contribute to permanent disability. Relapsing-remitting MS is the commonest clinical form. Treatment is aimed at the alleviation of acute relapses (new neurological symptoms or an exacerbation of old symptoms present for at least 24 h). Short courses of intravenous methylprednisolone, or high dose oral methylprednisolone, are as effective (and result in less side effects) than longer tapered courses. Attacks of demyelinating optic neuritis, transverse myelitis or disseminated encephalomyelitis are treated similarly.

Currently four treatments are available as disease modifying therapy in MS: Interferon IFNb-1b, IFNb-1a, copolymer 1 (glatiramer) and mitoxantrone. Each of the first three therapies reduces annual relapse rates by about one-third, but they are expensive and need to be given regularly (subcutaneous or intramuscular injections) on a long-term basis. Both intramuscular (IFNb-1a, Avonex) and subcutaneous injections (IFNb-1a, Rebif and IFNb-1b, 'Betaseron') are used. Most frequently reported side effects include irritation at injection sites (including skin necrosis), influenza-like symptoms and fatigue; rarely raised liver enzymes, hypersensitivity reactions, blood disorders, mood and personality changes, confusion and convulsions have been reported. Glatiramer is generally better tolerated, but has to be given as a daily injection. Mitoxantrone is a cytotoxic agent that has recently been studied in relapsing-remitting and relapsing-progressive forms of MS. Placebo-controlled trials have demonstrated its effectiveness, but its use is generally reserved for patients with aggressive forms of relapsing progressive MS, who may have failed on other therapies. It has significant side effects of myelosuppression and dose-related cardiotoxicity. For chronic progressive MS, there is little role for immunosuppression or interferon therapy—the pathological process at this stage is felt to be one of axonal degeneration. Symtomatic therapies are helpful, and Table 17.4 lists the symptomatic drugs available for patients with chronic neurological disability as seen in MS. These treatments can be delivered in any chronic

**Table 17.4** Symptomatic treatment of chronic neurological disability.

| Nature of symptoms | Drugs available |
| --- | --- |
| Spasticity | Oral and intrathecal baclofen (GABA agonist) |
| | Diazepam (GABA agonist) |
| | Dantrolene (direct effect on skeletal muscles) |
| | Tizanidine ($\alpha_2$-adrenoreceptor agonist) |
| | Botulinum toxin (local injections to spastic muscles) |
| Muscle spasms | Clonazepam |
| | Baclofen |
| Bladder symptoms | Antimuscarinics: flavoxate and oxybutinin for increased frequency; tolterodine, propiverine may also be effecive in urge incontinence: *all may cause retention and precipitate angle-closure glaucoma*; cholinergics (carbachol, bethanecol) for retention *in the absence of urinary obstruction*; adrenergic blockers (prazosin, doxazosin) improve urinary flow by reducing the tone of external uretheral sphincter |
| Nocturnal enuresis | Adults: desmopressin or propantheline |
| | Children: tricyclics (imipramine, amitriptyline) |
| Dysesthesia | Carbamazepine, lamotrigine |
| Pain | Tricyclics (amitriptyline, imipramine) |
| | Anti-epileptics (carbamazepine, gabapentin) |
| Fatigue | Amantadine or modafinil |
| Depression | SSRI (sertraline, citalopram) |
| Impotence | Sildenafil |

neurological disorder where similar symptoms emerge.

## Peripheral neuropathy

Acute and chronic inflammatory demyelinating polyneuropathies (AIDP, also termed Guillain–Barré syndrome, and CIDP) are rare disorders. They are treated with high doses (2 g/kg) of intravenous human IVIg or therapeutic plasma exchange. Oral corticosteroids (prednisolone) are also effective in CIDP but not in AIDP. Patients with CIDP usually require maintenance treatment with steroids or with pulses of IVIg or plasma exchange repeated at 1–6 monthly intervals. Some cases of CIDP may require additional immunosuppression (azathioprine or ciclosporin). Vasculitic peripheral neuropathy usually presents with multiple painful mononeuropathies. Often responsive to steroids (pulse methylprednisolone followed by oral prednisolone 1 mg/kg) alone, some cases may require the addition of cyclophosphamide, e.g. those with

an underlying systemic vasculitis. After maximal recovery of neurological deficit, steroids are tapered off and cyclophosphamide is continued, usually orally (2 mg/kg daily), for a period of 1 year.

## Muscle diseases

Polymyositis is a condition of presumed autoimmune aetiology in which the skeletal muscle is damaged by a lymphocytic inflammatory process. The term dermatomyositis is used when polymyositis is accompanied by characteristic skin changes. Both are treated with prednisolone (1–1.5 mg/kg/day), tapered after muscle strength improves and muscle enzymes (serum creatine kinase) decline. Approximately 75% of patients will have a good clinical response to steroids alone. The onset of steroid-induced myopathy may complicate therapy. Cytotoxic therapy should be considered for severe disease, inadequate response to steroids, relapsing disease and for steroid-induced complications. One of the three agents is used orally: methotrexate (7.5–15 mg/week), azathio-prine (2–2.5 mg/kg/day) and cyclophosphamide (1–2 mg/kg/day).

## Diseases of neuromuscular junction

In myasthenia gravis, there is an autoimmune attack by the complement system and antibodies are targeted to the nicotinic acetylcholine receptors in the post-synaptic neuromuscular junction. Typically, patients experience fluctuating symptoms of muscle weakness and fatigue provoked by exertion. Most forms of myasthenia are generalised and only 10% will have weakness restricted to the extraocular muscles (ocular myasthenia). Administration of drugs with neuromuscular blocking effects can dangerously exacerbate myasthenic symptoms. The thymus, which is abnormal in 75% of patients, plays a central role in sensitising lymphocytes to the acetylcholine receptors. Thymectomy offers the only possibility of a cure in this condition. Anticholinesterase drugs assist patients with short-term symptomatic improvement but overdose with cholinesterases can lead to weakness resulting from depolarising neuromuscular blockade ('cholinergic crisis'). Plasma exchange is probably superior to IVIg for rapid improvement in seriously weak patients with myasthenia ('myasthenic crisis') and to stabilise neuromuscular function prior to thymectomy or other major surgery.

Long-term treatment of acquired autoimmune myasthenia gravis requires immunosuppression, often started with a combinaton of corticosteroids and azathioprine. Low doses of corticosteroids are generally preferred (prednisolone 15 mg/day, then increased by 5 mg every third or fourth day until a dose of 1 mg/kg is reached). Larger doses of steroids can transiently worsen myasthenic symptoms, particularly bulbar weakness. Initial large doses of steroids (prednisolone 0.75–1 mg/kg) are only given to hospitalised patients, who can be closely monitored, or to the rare patient requiring ventilatory support as a result of myasthenic crisis. Azathioprine is usually introduced at a low daily dose and then increased to a maintenance dose of 2–2.5 mg/kg/day. Patients with ocular myasthenia are best maintained on cholinesterase inhibitors and/or low doses of steroids (prednisolone 5–10 mg) alone.

The principle of drug therapy in Lambert–Eaton myasthenic syndrome (LEMS) is broadly similar. In this condition, antibodies directed to the voltage-gated calcium channels in the presynaptic vesicles of the motor end plate affect acetylcholine release. LEMS may be associated with an underlying malignancy (small cell lung cancer) as a paraneoplastic syndrome. As compared to myasthenia gravis, response to treatment is far less satisfactory. 3,4-diaminopyridine, a potassium channel blocker, partially improves presynaptic transmission failure in LEMS.

## Drugs used for neuromuscular junction disorder

### Cholinesterase inhibitors

This class of drugs enhances neuromuscular transmission both in voluntary and involuntary muscles by increasing the intrasynaptic acetylcholine level as a result of the inhibition of cholinesterases, which normally terminate its action as a chemical transmitter. Muscarinic side effects (sweating, increased salivation, bradycardia, gastro-intestinal and uterine motility) are common to all members of this class. These parasympathomimetic effects are effectively antagonised by atropine. Edrophonium is extremely short-acting and is useful mainly for the diagnosis of myasthenia gravis or to determine whether or not a patient with myasthenia is receiving inadequate or excessive treatment with cholinergic drugs. It has to be given parenterally (i.v.). Neostigmine produces a therapeutic effect for 2–4 h and is available as 15 mg tablets (usual daily dose 120–180 mg). Pyridostigmine is less powerful than neostigmine but has a longer duration of action (3–6 h) and has relatively less gastrointestinal side effects. It is available as 60 mg tablets (usual daily dose 360–720 mg). Propantheline bromide (Pro-Banthine) is usually used as an antimuscarinic to minimise the side effects of cholinesterase inhibitors at a dose of 15 mg two or three times daily.

Cholinesterase inhibitors that cross the blood–brain barrier (donepezil, rivastigmine and galantamine) have been shown to improve symptoms of dementia in Alzheimer's disease. They are not used for peripheral neuromuscular disorders.

## Movement disorders

### Pathophysiology

The movement disorders can be broadly classified as: (i) hypo- or bradykinetic, causing poverty of movement and rigidity (parkinsonism); (ii) dystonic, focal or generalised, which are produced by involuntary spasm of the involved muscles and (iii) hyperkinetic, such as chorea and various dyskinesias. Parkinsonism is caused by many disorders and may be drug induced. Parkinson's disease (PD) is idiopathic parkinsonism that is characterised by bradykinesia, rigidity, tremor and gait disorder. PD is caused by loss of striatal dopaminergic projections from the substantia nigra pars compacta. The cause of neuronal death in PD is unknown but may result from the generation of free radicals and oxidative stress, perhaps by oxidation of dopamine itself. Levodopa, the aminoacid precursor of dopamine, acts mainly by replenishing striatal dopamine in PD. Parkinsonism caused by more diffuse degenerative brain disease (e.g. multiple system atrophy) does not normally respond to levodopa.

### Aim and principles of therapy

The goal of treatment in PD is to restore motor function. Levodopa improves bradykinesia and rigidity more than tremor. It is always given in combination with an extracerebral decarboxylase inhibitor (carbidopa or benserazide), which prevents peripheral degradation of levodopa to dopamine but, unlike levodopa, does not cross the blood–brain barrier. The advantages of using a decarboxylase inhibitor with levodopa are: (i) effective brain concentrations of dopamine can be achieved with lower doses of levodopa; (ii) reduced peripheral conversion to dopamine decreases cardiovascular side effects (hypotension and arrhythmia) and nausea; (iii) there is rapid

onset of therapeutic effect and (iv) a smoother clinical response. The main disadvantage of chronic levodopa therapy is the occurence of abnormal involuntary movements and motor complications on long-term therapy (>5 years).

## Drugs used for parkinsonism

See Table 17.5.

### Levodopa

It is always given in combination with one of the two extracerebral dopa-decarboxylase inhibitors: carbidopa (cocareldopa or 'Sinemet') and benserazide (cobeneldopa or Madopar) as fixed drug formulations. Sinemet is available in two formulations of levodopa : carbidopa (10 : 1 or 4 : 1); 1 part of benserazide is always combined with 4 parts of levodopa. When cocareldopa 100/10 is used, the dose of carbidopa may be insufficient to achieve full inhibition of the extracerebral decarboxylase system that usually requires a daily dose of carbidopa 75 mg. Treatment must be initiated with low doses (typical dose: 'Sinemet plus' 100/25 twice daily) and increased gradually. The final dose is usually balanced between the efficacy and side effects of treatment and the interval between doses may need to be individualised. Treatment should be taken before meals. As the patient ages, the maintenance dose may need to be reduced. Domperidone is useful in controlling nausea and vomiting if present. Other side effects, often dose related, include postural hypotension (rarely labile hypertension), arrhythmias, neuropsychiatric symptoms (insomnia, agitation, hallucinations) and dyskinesias.

### Dopamine agonists

Bromocriptine, cabergoline, pergolide and lisuride are ergot derivatives and act as direct agonists of dopaminergic receptors. Ropinirole and pramipexole are non-ergot derived dopamine agonists that do not cause fibrotic reactions (or require monitoring for fibrotic reactions). Trials have shown that, at least in younger patients with idiopathic

**Table 17.5** Commonly used anti-parkinsonian drug therapy.

| Drug | Dose | Side effects |
|---|---|---|
| *Levodopa* | | |
| Levodopa/carbidopa | | |
| Regular dose | 100/10 to 250/25, increase slowly to t.i.d. or q.i.d. | Orthostatic hypotension, gastrointestinal complaints, hallucinations, confusion, chorea, dyskinesias |
| Slow-release dose | 100/25 to 200/50 b.i.d. or t.i.d. | |
| *Dopamine agonists* | | |
| Bromocriptine | 7.5–30 mg daily in divided doses | Postural hypotension, nausea, vomiting, hallucinations, psychosis, dyskinesias |
| Pergolide | 0.05–3 mg daily in divided doses | Nausea, dizziness, hallucinations, confusion, constipation, postural hypotension, dyskinesias |
| Ropinirole | 0.5–9 mg daily in divided doses | Nausea, somnolence, leg oedema, abdominal pain, vomiting, syncope, dyskinesia, hallucinations |
| Pramipexole | 264 mcg – 3.3 mg (base) | Nausea, somnolence, drowsiness, confusion, insomnia, hallucinations, leg oedema |
| Amantadine (acts by NMDA-receptor blockade) | 100–200 mg | Livido reticularis, diarrhoea, depression |
| Apomorphine (subcutaneous injections) | 3–30 mg daily in divided doses | Nausea, vomiting, confusion, hallucination, postural hypotension, dyskinesias, local reaction to injections (nodule and ulcers) |
| *Enzyme inhibitors* | | |
| Selegeline (inhibits MAO-B) | 5 mg b.i.d. | Nausea, dizziness, insomnia, hallucination |
| Entcapone (inhibits COMT) | 200 mg with each dose of levodopa; maximum 2 g | Nausea, vomiting, abdominal pain, dizziness |
| *Antimuscarinics* | | |
| Trihexiphenidyl | 2–5 mg t.i.d. | Dry mouth, blurred vision, confusion |
| Benzatropine (benztropine) | 0.5–2 mg t.i.d. | Dry mouth, confusion |

PD, the use of dopamine agonists as initial therapy (as opposed to levodopa/dopa decarboxylase inhibitors) will lessen the incidence of motor complications (dyskinesias). This is at the expense of more adverse events and side effects, and possibly reduced efficacy. Levodopa is generally more effective in clinical practice, and is often introduced first line in the elderly. Dopamine agonists are useful in the advanced stages of PD as add-on therapy and also when response to levodopa therapy becomes less predictable and shows fluctuations with individual dosages ('on-off' phenomenon).

Apomorphine is a potent stimulator of dopamine receptors that is sometimes useful in stabilising PD patients experiencing frequent, unpredictable 'off' periods on levodopa treatment. It is essential to hospitalise such patients and commence domperidone 3 days before starting apomorphine (given by subcutaneous injections). Selegiline is a monoamine-oxidase B inhibitor used in the treatment of PD for its putative (unproven) neuroprotective effect and in conjunction with levodopa to reduce 'end of dose' deterioration. Entacapone, a catechol-*o*-methyl-transferase inhibitor,

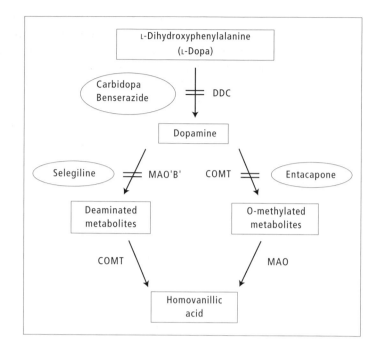

**Figure 17.1** Sites of action of anti-parkinsonian drugs. COMT, catechol-*o*-methyl transferase; DDC, dopa carboxylase; MAO, monoamine oxidase.

is also prescribed for the latter indication–combination therapies (levodopa with entacapone) that have recently become available. Amantadine (first introduced for its antiviral activity) has modest anti-parkinsonian effects and improves mild bradykinetic disabilities, rigidity and tremors. Although initially believed to be a dopamine agonist, its anti-parkinsonian effect is probably a result of NMDA-receptor blockade.

## Anticholinergics

The role for antimuscarinic drugs (less appropriately called anticholinergics) in the treatment of PD is probably restricted to patients with predominant tremors or mild symptoms. The use of these agents has lessened in recent years because of concerns about their longer-term effects on cognition. They have a worse adverse event profile than levodopa, particularly in the elderly. They are believed to exert their anti-parkinsonian effect (mainly on tremor and rigidity with no effect on bradykinesia) by correcting the relative cholinergic excess that occurs in the striatal network as a result of dopamine deficiency. Antimuscarinics are also useful in reducing sialorrhoea and are indicated as the first-line therapy in drug-induced parkinsonism. However, tardive dyskinesia does not respond to antimuscarinics and may actually be made worse. No important differences exist in the efficacy or side effects between the many synthetic antimuscarinics that are available. Those most commonly used are orphenadrine, trihexyphenidyl, benzatropine and procyclidine.

A summary of the sites of action of anti-parkinsonian drugs is given in Fig. 17.1.

## Dystonia and other movement disorders

Drug therapy for generalised dystonia is often empirical. Because some forms of generalised dystonia are levodopa responsive, it is mandatory to offer a trial of levodopa in all cases. Nonresponders are treated with antimuscarinics, carbamazepine or tetrabenazine, which acts by depleting nerve endings of dopamine. Tetrabanazine is also effective in Huntington's chorea and related disorders. Haloperidol, pimozide and clozapine are used to treat complex motor tics and symptoms of Gilles de la Tourette syndrome. Small doses of haloperidol alone are remarkably effective in Sydenham's chorea; valproate is an alternative. Essential tremors are treated with propranolol or primidone. Focal dystonias (blepharospasm and torticollis) are best treated with botulinum toxin injected periodically in small amounts locally to the involved muscles.

## Wilson's disease

This is an autosomal recessive disease of brain and liver that presents between 10 and 30 years of age with a syndrome of tremor, extrapyramidal rigidity, dystonia, dysarthria and cerebellar ataxia. The fundamental defect is probably hepatic failure to incorporate copper into ceuloplasmin, the copper-binding protein in serum. There are deposits of excess copper in liver that may cause cirrhosis; the presence of rings of copper pigment in the cornea (Kayser–Fleischer or KF rings) is diagnostic. Treatment consists of reducing dietary copper, taking oral zinc to reduce copper absorption in the gut and eliminating tissue-bound copper by using a specific chelator, D-penicillamine. Penicillamine is used for copper and lead poisoning, in the treatment of cystinuria and as disease-modifying therapy in rheumatoid arthritis and in chronic active hepatitis (anti-inflammatory effect). In Wilson's disease, penicillamine is started at a small dose (250 mg twice daily) and then slowly increased to a maximum daily dose of 1.5–2 g in adults (20 mg/kg in children). The serious side effects are hypersensitivity, pemphigus, erythema multiforme, drug-induced lupus erythematosus, myasthenia gravis (with positive autoantibodies), polymyositis, dermatomyositis, nephrotic syndrome, Goodpasture's syndrome, agranulocytosis, aplastic and haemolytic anaemia. Patients on penicillamine must have periodic blood counts, urine tests and renal clearance estimated. Appearance of any of the above side effects must lead to permanent discontinuation of the therapy. A proportion of patients

with Wilson's disease may actually deteriorate on penicillamine therapy that may be irreversible in some cases, even on drug withdrawal. Trientine is an alternative to D-penicillamine but it acts differently.

## Drug-induced neurological disorders

See Table 17.6.

**Table 17.6** Drug-induced common neurological disorders.

| | |
|---|---|
| *Exacerbation of myasthenia* | *Peripheral neuropathy* |
| Aminoglycosides | Amiodarone |
| Erythromycin | Chlorpropamide |
| Phenytoin | Clofibrate |
| Polymyxin | Ethambutol |
| | |
| *Extrapyramidal effects* | Ethionamide |
| Butyrophenones, e.g. | DDC and DDI |
| haloperidol | |
| Methyldopa | Isoniazid |
| Metoclopramide | Metronidazole |
| Phenothiazines | Nalidixic acid |
| | |
| *Myopathy* | Nitrofurantoin |
| Colchicine | Vincristine |
| Corticosteroids | *Optic neuritis* |
| Penicillamine | Aminoquinolenes |
| Quinine | Ethambutol |
| | |
| *Headache* | Isoniazid |
| Ergotamine (withdrawal) | Phenothiazines |
| Nitrites | *Sleep disturbances* |
| Vasodilators | Dopamine agonists |
| (e.g. hydralazine) | /levodopa |
| Drugs causing benign | MAO inhibitors |
| intracranial hypertension | |
| (hypervitaminosis A, | |
| corticosteroids, tetracycline) | |
| | |
| *Seizures* | *Stroke* |
| Amfetamines | Oral contraceptives |
| (amphetamines) | |
| Ciclosporin (cyclosporin) | |
| Isoniazid | |
| Lidocaine | |
| Lithium | |

## Neuroleptic malignant syndrome

A small percentage (1–2%) of patients exposed to neuroleptics develop neuroleptic malignant syndrome (NMS), a serious and potentially fatal (mortality rate up to 25%) condition. Hyperpyrexia, muscle rigidity, agitation and autonomic hyperactivity that may progress to mental obtundation, raised muscle enzymes (serum creatine kinase) and leukocytosis are characteristic. Treatment includes immediate discontinuation of neuroleptics, supportive care and use of dantrolene and bromocriptine. A similar condition may be reproduced by abrupt discontinuation of levodopa in PD patients.

## Malignant hyperthermia

The malignant hyperthermia (MH) syndrome is distinct from NMS but shares similar features with it. In susceptible individuals (those with genetic disorder of calcium channels or neuromuscular diseases such as central core disease and other myopathies), fever, muscle rigidity (with raised serum creatine kinase), metabolic and respiratory acidosis occur soon after exposure to halogenated inhaled anaesthetics and/or depolarising muscle relaxants such as succinylcholine.

Vulnerability to this syndrome can be evaluated by *in vitro* testing of biopsied muscle for a hypercontractile response to caffeine and/or halothane.

## Serotonin syndrome

This syndrome consists of altered mental status, autonomic dysfunction and disordered motor function that typically occur within minutes to hours of initiating or increasing the dose of a serotoninergic agent or combining a serotoninergic agent with MAO inhibitors. Hyperstimulation of brainstem and spinal cord $5-HT_{1A}$-receptors is the presumed mechanism. Treatment consists of withdrawal of the offending agent, supportive care and use of a serotonin antagonist like cyproheptadine or methylsergide.

## Drug used in NMS and MH

### Dantrolene

It acts on the skeletal muscle by interfering with the calcium influx in the muscle cell and stopping the contractile process. Because of its muscle relaxant effect, dantrolene is used commonly as an antispasticity agent (initial oral dose 25 mg daily, slowly increased to a maximum of 100 mg 3–4 times daily). It is the drug of choice for NMS and malignant hyperthermia, and dantrolene in these emergent circumstances must be given as rapid i.v. injection, 1 mg/kg, repeated as required to a cumulative maximum of 10 mg/kg. Side effects are drowsiness, fatigue, weakness, liver enzyme rises (occasionally fatal dose-related hepatotoxicity), diarrhoea, urinary symptoms, seizures, pleurisy and pericarditis.

# Chapter 18

# Drugs and endocrine disease

## Diabetes mellitus

### Pathophysiology

Diabetes mellitus is a group of metabolic disorders characterised by hyperglycaemia. This can be due to abnormalities of insulin secretion, insulin action or both. The WHO classification of diabetes mellitus reflects the underlying aetiology (Table 18.1).

Diabetes mellitus causes premature mortality and increased morbidity. Sustained hyperglycaemia is associated with both microvascular complications (retinopathy, nephropathy and neuropathy) and macrovascular complications especially coronary heart disease, stroke and peripheral vascular disease.

**Table 18.1** Aetiological classification of diabetes mellitus.

| Type 1 | Pancreatic β-cell destruction, usually leading to absolute insulin deficiency |
| --- | --- |
| Type 2 | May range from predominantly insulin resistance with relative insulin deficiency to a predominant secretory defect with or without insulin resistance |
| Type 3 | Other specific types, e.g. genetic defects, endocrinopathies |
| Type 4 | Gestational diabetes |

Type 1 diabetes mellitus—previously known as insulin-dependent diabetes mellitus or juvenile onset diabetes mellitus—accounts for approximately 5% of cases. It usually presents in childhood or adolescence but can occur at any age. The majority of cases arise through a cellular-mediated autoimmune destruction of pancreatic β-cells. The resulting insulopaenia results in hyperglycaemia and ketoacidosis. Patients depend on exogenous insulin for survival.

Type 2 diabetes mellitus—previously referred to as non-insulin-dependent diabetes mellitus or maturity onset diabetes—accounts for approximately 95% of cases. It usually presents in later adult life, most cases are obese and there is a strong genetic predisposition. Weight loss improves the metabolic abnormalities but the disease is progressive and patients usually need to be treated with a combination of one or more oral hypoglycaemic agent, and ultimately insulin treatment may become necessary.

### Aims of treatment

The aims of treatment are the relief of the symptoms of hyperglycaemia and the prevention of diabetic complications. Strict glycaemic control in both type 1 and type 2 diabetes mellitus has been shown to reduce the onset and progression of diabetic complications in the Diabetes Control and Complications Trial and UK Prospective Study in

**Table 18.2** Aspects for consideration in the management of diabetes.

| |
|---|
| Glycaemic control optimisation |
| Blood pressure management |
| Weight loss/treatment of obesity |
| Smoking cessation |
| Treatment of hyperlipidaemia |
| Anti-platelet agents |

Diabetes trials. Glycaemic control is monitored by measuring glycated haemoglobin levels (usually HbA$_{1c}$). A target HbA$_{1c}$ level of less than 7% is usually set but this should be adjusted to individual patient circumstances.

There is also good evidence supporting aggressive treatment of hypertension. Angiotensin-converting enzyme (ACE) inhibitors or angiotensin receptor antagonists should be considered as first-line treatment, especially in those with microalbuminuria or proteinuria. Other aspects for consideration in the management of diabetes are summarised in Table 18.2.

## Non-pharmacological therapy

In type 2 diabetes mellitus, weight loss, nutrition and exercise should be used as first-line management. In type 1 diabetes, nutrition and exercise should be used as an adjunct to insulin therapy.

## Drug treatments in diabetes mellitus

Pharmacological therapies used in the treatment of diabetes mellitus are shown in Table 18.3.

**Table 18.3** Drug treatment of diabetes mellitus.

| Class of diabetes | Drug |
|---|---|
| Type 2 | Oral hypoglycaemic agents |
| | Biguanides |
| | Sulphonylureas |
| | Meglitinide analogues |
| | Thiozolidinediones |
| | Glucosidase inhibitors |
| Type 1 and type 2 | Insulin |

## Insulin

### Mechanism

Insulin is a peptide hormone. Endogenous insulin is synthesised in the pancreatic β-cells and secreted into the portal circulation. The main actions of insulin are shown in Table 18.4.

**Table 18.4** Main actions of insulin.

| |
|---|
| 1 Glucose transport into muscle and fat cells |
| 2 Increased glycogen synthesis |
| 3 Inhibition of gluconeogenesis |
| 4 Inhibition of lipolysis and increased formation of triglycerides |
| 5 Stimulation of membrane-bound energy-dependent ion transporters (e.g. sodium/potassium ATPase) |
| 6 Stimulation of cell growth |

### Pharmacokinetics and insulin preparations

Insulin is destroyed in the gastrointestinal tract and must be given parenterally. Once absorbed it is inactivated enzymically in the liver and kidney and has a half-life of approximately 9 min. Therapeutic insulin (subcutaneous or intravenous) is delivered into the systemic circulation, resulting in an unphysiological situation with high insulin levels in both the systemic and the portal circulation, rather than in the portal circulation alone.

Therapeutic insulin is usually human insulin synthesised using recombinant DNA technology or genetically engineered insulin analogues in which the human amino acid sequence is altered to modify its properties. Animal insulin extracted from bovine or porcine pancreas is still available but is rarely used.

Subcutaneous injection of insulin slows its rate of delivery to the circulation, and different insulin formulations are available with varying onset and duration of action. Insulin is usually broadly classified into five categories based on these properties: rapid, short, intermediate, long and mixed (Table 18.5). Precipitating insulin with protamine (a basic protein), zinc or both slows absorption by the formation of amorphous solid or relatively insoluble crystals. In the rapid-acting insulin

**Table 18.5** Insulin formulations.

| Type of insulin | Examples | Peak activity (h) | Duration of action (h) |
|---|---|---|---|
| Rapid-acting analogue | Insulin lispro (Humalog) | 0.5–1.5 | 3–5 |
| | Insulin aspart (Novorapid) | | |
| Short acting (soluble) | Human Actrapid | 1–3 | 4–8 |
| | Humulin S | | |
| Intermediate acting (isophane) | Human Insulatard | 4–8 | 12–18 |
| | Humulin I | | |
| Long acting | Human Ultratard | 6–16 | 24–30 |
| Long-acting analogue | Insulin glargine | Smooth profile | 18–26 |
| | Insulin detemir | | |
| Mixed short/rapid with intermediate acting | Novomix 30 | Biphasic profile | 12–18 |
| | Mixtard 10–50 | | |
| | Humulin M1–M5 | | |

analogues, insulin lispro and aspart, one or two amino acid substitutions reduce the tendency of the molecules to form dimers and hexamers and speed absorption from the subcutaneous tissue.

Recently, two long-acting soluble insulin analogues have become available. The first, insulin glargine, has an altered isoelectric point, which causes insulin to precipitate on injection into the subcutaneous tissue. This forms a depot from which insulin is slowly released. In the second, insulin detemir, the addition of a fatty acyl chain promotes the formation of insulin hexamers and its binding to albumin prolongs the duration of action.

### Dose and regimes

In the United Kingdom, all insulin preparations are available in a uniform strength of 100 units/ml. The dose and insulin regime should be tailored to the individual. It can be monitored and adjusted by the patient, if educated, on a daily basis according to capillary blood glucose levels.

An ideal regime mimics physiological insulin secretion, with low, basal level between meals and increased secretion at meal times. Regimes in common use include injection of a short- or rapid-acting insulin with meals and a longer acting insulin once or twice daily (basal-bolus regime); alternatively, a twice daily injection of an intermediate acting or a mixed insulin might be appropriate.

Insulin delivery can be via needle and syringe, using pen injector devices or, in selected patients, by continuous subcutaneous infusion.

### Adverse effects

1 Hypoglycaemia is a common side effect. It is usually a result of decreased carbohydrate intake, unaccustomed exercise, administration of too much insulin or ingestion of alcohol. Symptoms and signs are those of adrenergic activation (sweating, tachycardia, systolic hypertension and hunger) and of neuroglycopaenia (visual disturbance, drowsiness, seizures and coma). The patient is usually alerted by the adrenergic symptoms and can take corrective action before neuroglycopaenic symptoms ensue.

2 Weight gain is commonly seen on insulin initiation. This is a particular problem in patients with type 2 diabetes mellitus in whom weight loss is recommended. It is thought to be due to reduced urine glucose loss and the general anabolic effects of insulin.

3 Local effects of subcutaneous insulin injection are hypertrophy of fat (lipohypertrophy) or loss of fat (lipoatrophy). Injection into areas of lipohypertrophy increases the variability of insulin absorption. Lipoatrophy is uncommon since the advent of human or highly purified animal insulins.

**4** Antibodies may develop to insulin, resulting in prolongation or attenuation of the action of insulin. They are not usually seen with human insulin.

## Oral hypoglycaemic agents

### Biguanides

*Mechanisms*

The mechanism of action is not completely understood. Biguanides have many metabolic effects, including reduced hepatic glucose production (gluconeogenesis) and increased glucose uptake and oxidation by skeletal muscle. They reduce insulin resistance.

*Pharmacokinetics*

Metformin is rapidly absorbed and has a half-life of 2–5 h. It is excreted unchanged by the kidney.

*Clinical use and dose*

Metformin is considered the drug of first choice in overweight or obese patients with type 2 diabetes. It is also used extensively as first-line monotherapy in patients of normal weight. The dose should be titrated up from a starting dose of 500 mg daily to a maximum dose of 3000 mg/day in divided doses. Metformin does not lead to weight gain or hypoglycaemia. Metformin can be used in combination with all other classes of oral hypoglycaemic agents and with insulin.

*Adverse effects*

The most frequent adverse effects are abdominal discomfort and gastrointestinal upset (e.g. nausea, diarrhoea, anorexia). It is dose related and can be minimised by gradual dose titration. Lactic acidosis is the most serious adverse event. It is rare but carries a high mortality, and metformin should not be given to patients with renal, hepatic, hypoxic respiratory or cardiac disease, or who are shocked.

### Sulphonylureas

*Mechanism*

Sulphonylureas stimulate insulin secretion by a direct effect on pancreatic β-cells. They bind to sulphonylurea receptors on these cells, resulting in release of insulin granules. Functioning pancreatic tissue is therefore necessary for their action.

*Pharmacokinetics*

All sulphonylureas are well absorbed and reach peak plasma concentrations within 2–4 h. Their duration of action is variable (Table 18. 6). All are metabolised by the liver but routes of elimination differ. All bind strongly to albumin and can interact with other highly protein-bound drugs (e.g. warfarin, sulphonamides).

*Clinical use and dose*

Sulphonylureas are used as first-line agents in patients who are not overweight, or in patients who have contraindications or intolerance to other agents. Patients should start at a low dose, which should be gradually titrated up.

A sulphonylurea with a shorter duration of action and without active metabolites (e.g. glipizide or tolbutamine) should be used in the elderly or those with renal or hepatic impairment to reduce risk of hypoglycaemia. Sulphonylureas can be combined with metformin, acarbose or the thiozolidinediones to optimise glycaemic control. They

**Table 18.6** Sulphonylureas—pharmacokinetic properties.

| Drug | Daily dose (mg) | Duration of action (half-life) in hours | Metabolites |
|---|---|---|---|
| Glibenclamide | 2.5–15.0 | up to 24 (10) | Active |
| Gliclazide | 40–320 | up to 24 (12) | Inactive |
| Glipizide | 2.5–20.0 | 6–12 (3) | Inactive |
| Chlorpropamide | 100–500 | 24–72 (35) | Active |
| Tolbutamide | 500–2000 | 6–12 (4) | Inactive |
| Glimepiride | 1–6 | up to 24 (9) | Active |

can also be combined with insulin but this option is rarely used in the United Kingdom.

*Adverse effects*

All sulphonylureas can cause hypoglycaemia which can be severe and prolonged. It is more likely with the long-acting agents and chlorpropamide is no longer recommended for this reason. Sulphonylurea therapy is also associated with weight gain. Other adverse effects include allergic reactions (mainly rashes), gastrointestinal symptoms and, rarely, bone marrow suppression or cholestatic jaundice.

### Glucosidase inhibitors (acarbose)

Inhibition of α-glucosidase activity in the gastrointestinal tract reduces breakdown of more complex sugars to glucose. This reduces post-prandial hyperglycaemia. Acarbose can be given as monotherapy or in combination with other oral hypoglycaemic agents or insulin. Unfortunately, failure to adequately digest carbohydrate results in bacterial fermentation within the gut, resulting in excessive flatus production, and many patients do not tolerate the treatment. The α-glucosidase inhibitors do not cause weight gain and are unlikely to cause hypoglycaemia.

### Meglitinide analogues (repaglinide and nateglinide)

*Mechanism*

The meglitinides are rapid-acting insulin secretagogues. Like sulphonylureas they act at the sulphonylurea receptor of pancreatic β-cells but they bind at a different site.

*Pharmacokinetics*

They are rapidly absorbed and eliminated, peak plasma concentrations are reached within 1 h and the half-life is approximately 3 h.

*Clinical use and dose*

The meglitinides should be given 30 min before meals and started at a low dose. The indications and adverse event profile are similar to the sulphonylureas. They have a lower risk of hypoglycaemia and potentially cause less weight gain. They may suit individuals with an irregular lifestyle (e.g. shift workers).

### Thiozolidinediones (glitazones)

*Mechanism*

Two thiozolidinediones, rosiglitazone and pioglitazone, are currently marketed. Troglitazone was withdrawn following reports of idiosyncratic hepatotoxicity. They are insulin-sensitising drugs. They activate nuclear receptors (peroxisome proliferator-activated receptor-γ or PPARγ) that increase the transcription of insulin-sensitive genes. PPARγ is predominantly expressed in adipose tissue and also in skeletal muscle and liver. The effect of thiozolidinediones on glucose lowering is slow and maximal effect may be achieved only after 2–3 months.

*Pharmacokinetics*

Both rosiglitazone and pioglitazone are rapidly and almost completely absorbed (Table 18.7). They are highly protein bound but their concentrations are generally low. Both agents undergo extensive hepatic metabolism. Rosiglitazone is excreted mainly in urine and pioglitazone mainly in bile. No significant drug interactions have been reported.

*Clinical use and dose*

Rosiglitazone has a starting dose of 4 mg/day (maximum 8 mg/day) and pioglitazone 15–30 mg/day (maximum 45 mg/day). The dose should be titrated gradually. They can be used as monotherapy or in combination with metformin or a sulphonylurea. In the United Kingdom, combination with insulin therapy is contraindicated due to concerns about fluid retention; however, this combination is being widely used in the United States.

**Table 18.7** Thiozolidinediones—pharmacokinetic properties.

| Drug | Half-life parent drug (h) | Half-life metabolite (h) | Elimination |
|---|---|---|---|
| Rosiglitazone | 3.5 | 100–150 | Mainly urine |
| Pioglitazone | 3–7 | 16–24 | Mainly bile |

*Adverse effects*

The commonest adverse effects are weight gain, fluid retention, increased plasma volume and a reduced haematocrit. Contraindications are heart failure and hepatic impairment. Precautionary monitoring of liver function is currently recommended, although to date the hepatotoxicity seen with troglitazone has not been observed.

## Diabetic emergencies

### Hypoglycaemic coma

**Causes**

Coma is usually precipitated by missing a meal, unaccustomed exercise or taking too much insulin or sulphonylurea.

**Clinical features**

Coma can present with a wide range of neurological signs. Every medical emergency arriving with mental impairment, coma or other neurological signs must have capillary glucose checked on arrival.

**Treatment**

A 50-ml dose of 50% dextrose is given intravenously and repeated as necessary. Alternatively, 1-mg glucagon is given intravenously or intramuscularly, which is useful if the patient is difficult to restrain. Glucagon may be given to patients for administration by relatives as emergency treatment for hypoglycaemia.

### Ketoacidosis

**Causes**

Infections are the most common identifiable cause. Myocardial infarction, trauma and inadequate insulin dosage are other causes.

**Clinical features**

Typically these patients are dehydrated, hyperventilating and may have impaired consciousness. Blood glucose is usually markedly elevated, ketones are present (measured in the urine or blood) and there is acidosis. Venous bicarbonate measurement is used to assess severity. Total body potassium stores are always depleted largely due to the osmotic diuresis. However, the plasma potassium is usually high normal or slightly elevated because insulin deficiency prevents entry of potassium into cells and there is extracellular potassium shift in response to the acidosis.

**Treatment**

This is based on replacement of fluid, electrolytes and insulin.

1 Fluid replacement. The free water deficit averages 5–7 l in diabetic ketoacidosis (DKA). Isotonic saline should be used in most cases. A suggested regime over the first hours of treatment is shown below.

    1000 ml isotonic saline in 30 min

    1000 ml isotonic saline in 1 h (with added potassium—see Table 18.8)

    1000 ml isotonic saline in 2 h (with added potassium—see Table 18.8)

Subsequent fluid should be tailored to the patient, e.g. 1000 ml isotonic saline 4- to 8-hourly until the fluid deficit is corrected. Use a central venous pressure line in the elderly or those with cardiac disease. If serum sodium rises above 150 mmol/l (mEq/l), use half normal saline instead.

2 Insulin. In DKA, insulin is given intravenously and the infusion rate adjusted according to blood glucose. A typical starting rate is 5 units/h. An initial dose of 10 units of soluble insulin can be given intramuscularly if there is a delay in initiating intravenous treatment.

When blood glucose is <15 mmol/l (270 mg/100 ml), change the infusion fluid to 5% glucose with potassium replacement and continue the insulin infusion.

**Table 18.8** Suggested potassium regimen in patients with diabetic ketoacidosis.

| Plasma potassium (mmol/l) | Potassium added (mmol/l) |
| --- | --- |
| >5.5 | None |
| 3.5–5.5 | 20 |
| <3.5 | 40 |

**3** Potassium replacement. The total body potassium deficit ranges from 3 to 12 mmol/kg (mEq/kg). With insulin and fluid replacement, serum potassium concentrations fall and early potassium replacement is vital. Replacement should begin with the second and subsequent bags of fluid, adjusting as shown in Table 18.8.

The use of sodium bicarbonate in treating acidosis in DKA is controversial. It has been associated with serious fluid disequilibrium and development of cerebral oedema. The use of bicarbonate is therefore not routinely recommended. The majority of cases respond to the treatments above and bicarbonate should be considered only in patients who remain hypotensive and have severe acidosis (pH <6.9).

*Comment.* Patients require frequent observations and glucose and electrolyte monitoring. Remember that there is often an underlying cause. If you suspect infection, treat with antibiotics after relevant culture specimens have been obtained.

## Hyperosmolar, non-ketotic hyperglycaemic coma

### Cause

It usually occurs in patients older than 60 years and may be the first presentation of type 2 diabetes mellitus. The cause is obscure.

### Features

The patient is often drowsy and is dehydrated. Typical laboratory findings are very high blood glucose, raised urea, raised sodium and a high plasma osmolality.

### Treatment

Isotonic saline is given, or half normal if plasma sodium is >150 mmol (mEq)/l. Fluid replacement is otherwise similar to DKA, and a central venous pressure line may be required. Intravenous insulin is given; insulin sensitivity is greater in these patients due to lack of severe acidosis. Patients are at risk of thrombosis, and unless contraindicated, full anticoagulation with heparin should be given.

## Thyroid disease

### Thyrotoxicosis (hyperthyroidism)

### Pathophysiology

Thyrotoxicosis results from the actions of excess thyroid hormone on target tissue. Typical features are caused by stimulation of metabolism and effects on catecholamines. They include weight loss with increased appetite and heat intolerance, palpitations, tremor, nervousness. It is more common in females.

Hyperfunction of the thyroid gland can be caused by

**1** Graves' disease
**2** Toxic multi-nodular goitre
**3** Toxic solitary nodule.

Graves' disease is an organ-specific autoimmune disease. Stimulating antibodies to the thyroid-stimulating hormone (TSH) receptor can be detected in the majority of cases. The disease can relapse and remit. Following a course of anti-thyroid drugs, 30–40% of cases enter long-term remission.

Patients with toxic multi-nodular goitres or a toxic solitary nodule do not enter remission with anti-thyroid drugs, and definitive treatment is with radioiodine or surgery.

### Aims of treatment

Treatment of thyrotoxicosis is dependent upon the underlying aetiology and is summarised in Table 18.9. In general, the aims of treatment are symptom relief, control of the disease and if appropriate definitive treatment with radioiodine or surgery. Thiourylene anti-thyroid drugs are often used to achieve a euthyroid status prior to definitive treatment.

### Drug treatments in thyrotoxicosis

#### Thiourylene anti-thyroid drugs
*Mechanism*
These drugs (carbimazole, methimazole, propylthiouracil) all share a similar chemical structure. Methimazole is a product of carbimazole metabolism and is the active compound. Methimazole is

239

**Table 18.9** Treatments used in the management of thyrotoxicosis.

| Treatment | Example | Indication |
|---|---|---|
| β-Adrenoreceptor blockade | Propanolol | Symptom relief only |
| Thiourylene antithyroid drugs | Carbimazole, methimazole, propylthiouracil | Control of throtoxicosis, induction of remission in Graves' disease |
| Radioactive iodine | Iodine-131 | Definitive treatment of relapsed Graves' disease, toxic multi-nodular goitre and toxic solitary nodule |
| Potassium iodide | | Preparation for surgery and treatment of thyrotoxic crisis (thyroid storm) |
| Surgery | Total or subtotal thyroidectomy | Definitive treatment as per radioactive iodine. Often reserved for cases with local compressive symptoms |

widely used in the United States and Europe, while carbimazole is available in the United Kingdom.

Their exact mode of action is unclear but is thought to involve reduced thyroid hormone synthesis by:

1 Inhibition of iodide oxidation.

2 Inhibition of iodination of tyrosine.

3 Inhibition of coupling of iodotyrosines.

Propylthiouracil also reduces the conversion of $T_4$ to $T_3$ in the peripheral tissues, which may have additional therapeutic benefit.

As anti-thyroid drugs do not alter the secretion of pre-formed thyroid hormone, the effects on circulating thyroid hormone levels and on the symptoms of thyrotoxicosis are not apparent for some time (2–4 weeks).

*Pharmacokinetics*

The thioureylenes are given orally. Carbimazole is rapidly hydrolysed in plasma to methimazole. Methimazole has a plasma half-life of 12–15 h.

*Clinical use and dose*

*Carbimazole*: A starting dose of 20–40 mg daily is normally used in adults. Once a euthyroid state has been achieved, one of two regimes to prevent hypothyroidism can be used—either dose titration or a block and replace regime. In the dose titration regime the dose of carbimazole is gradually reduced to reach a maintenance (usually 5–10 mg/day). In the block and replace regime, carbimazole is continued at 40 mg daily together with levothyroxine sodium (100–150 μg).

*Propylthiouracil*: A starting dose of 200–400 mg daily is used in adults. Once euthyroid, the dose is gradually reduced to a maintenance of 50–100 mg.

Patients with Graves' disease who may enter remission are often given anti-thyroid drugs for up to 18 months. If remission seems likely at that point, treatment may be withdrawn and the patients monitored to detect relapse. This approach is not appropriate for patients whose disease will not enter remission (e.g. multi-nodular goitre).

*Adverse effects*

1 All the drugs will cause hypothyroidism and goitre enlargement, when given chronically. This can be prevented by using the dosing regimes described above.

2 Agranulocytosis is the most serious side effect. It is rare and generally resolves on stopping therapy. Patients should be given a written warning at the start of treatment about this and should be instructed to report any sore throat or fever immediately.

3 The most common side effects are skin rashes and pruritus. A substantial proportion of patients

who develop a rash when on carbimazole will also do so on propylthiouracil.

**4** Arthralgia, hepatitis and serum sickness type reactions are all rarely seen with these drugs.

**5** Carbimazole/methimazole and propylthiouracil cross the placenta and can cause fetal hypothyroidism and goitre. Pregnant patients should therefore be given the lowest possible dose to control the disease. Use of carbimazole in pregnancy has been associated with a very rare occurrence of aplasia cutis, a congenital abnormality of scalp skin development. The drugs are secreted in breast milk (propylthiouracil to a lesser extent than carbimazole/methimazole), and this can result in neonatal hypothyroidism. Propylthiouracil is considered the drug of choice during pregnancy and lactation.

### Radioactive iodine

The indications for using radioiodine are shown in Table 18.9. It is well absorbed orally and is given as a single dose. It is taken up by the thyroid where it causes localised destruction by a radiation thyroiditis. There is little radiation dose to other tissues. The iodine-131 has a half-life of 8 days. The effects on the thyroid take several weeks with the maximal effect occurring approximately 2 months later.

The advantages of radioactive iodine are its simplicity, low cost and safety. The major disadvantage is the occurrence of hypothyroidism. Early hypothyroidism (within a few months) is a dose-related phenomenon. Thereafter, late hypothyroidism will affect between 2 and 4% of patients per year. This is an inexorable phenomenon and the incidence of hypothyroidism is approximately 50% at 10 years.

There is no evidence of any carcinogenic risk following radioactive iodine treatment. There is no evidence of any harm to germinal tissue; however, patients are advised to avoid conception for a minimum of 4 months following radioactive iodine therapy (male patients are advised not to father children for a similar period of time).

### Potassium iodide

Iodide has multiple actions on the thyroid. The most important is an immediate reduction in thyroid hormone release and for this reason potassium iodide is used in thyroid crisis. The drug will also inhibit thyroid hormone formation and iodide trapping and reduces gland vascularity. With regular dosing it has a maximal effect at 10–15 days, its effects then diminish because of loss of its inhibitory effects on the thyroid.

### β-Adrenoreceptor blockade

Propranolol reduces peripheral conversion of $T_4$ to $T_3$, and also provides some symptomatic relief. It should be emphasised that beta-blockers have no effect on the underlying process of Graves' disease or on thyroid hormone secretion.

## Thyroid crisis

This condition has a high mortality and is characterised by fever, tachycardia, dehydration and confusion. It is treated with potassium iodide and carbimazole. Patients also require general supportive measures, including rehydration, intravenous beta-blocker therapy and steroids.

## Hypothyroidism

### Pathophysiology

Hypothyroidism results from insufficient secretion of thyroid hormones; classical features include lethargy, weight gain, dry skin and cold intolerance. It is most commonly due to an autoimmune thyroiditis (Hashimoto's thyroiditis) but has a variety of other causes including congenital dysfunction, iodine deficiency and following treatment of thyrotoxicosis.

### Treatment—thyroid replacement therapy

Treatment is directed at replacing thyroid hormone levels in the circulation. Two thyroid hormone preparations are available: levothyroxine sodium (thyroxine, $T_4$) and liothyronine sodium ($T_3$), although the latter is rarely used.

## Mechanism

$T_4$ is converted to $T_3$ in cells by a deiodinase enzyme. $T_3$ binds to nuclear receptors and regulates gene transcription. This leads to multiple metabolic actions. In some tissue (e.g. the pituitary) there is an obligatory requirement for a high percentage of $T_3$ to be derived from intracellular $T_4$ conversion. For this reason, $T_4$ is a more effective hormone in suppression of TSH than is $T_3$ and is therefore the preferred thyroid hormone for replacement.

## Pharmacokinetics

Both $T_4$ and $T_3$ are adequately absorbed following oral administration. $T_4$ has a half-life of about a week and $T_3$ about 2 days. Both undergo conjugation in the liver and enterohepatic circulation.

## Clinical use and dose

The doses of thyroid hormone required for adequate replacement are assessed by measurement of serum TSH concentrations unless there is underlying pituitary disease.

Levothyroxine sodium is started at a dose of 50–100 µg/day (25 µg/day if elderly or with heart disease), with dose increments every 4 weeks, depending on thyroid function. The usual maintenance dose is 100–200 µg/day. Liothyronine sodium can be used to achieve a more rapid response and is given intravenously in hypothyroid coma; 20 µg is equivalent to 100 µg of levothyroxine.

Levothyroxine sodium is also used postoperatively in thyroid carcinoma to replace endogenous thyroxine and to suppress TSH, as many tumours are TSH dependent. The dose of levothyroxine used under these circumstances is higher than that given as replacement therapy, and is normally in the region of 200 µg/day.

## Adverse effects

These are related to the physiological and pharmacological actions of thyroid hormone. Elderly patients, or those known to have ischaemic heart disease, are given low initial doses with slow increments because angina or myocardial infarction can be precipitated. Thyroid hormone excess produces the usual clinical features of thyrotoxicosis.

# Obesity

## Pathophysiology

Obesity is increasing in prevalence amongst both the developed and the developing world. In Europe, approximately 15–20% of the middle-aged population are obese. Obesity is a risk factor for serious diseases including ischaemic heart disease, hypertension, type 2 diabetes mellitus, stroke and certain malignancies (e.g. breast, ovary, colon, prostate, endometrial). It is also associated with obstructive sleep apnoea, osteoarthritis, gallstones and varicose veins.

Most patients have 'simple' obesity although it is a feature of certain conditions, e.g. Prader–Willi syndrome. It results from energy intake in excess of energy expenditure over a prolonged period of time. Genetic factors, environmental change (sedentary lifestyle with an abundance of energy-rich foods) and potentially, alterations in neurotransmitters that influence appetite, e.g. leptin, contribute to the tendency to develop obesity.

## Aims of treatment

Treatment should aim for realistic weight loss (e.g. 0.5–1 kg/week) which is then maintained. A 10% weight loss is a reasonable initial aim and is associated with a reduction in mortality and morbidity.

## Non-pharmacological therapy

A reduction in dietary calorie intake, increased energy expenditure through exercise and behavioural modification are fundamental aspects of obesity management.

## Drug treatments of obesity

Drug treatment can be used as an adjunct to diet and exercise in patients who are obese or overweight with significant co-morbidity.

## Pancreatic lipase inhibitors (Orlistat)

### Mechanism

Orlistat binds to the active site of pancreatic lipases and slows the breakdown of dietary fat in the gastrointestinal tract. It can reduce the amount of fat absorbed by up to 30%.

### Pharmacokinetics

Orlistat is excreted in the faeces.

### Clinical use and dose

When used as part of a weight-control program, average weight loss of 10% in a year has been observed. A dose of 120 mg is taken immediately before or within an hour of each main meal (up to a maximum of 360 mg daily). It is contraindicated in patients with chronic malabsorption and cholestasis.

### Adverse effects

The most frequent adverse effects are loose oily stools and faecal urgency, and oily rectal discharge. The potential for impaired absorption of fat-soluble vitamins and concomitant medications, e.g. oral contraceptive pills, should be considered.

## Sibutramine

### Mechanism

Sibutramine is a centrally acting anti-obesity drug. It blocks the re-uptake of noradrenaline and serotonin. It causes dose-dependent weight loss by reduced food intake and increased satiety.

### Pharmacokinetics

Sibutramine is well absorbed after oral administration. It undergoes extensive first-pass metabolism and the metabolites are pharmacologically active. The active metabolites are inactivated in the liver and are excreted in the urine and faeces.

### Clinical use and dose

The starting daily dose is 10 mg; this can be increased up to 15 mg if target weight loss is not achieved.

### Adverse effects

In some individuals, sibutramine may cause a rise in blood pressure and pulse rate, and its use is contraindicated in patients with uncontrolled hypertension and cardiovascular disease. Dry mouth, constipation and insomnia are common adverse effects.

# Bone metabolism

The drugs described in this section are used in the management of disorders of bone structure, e.g. osteoporosis and osteomalacia, and disorders of calcium metabolism, e.g. hypoparathyroidism and hyperparathyroidism.

## Calcium salts

Calcium salts are used in the management of
1 Dietary deficiency
2 Prevention and treatment of osteoporosis
3 Hypocalcaemia due to malabsorption or hypoparathyroidism
4 Hyperphosphataemia
5 Cardiac dysrhythmias associated with hyperkalaemia.

Dietary deficiency is more likely during childhood, pregnancy and breast feeding, due to increased demand, and in the elderly, due to reduced absorption.

## Calcium preparations

Calcium salts are given orally in divided doses. Calcium salts used include calcium gluconate, calcium lactate and calcium carbonate. A daily calcium dose of 1000–1500 mg is recommended in osteoporosis. The main adverse effect is gastrointestinal disturbance.

Calcium carbonate binds phosphate in the gut and is used to treat the hyperphosphataemia seen in renal failure. Calcium gluconate is given intravenously in the treatment of hypocalcaemic tetany and in the treatment of cardiac dysrhythmias caused by severe hyperkalaemia.

## Vitamin D compounds

Vitamin D is a prehormone. In humans, the main source of vitamin D (cholecalciferol/calciferol) is from the photoactivation of 7-dehydrocholesterol in the skin. This undergoes hydroxylation in the liver to 25-hydroxycholecalciferol and in the kidneys to the active metabolite 1,25-dihydroxycholecaciferol (calcitriol). Some vitamin D (ergocalciferol) is derived from the diet.

A range of vitamin D compounds are available for therapeutic use, including ergocalciferol, calciferol, alfacalcidol (1α-hydroxycholecalciferol) and calcitriol (1,25-dihydroxycholecalciferol).

## Mechanism

The main action of vitamin D compounds is to facilitate intestinal absorption of calcium and phosphate. They also promote calcium mobilisation from bone and increase calcium reabsorption in the kidney tubules.

## Pharmacokinetics

All vitamin D compounds are given orally and are well absorbed. Vitamin D is fat soluble and bile is necessary for absorption. Vitamin D undergoes enterohepatic circulation and is largely eliminated in the faeces.

## Clinical use and dose

The indications and dosages of the commonly used vitamin D compounds are shown in Table 18.10.

## Adverse effects

Hypercalcaemia is the main complication of vitamin D therapy. All patients receiving pharmacological doses should have monitoring of their serum calcium. Some anti-convulsants induce the enzymes that metabolise vitamin D and cause increased requirements.

## Bisphosphonates

### Mechanism

Bisphosphonates are a family of carbon-substituted pyrophosphates that bind avidly to bone. They have an inhibitory action on osteoclasts and therefore reduce bone resorption. Substitution of different chemical moieties at the carbon atom produces compounds with differing potencies (Table 18.11).

### Pharmacokinetics

When administered orally, bisphosphonates are poorly absorbed. Between 20 and 50% of the absorbed drug binds to bone within 24 h where it remains for many months, possibly years, until the bone is resorbed. Unbound (free) drug is excreted unchanged by the kidneys. Calcium and other chelating agents reduce the absorption of bisphosphonates from the gastrointestinal tract. Bisphosphonates should be taken with plain water on an empty stomach first thing in the morning at least 30 min before breakfast or, if taken at

**Table 18.10** Vitamin D preparations and their use.

| | Ergocalciferol, calciferol (IU/day) | Alfacacidol (μg/day) | Calcitriol (μg/day) |
|---|---|---|---|
| Vitamin D deficiency | | | |
| Dietary deficiency | 400–5000 | | |
| Malabsorption | | | |
| Chronic liver disease | Up to 40,000 | | |
| Hypoparathyroidism | 25,000–100,000 | 0.5–2.0 | 0.25–1.00 |
| Renal osteodystrophy | | 0.5–2.0 | 0.25–1.00 |
| Osteoporosis | | | 0.5 |

**Table 18.11** Bisphosphonates.

| Drug | Relative potency | Indications (*current licensed indications in the United Kingdom*) |
|---|---|---|
| *First generation (short alkyl or halide side chain)* | | |
| Etidronate | 1 | Osteoporosis, Paget's disease |
| Clodronate | 10 | Hypercalcaemia, metastatic bone disease |
| *Second generation (generally with amino terminal group)* | | |
| Tiludronate | 10 | Paget's disease |
| Pamidronate | 100 | Paget's disease, hypercalcaemia, metastatic bone disease |
| Alendronate | 100–1000 | Osteoporosis |
| *Third generation (cyclic side chain)* | | |
| Risendronate | 1000–10,000 | Osteoporosis, Paget's disease |
| Ibandronate | 1000–10,000 | Hypercalcaemia, metastatic bone disease |
| Zolendronate | 10,000+ | Hypercalcaemia, metastatic bone disease |

any other time of day, food and drink should be avoided for 2 h before and after the dose.

## Clinical use and dose

The indications are summarised in Table 18.11.

1 *Treatment and prevention of osteoporosis.* Bisphosphonates are associated with an increase in bone mineral density and a significant reduction in risk of vertebral fractures (etidronate, alendronate, risendronate, ibandronate) and hip and other fractures (alendronate, risendronate, ibandronate) when given orally in association with calcium supplementation. Etidronate is given in 14-day cycles followed by 76 days of calcium carbonate. Alendronate and risendronate are given as a once-daily or once-weekly regimen and oral ibandronate has a daily or monthly dosing schedule.

2 *Paget's disease.* In Paget's disease, bisphosphonates are used to suppress disease activity, aiming for an alkaline phosphatase in the normal range, and in the treatment of bone pain.

3 *Hypercalcaemia.* Intravenous bisphosphonates (pamidronate, clodronate and zolendronate) are used in the treatment of severe hypercalcaemia. They should not be used until there has been adequate intravenous saline rehydration (with furosemide diuresis if salt and water retention occurs). The dose should be reduced if there is renal impairment. Plasma calcium usually falls by 72 h.

4 *Metastatic bone disease.* Bisphosphonates have been found to reduce complications (including pathological fracture) associated with advanced multiple myeloma and metastatic bone disease (e.g. breast cancer).

## Adverse effects

Bisphosphonates are generally well tolerated. They have a number of gastrointestinal side effects including nausea, diarrhoea, and oesophageal irritation and ulceration. Intravenous use of bisphosphonates can be associated with transient pyrexia and flu-like symptoms.

## Hormone replacement therapy

### Mechanism

Oestrogen suppresses osteoclast-mediated bone resorption. Hormone replacement therapy (HRT) prevents menopause-associated bone loss, and an increase in bone mineral density is seen. HRT use is associated with a reduction in hip, vertebral and forearm fractures.

### Pharmacokinetics

Orally administered oestrogens undergo extensive first-pass metabolism by the liver. They have a half-life of 10–18 h.

## Clinical use

Due to the risk of serious adverse events (see below), HRT is no longer recommended as first line in the prevention and treatment of post-menopausal osteoporosis. Short-term use of HRT is still appropriate for women with menopausal symptoms, e.g. vasomotor instability, where benefits outweigh the risks.

## Adverse effects

HRT is associated with a slight increase in stroke and an increase in thromboembolic disease, breast cancer and endometrial cancer. HRT does not prevent coronary heart disease. Common side effects include breast tenderness, fluid retention and weight gain.

## Selective oestrogen-receptor modulators

### Mechanism

Selective oestrogen-receptor modulators (SERMS) are non-hormonal agents that bind to oestrogen receptors. Raloxifene is the only SERM currently available. Depending on the target tissue, SERMS have agonist or antagonist action. Raloxifene has agonist action on bone and cardiovascular system and antagonist action on mammary tissue and the uterus. Their action on bone causes a reduction in osteoclast activity and an increase in bone mineral density.

### Pharmacokinetics

Approximately 60% of an oral dose is absorbed. Raloxifene undergoes extensive first-pass metabolism and has a bioavailability of around 2%. It has a half-life of approximately 32 h and after metabolism is excreted in the faeces. Cholestyramine reduces its absorption due to reduced enterohepatic cycling.

### Clinical use and dose

Raloxifene is used in the treatment and prevention of post-menopausal osteoporosis at a daily dose of 60 mg. Raloxifene does not reduce menopausal vasomotor symptoms.

## Adverse effects

Hot flushes and leg cramps are common side effects. SERMS are associated with an increased risk of thromboembolic disease similar to that observed with HRT.

## Calcitonin

### Mechanism

Calcitonin is a peptide hormone synthesised by the parafollicular cells within the thyroid gland. Synthetic forms (salmon, porcine) are available for therapeutic use. Calcitonin reduces bone resorption by decreasing the number and activity of osteoclasts.

### Pharmacokinetics

Administration is by subcutaneous or intramuscular injection or nasal spray (licensed for osteoporosis in the United Kingdom). Calcitonin has a short half-life (4–40 min according to preparation) but its duration of action is several hours. It is metabolised by the kidneys.

### Clinical use and dose

1 *Treatment and prevention of osteoporosis.* Calcitonin is associated with a reduction in the incidence of osteoporotic vertebral fractures. It is less efficacious than bisphosphonates and HRT. Patients should also be prescribed calcium and vitamin D supplements. A daily dose of 100 units (subcutaneous or intramuscular injection) or 200 units (intranasally) is used. Calcitonin has potent analgesic properties and can be used in the management of acute fracture pain.

2 *Paget's disease.* Calcitonin is effective in relieving bone pain in Paget's disease and can suppress disease activity. The dose ranges from 50 units three times weekly to 100 units daily.

3 *Hypercalcaemia.* Calcitonin can be used to treat severe hypercalcaemia following saline rehydration and furosemide diuresis. High doses are required (up to 400 units 6 hourly). It is usually reserved for cases who have not responded to intravenous bisphosphonates.

4 *Bony metastases.* Bone pain in neoplastic disease can be treated with 200 units of calcitonin 6 hourly or 400 units 12 hourly.

## Adverse effects

Nausea, vomiting and flushing are common side effects. Local discomfort can occur at injection sites. Nasal spray can cause local irritation and ulceration. Antibodies may develop with long-term use, which attenuate its action. Allergic reactions rarely occur.

## Teriparatide

### Mechanism

Teriparatide is a recombinant peptide composed of 34 amino acids identical to the active region of parathyroid hormone. It stimulates osteoblasts, and increased bone formation and improved bone architecture are seen. A reduction in fractures has been demonstrated in post-menopausal patients with established osteoporosis.

### Pharmacokinetics

It is given by daily subcutaneous injection. It has a half-life of approximately 1 h and is thought to be metabolised by the liver and excreted by the kidneys.

### Clinical use and dose

Teriparatide is used in the treatment of established osteoporosis. A daily dose of 20 µg is given by subcutaneous injection.

### Adverse effects

Teriparatide is generally well tolerated. A transient increase in serum calcium is seen. Preclinical toxicology data showed a high incidence of osteosarcoma in rats given high doses of the drug. To date, development of osteosarcoma has not been reported in the clinical trials of teriparatide.

## Strontium ranelate

Strontium ranelate promotes bone formation by stimulating osteoblast activity and inhibiting osteoclasts. It is associated with a reduction in vertebral and non-vertebral fractures in established osteoporosis. An oral daily dose of 2 g is used in the treatment of osteoporosis.

## Pituitary and adrenal cortex disease

### Hypopituitarism

Partial or complete deficiency of anterior pituitary hormones arises from conditions including pituitary tumours, pituitary infarction and radiotherapy. It can result in inadequate production of thyroid hormones, adrenal steroids, sex steroids and growth hormone.

Treatment is with hormone replacement. Replacement of thyroid hormone, adrenal and sex steroids is considered elsewhere. Treatment of growth hormone deficiency depends on whether it is of childhood or adult onset. In childhood, growth hormone deficiency requires replacement. In adults, there is evidence that replacement improves quality of life and has favourable effects on lipid profile, bone mineral density and lean body mass. Growth hormone replacement for adults has now been approved in many countries. Synthetic human growth hormone, manufactured using recombinant DNA technology, is given by daily subcutaneous injection. In childhood, the dose is determined by body weight and surface area. Adults are started at a dose of 100–300 µg daily, which is titrated up to a usual maintenance dose of 200–600 µg.

## Cranial diabetes insipidus

Cranial diabetes insipidus is due to deficiency of circulating arginine vasopressin (anti-diuretic hormone). It arises due to hypothalamic or posterior pituitary dysfunction. In patients with an intact thirst mechanism, it presents with polyuria and polydipsia. In patients with an absent thirst mechanism (sometimes seen in head injury and hypothalamic syndromes) polyuria is seen without polydipsia, which can result in severe hypernatraemia.

Treatment is with synthetic vasopressin analogue (desmopressin). Treatment is given in divided doses, intranasally (10–40 μg/day), by parenteral injection (1–4 μg/day) or orally (100–1000 μg/day). There is wide variation in the doses required, and monitoring of the serum sodium and osmolality is essential. Desmopressin is broken down by vasopressinase. The activity of this enzyme increases during pregnancy and dose requirements increase in pregnancy.

## Drug treatment of pituitary tumours

### Dopamine agonists

**Mechanism**

Dopamine agonists cause activation of D2 receptors. Bromocriptine is short acting and is taken daily. Cabergoline is long acting and is taken once or twice weekly.

**Clinical use**

1 Hyperprolactinaemia/prolactinoma—D2 receptor stimulation inhibits prolactin secretion and leads to tumour shrinkage.
2 Growth-hormone-secreting tumours—A fall in growth hormone is seen in approximately half of patients with growth-hormone-secreting tumours given dopamine agonists. Dopamine acts directly on the tumours to inhibit growth hormone release. Tumour shrinkage can be seen and is more likely if the tumour co-secretes prolactin.

**Adverse effects**

Nausea and postural hypotension are common side effects. They may be minimised by slow initiation of therapy. Cabergoline is often better tolerated than bromocriptine.

### Somatostatin analogues

**Mechanism**

Somatostatin is released from the hypothalamus and inhibits the secretion of growth hormone and TSH. It is also produced in neuroendocrine cells in the gastrointestinal tract where it inhibits the release of numerous gut peptides including gastrin, glucagon and insulin. Ocreotide and lanreotide are synthetic analogues of somatostatin.

**Clinical use**

1 Growth-hormone-secreting tumours—somatostatin analogues can be used as initial therapy or as an adjunct to surgery and radiotherapy. A reduction in growth hormone is seen in approximately 60% of patients and tumour shrinkage can occur.
2 Neuroendocrine tumours—somatostatin analogues are used in the treatment of several neuroendocrine tumours including glucagonomas and VIPomas. They are also used in the management of carcinoid syndrome.

Octreotide is a short-acting formulation that is given by subcutaneous injection (50–100 μg three times a day). Long-acting preparations of lanreotide and octreotide are available, which are given by intramuscular injection on a 1–6 weekly regime dependent on the preparation and response.

**Adverse effects**

Gastrointestinal side effects are common and include nausea, abdominal pain and mild steatorrhoea. Gallstones have been reported after long-term treatment. Pain may occur at injection sites.

## Adrenal steroid replacement

Adrenal steroid deficiency occurs in primary adrenal failure (Addison's disease) or can be secondary to adrenocorticotropic hormone (ACTH) deficiency in pituitary disease. In primary adrenal failure there is deficiency of the glucocorticoid, cortisol and also the mineralocorticoid, aldosterone. In secondary adrenal failure there is only glucocorticoid deficiency because aldosterone secretion is regulated by the renin–angiotensin system.

Glucocorticoid replacement is usually with hydrocortisone although prednisolone or dexamethasone can be used. The replacement dose of hydrocortisone is usually 15–30 mg/day. The dose is divided to mimic the normal diurnal pattern of cortisol production; a typical regimen would be 10 mg on waking, 5 mg at midday and 5 mg at 6 p.m. The replacement dose needs to be increased during times of intercurrent illness, surgery or major physiological stress. All patients taking steroid replacement should carry a form of identification (e.g. medic alert) that gives details of their medical condition and current therapy.

Mineralocorticoid replacement is with fludrocortisone. Fludrocortisone is a synthetic steroid that has high affinity for the mineralocorticoid receptor. The usual dose is 100 μg/day (range 50–300 μg): the dose is titrated against blood pressure and plasma electrolytes.

# Chapter 19

# Travel medicine and tropical disease

Over 45 million Britons travel abroad each year. Many travelling to Europe, the United States and Australia require no special prophylaxis against infections different to those in Britain as the risks and public health are similar. However, travel to many other countries, especially in the tropics and subtropics, can expose the traveller to new health risks. Making a sound risk assessment for each traveller is the first stage of any pre-travel consultation.

It must be remembered that most illness encountered by travellers is not preventable by prophylaxis and much morbidity and mortality encountered abroad is not infection-related (e.g. sunburn, dehydration, alcohol excess and road-traffic accidents). To prevent infections it is always important to emphasise other health precautions, including care with food and water hygiene, safe sex and the avoidance of mosquito bites through repellents and impregnated bed nets when appropriate.

Those planning to work or travel in Africa or Asia should be aware of the high prevalence of HIV infection in these regions and the ways in which risk of infection can be minimised. Health-care workers who may be carrying out exposure-prone procedures may consider a post-exposure prophylaxis pack containing three antiretroviral agents to be administered if there is mucosal exposure or a penetrating needle stick injury with HIV-infected body fluids.

There are a number of sources of continually updated information on disease prevalence within different countries combined with other information necessary to make these risk assessments. The TRAVAX (A–Z of Healthy Travel) database is provided within the NHS by Health Protection Scotland (http://www.travax.scot.nhs.uk) and it is available through the NHS Net. A public site is also available (http://www.fitfortravel.scot.nhs.uk).

## Assessing the need for prophylaxis

- The significance to the individual traveller relates to the potential seriousness of the disease itself but it must not be forgotten that infected asymptomatic carriers can often, after the traveller returns home, transmit serious illness to other family members and close contacts (e.g. hepatitis A, HIV infection).
- The likelihood of contracting any infection depends upon multiple factors including the prevalence of the infection in the countries being visited, the length of time abroad and activities to be undertaken (e.g. rural or safari trips where malaria and rabies need to be given extra consideration and sporting activities such as rugby football where injury, with bleeding and the possibility of blood-borne infection, is common).
- The value of any immuno- or chemoprophylaxis depends upon the level of protection it provides,

ease of administration (e.g. number of doses) and cost in relation to the protection provided.

• Sometimes peer pressures and less logical considerations enter into the decision-making process and these cannot be ignored. For example, there is a lot of understandable and sometimes exaggerated fear over the risk of contacting rabies, and while the risk of yellow fever in East Africa is negligible for the package tourist the vaccine is usually given in line with national directives. The media can also have a positive role to play in increasing the traveller's awareness of real risks such as the recent increase in diphtheria in countries of the former Soviet Union or the risk of food- and water-borne diseases following natural disasters such as earthquakes.

These points are shown schematically below in Table 19.1. They can help the advisor and traveller make decisions only after balancing these various factors. A high score makes it likely that a particular form of prophylaxis will be worthwhile and a low score makes it questionable.

The decision whether to give a particular traveller prophylaxis should be the result of an informed decision and this may also involve the patient and when appropriate parents or other family and party members or group leaders.

## Principles of immunisation

### Passive immunisation

Passive immunisation uses existing antibodies in human immunoglobulin, prepared from pooled human blood donations, to provide protection.

*Human normal* pooled immunoglobulin (HNIG) is almost entirely IgG, and can provide pre-exposure protection against diseases prevalent in the blood-donating population such as hepatitis A.

*Human-specific* immunoglobulin is obtained from convalescent patient sera or taken from those recently actively immunised. This is used as post-exposure treatment for rabies, tetanus and hepatitis B to prevent or modify any subsequent illness. It should always be given as soon as possible following exposure.

Occasionally HNIG, against hepatitis A, and specific hepatitis B immunoglobulin are given to those going to be a high risk when there is no time to give effective active vaccination. However, the indications for this are now few with more rapidly effective, and often single dose, active vaccines.

Passive immunity following the administration of HNIG wanes within a few months related to the half-life of the product. Thus, it should be given close to the date of travel.

Live vaccinations should ideally be given 3 weeks before or 3 months after normal human immunoglobulin, which may contain antibodies to the relevant live vaccine, preventing an optimal vaccine response. Yellow fever vaccine is an exception to this rule, because HNIG does not contain significant specific antibodies to yellow fever.

## Active immunisation

Active immunisation is achieved when the immune system is challenged by immunogens to produce humoral or cellular responses. Should infection subsequently rechallenge the immune 'memory', it will provoke a rapid and specific response to that antigen.

• Active immunisation may be induced by inactivated organisms, inactivated toxins (toxoids), immunogenic components of organisms or live attenuated organisms (Table 19.2).

• Active vaccines can be absorbed onto an adjuvant such as aluminium salts to increase their immunogenicity.

• Oral vaccines can provide gut immunity through stimulating IgA in enteral secretions.

• The length of protection of active vaccination varies but is usually longer with live vaccines.

Most active vaccines induce humoral (antibody-related) immunity; however, intradermal attenuated mycobacterium, bacillus Calmette–Guérin (BCG), provides protection against *Mycobacterium tuberculosis* infection by inducing cell-mediated immunity.

Following administration of a live or inactivated vaccine, there is a primary delay before appreciable levels of antibody are manufactured by the

**Table 19.1** Scheme for helping to make risk assessments on the need for prophylaxis for a traveller.

| Grade | Qualifier | Description |
|---|---|---|
| **1** | | Significance to the individual traveller |
| *How serious could the specific infection be for the individual if infected?* | | |
| 0 | Minor | Rarely a severe illness |
| 1 | Moderate | Serious illness, complete recovery usual, rare death |
| 2 | Major | Severe illness, complications and death possible |
| 3 | Critical | Severe illness, serious or long-term complications common |
| 4 | Grave | Severe illness, complications and death are usual |
| **2** | | Significance to the community |
| *How serious are the public health implications if the traveller was to be infected?* | | |
| 0 | Minor | Minimal or no risk to public health |
| 1 | Moderate | Potential for spread to close contacts but usually confinable |
| 2 | Major | Potential for spread within the population |
| 3 | Critical | High probability of spread within a population |
| 4 | Grave | Certainty of spread within the exposed population |
| **3** | | Likelihood of exposure |
| *How likely is the traveller to become infected—considering destination and intended lifestyle?* | | |
| 0 | Very unlikely | Disease not normally present at destination |
| 1 | Unlikely | Disease present, intended lifestyle makes infection unlikely |
| 2 | Possible | Disease widespread but traveller likely to be able to avoid infection |
| 3 | Probable | Disease widespread; traveller's lifestyle makes avoiding infection difficult |
| 4 | Almost certain | Disease widespread and highly contagious |
| **4** | | Evaluation of active intervention |
| *How effective and practical is the available prophylaxis (vaccine or tablets) also considering side effects, cost and time available for completing optimal schedule?* | | |
| 0 | Passable | Marginal benefits, acceptable side effects, may be difficult to deliver |
| 1 | Satisfactory | Significant benefits, possible side effects, may be difficult to deliver |
| 2 | Useful | Useful and feasible intervention with some measurable benefits and few adverse side effects |
| 3 | Effective | Useful and feasible intervention with significant measurable benefits and few or no adverse side effects |
| 4 | Ideal | Highly effective and feasible intervention with side effects very unlikely |
| **5** | | Context |
| *Could the 'best' decision about prophylaxis be influenced by current public concerns, peer or media pressure?* | | |
| 0 | Indifferent | Little public interest or likely media response |
| 1 | Unsettled | Some public or media unease. Potential for repercussions if intervention fails |
| 2 | Sensitive | A publicly sensitive issue, press interest. Risk of serious repercussions if intervention fails |
| 3 | Adverse | Considerable public concern, political and emotional pressure, unhelpful and antagonistic media reports |
| 4 | Hostile | A lot of public and media interest, political involvement. Inappropriate demands may lead to inappropriate responses |

**Table 19.2** Current vaccines available in Britain.

|  | **Viral** | **Bacterial** |
|---|---|---|
| Live attenuated vaccines | Oral polio<br>Measles<br>Mumps<br>Yellow fever | BCG<br>Rubella |
| Inactivated organisms | Inactivated polio<br>Hepatitis A<br>Rabies<br>Japanese B encephalitis (not<br>licensed in the UK)<br>Tick-borne encephalitis (not<br>licensed in the UK) | Pertussis<br>Typhoid<br>Cholera |
| Immunogenic<br>components of<br>organisms | Influenza<br>Hepatitis B | *Haemophilus influenzae*<br>type B<br><br>Pneumococcal (polysaccharide)<br>Quadravalent<br>Meningococcal vaccine<br>(A, C, W135 and Y)<br>Typhim Vi (polysaccharide) |
| Inactivated toxoids |  | Tetanus<br>Diphtheria<br>Cholera |

immune system. Therefore, for maximum protection, primary active immunisation courses require to be in advance of possible exposure, and in some instances quite long periods (e.g. toxoids of diphtheria and tetanus) and with rabies (see Table 19.3).

If a definite exposure occurs before these intervals have passed, extra immediate doses of vaccine may have to be considered (e.g. following a potentially rabid bite) or a dose of specific immunoglobulin (e.g. after a tetanus-prone wound or exposure to hepatitis B).

In time, most vaccine-induced antibody responses decline and may require to be boosted. These intervals can vary greatly (e.g. a few years with typhoid and more than 10 years with hepatitis A). Increasingly it is being recognised that real protection can be achieved for much longer than the detectable presence of antibodies because a very rapid amnestic response can still occur after exposure to infection.

**Table 19.3** Approximate time interval required for maximum protection after primary course of vaccination.

| Vaccine | Interval required primary course for maximum protection |
|---|---|
| Poliomyelitis (oral) | 1–2 weeks after three doses |
| Poliomyelitis (parenteral) | 1–2 weeks after three doses |
| Tetanus | 1–2 weeks after three doses |
| Diphtheria | 1–2 weeks after three doses |
| BCG | 6 weeks after one dose |
| Typhoid Vi | 2 weeks after one dose |
| Hepatitis A | 2 weeks after one dose |
| Immunoglobulin | Immediate |
| Hepatitis B | 1 month after three doses |
| Japanese B encephalitis | 1–2 weeks after three doses |
| Rabies intramuscular | 1–2 weeks after three doses |
| Rabies intradermal | 4 weeks after three doses |
| Tick-borne encephalitis | 2 weeks after two doses |
| MMR | 2 weeks after one dose |
| Yellow fever | 10 days after one dose |

Boosters normally give maximum protection after a few days, although this may be longer with intradermal vaccinations. If the booster dose interval has been substantially delayed, the interval may be longer.

## Live vaccines

Live vaccines are usually best stored at cool temperatures (0–5°C) and are heat- and light-labile once reconstituted. Thus, provision of a 'cold chain' of refrigeration is important but may be difficult, especially in poorer and tropical developing countries.

When more than one live vaccine is required, they are best given simultaneously or at least 3 weeks apart to prevent the interferon response from the first vaccine reducing the effectiveness of subsequent vaccines.

## Vaccine contraindications

Live vaccines should usually be avoided in pregnancy and also in patients who are significantly immunosuppressed from either illness or medication. Manufacturers often also advise that inactivated vaccines are best avoided in pregnancy, although there is little evidence of them causing any harm to the fetus. They can be administered if the risk of infection is substantial. Febrile reactions can sometimes precipitate a miscarriage.

During an acute febrile illness, vaccination should be postponed, as it will be difficult to recognise a vaccine 'reaction'. Mild afebrile or non-systemic illnesses are not normally contraindications.

If there has been a severe local or systemic reaction such as anaphylaxis, to a previous dose of vaccine then further doses of that vaccine must be avoided.

Some vaccines contain traces of egg proteins or antibiotics and should be avoided in those who have serious allergy to these components.

As vaccines may induce severe allergic reactions, all vaccination centres should have facilities for dealing with anaphylaxis. Vaccinated patients should ideally be observed in the vaccination centre for 30 min. Vasovagal reactions are much more common and these can be quite alarming, sometimes with anoxic convulsions. A previous history of faints should alert the advisor to this possibility.

## Vaccines used for preventing infection in travellers

### Poliomyelitis

Poliomyelitis is an enterovirus spread by the faecal–oral route and is associated with poor sanitation. It is a hardy virus, resistant to lower concentrations of chlorine and can survive for long periods outside the host. The virus has a predilection for central nervous system (CNS) tissue. There are three strains of poliovirus.

*Disease risk areas.* Poliomyelitis used to be of worldwide distribution but intensive immunisation campaigns supported by the World Health Organization (WHO) have resulted in the disease being eliminated from the Americas, and the Far East is close to being declared infection-free. Main foci are now the Indian subcontinent and parts of Africa.

### Vaccines

Oral polio vaccine (OPV) is included in the British vaccination schedule. Booster doses should be given to travellers to risk areas who have not had OPV for more than 10 years. OPV is a live vaccine and contains all three viral types. Attenuated strains of OPV may rarely revert to pathological 'wild' virus after transit through the bowel and cause a polio-like illness. Therefore, scrupulous attention to hygiene following toileting or nappy changes should be practiced when children have received the vaccine and close contacts should receive a booster dose of OPV at the same time. OPV drops are often given on sugar lumps to disguise its oily taste.

Inactivated polio vaccine (IPV) is a whole cell virus vaccine inactivated by formaldehyde. It is given by intramuscular or subcutaneous injection; booster doses are required at 10-yearly intervals.

If oral polio is contraindicated (immunosuppression or pregnancy) IPV may be given instead. Some countries now give IPV (often in combination with other childhood vaccines) instead of OPV to try and eliminate the rare cases of vaccine-associated disease.

## Tetanus

*Clostridium tetani* is a Gram-positive anaerobe that lives in soil and arises from bird and animal faecal contamination. Contaminated wounds, which may often be minor such as from thorns, lead to muscular spasms secondary to CNS changes induced by tetanus toxin. It is the toxin, not the organism itself, which leads to disease.

*Disease risk areas.* Worldwide. Herd immunity is not helpful since the disease is not spread from person to person and every individual must be vaccinated. In countries where childhood vaccination schedules have been introduced recently it has become a disease of unimmunised adults. While 10-yearly boosters are not currently advised in Britain, after the full five doses have been received in childhood and adolescence, extra boosters for travellers going to countries with poor hygiene can be given.

## Vaccine

Tetanus toxoid vaccine is tetanus toxin inactivated by formaldehyde and adsorbed on aluminium phosphate or aluminium hydroxide. Medical attention should be sought for a wound possibly contaminated by tetanus when tetanus toxoid boosters or tetanus-specific immunoglobulin may be required. Local reactions may occur, but systemic febrile reactions are rare. Their incidence increases, however, if fully immune individuals have been given unnecessary extra doses of vaccines (e.g. for repeated wounds requiring attention in accident and emergency departments). Vigorous local inflammatory reactions at the site of injection suggest that the individual may be becoming hypersensitive.

## Typhoid

*Salmonella typhi* is a Gram-negative bacillus that causes a septicaemic illness. Untreated illnesses can lead to serious complications and death in around 10% of instances. Spread is through the faecal–oral route from contaminated food or water and occasionally from person to person. Typhoid vaccines do not protect against other enteric fevers, including *S. paratyphi*.

*Disease risk areas.* Typhoid is endemic in developing countries with poor sanitation.

## Vaccine

Typhoid Vi polysaccharide capsular vaccine (typhim Vi) contains the Vi antigen of the *S. typhi* capsule and is preserved with phenol. One dose is given intramuscularly or subcutaneously with 3-yearly boosters.

It should only be used in pregnancy when the risk of infection is high and there is often a suboptimal response in children younger than 18 months. Local and febrile reactions lasting 24 h are much less marked with typhoid Vi capsular vaccine than with a previously available injectable heat-killed vaccine.

This vaccine is now available combined with one for hepatitis A.

*An oral* live attenuated vaccine is no longer available in the United Kingdom.

## Cholera

Cholera is characterised by profuse watery non-bloody diarrhoea and is caused by the enterotoxin of *Vibrio cholerae*. A high infective dose of organisms is required and it is rare in travellers taking sensible precautions with their water hygiene. Disease is spread through contaminated water and less commonly, food. Those unable to take effective precautions or at particular risk, for example, health-care workers, during wars and when working in refugee camps or slums, may consider vaccination when outbreaks are reported.

*Disease risk areas*. India, South-east Asia, Africa and Central and South America.

## Vaccine

The cholera vaccine (Dukoral) was licensed in the United Kingdom in 2004 and consists of killed whole V. cholerae O1 bacteria and the recombinant non-toxic B-subunit of the cholera toxin. Bacterial strains of all the common biotypes are included in the vaccine. Two oral doses at an interval of at least one week should be administered to those aged over 6 years. Three doses should be given to those aged 2–6 years. Yearly boosters are required for adults and 6-monthly for those aged 2–6 years. The vaccine should be postponed in those with a gastrointestinal or acute febrile illness. Food, drink and other medication should be avoided for the hour prior to and following the vaccine's administration. No country officially requires cholera certificates for entry; however, these may be requested by travellers. The cholera vaccine is also effective in reducing the risk of travellers' diarrhoea which is predominantly caused by enterotoxigenic *Escherichia coli*, which produces a heat-labile toxin. Vaccine side effects include gastrointestinal upset and headache.

## Hepatitis A

Hepatitis A is a hepatotropic virus spread by the faecal–oral route and also from person to person when hygiene is poor. Asymptomatic infections are common, especially in children. In countries with poor hygiene, 90% of children have been naturally infected by the age of 10 years.

Hepatitis IgG antibodies from natural infection confer life-long immunity. Therefore it is worthwhile checking the immune status of older people (above 60 years), those with a previous history of unexplained jaundice and those who have lived in endemic areas before immunisation.

*Disease risk areas*. Worldwide but greater risk in developing countries with poor sanitation.

## Vaccine

Hepatitis A vaccine is a whole cell virus vaccine inactivated with formaldehyde and is given intramuscularly.

A single monodose vaccine is available for primary immunisation, with a booster in 6 months to 1 year conferring protection for at least 10 years. Following immunisation, transient local reactions rarely occur and less commonly fever, fatigue or loss of appetite.

If vaccine is contraindicated, passive immunity can be conferred using human normal immunoglobulin. This will protect for 2–6 months depending on the dose.

Hepatitis A vaccine is also available either combined with hepatitis B vaccine or with the typhim Vi vaccine.

## Diphtheria

Diphtheria is caused by toxin-producing *Corynebacterium diphtheriae* and is spread by respiratory droplets.

It causes upper respiratory tract symptoms characterised by the development of a thick grey membrane over the tonsils and pharynx and marked lymphadenopathy, which may lead to respiratory obstruction. Toxin-mediated damage affects the myocardium and nervous system.

*Disease risk areas*. Worldwide but particularly sub-Saharan Africa, South-east Asia and South America. Diphtheria is becoming rarer as vaccination of children becomes more widespread. If vaccination coverage declines, large outbreaks can follow as has been seen in the former Soviet Union.

## Vaccine

Diphtheria vaccine is prepared from formaldehyde-inactivated diphtheria toxin adsorbed onto aluminium phosphate or aluminium hydroxide. The primary course is three doses and low-dose vaccine is used for primary and booster doses in adults. Boosters are required 10-yearly.

Vaccination is recommended especially for those likely to be mixing with the local population (e.g.

health-care workers, aid workers and teachers) in risk areas.

Swelling and redness may occur at the injection site, with fever and headache occurring less frequently.

## Yellow fever

Yellow fever is a mosquito-borne arbovirus infection. The responsible mosquito is *Aedes aegypti* which, in contrast to the *Anopheles* mosquito responsible for transmitting malaria, takes a blood meal during daylight hours. It causes high fever, widespread haemorrhage, jaundice and death around 50% of cases. Precautions against mosquito bites should be taken.

*Disease risk areas.* Sub-Saharan Africa and South America. The disease is not present in Asia.

### Vaccine

Yellow fever vaccine is a very effective live attenuated vaccine containing the 17D strain of yellow fever, grown within live chick embryos.

A single subcutaneous dose is given. A vaccination certificate is issued for immigration purposes, which is valid 10 days after vaccination or immediately after boosters. Booster doses are required 10-yearly.

Yellow fever vaccination is recommended and is sometimes mandatory for entering countries with yellow fever. A certificate may also be required if travelling from a yellow fever area to an uninfected country that has *Aedes* mosquitoes. Vaccination is only administered in WHO-designated centres.

Mild local or systemic reactions may appear 5–10 days post-vaccination. Severe reactions are rare.

Yellow fever vaccine contains live attenuated virus and is contraindicated in pregnancy, immunocompromised people, children under 6 months of age (encephalitis may occur in young infants) and in patients with serious egg allergy.

## Japanese B encephalitis

Japanese B encephalitis is a *Culicine* mosquito-borne flavivirus. The mosquito usually breeds in rice paddies. Pigs and some bird species act as intermediate hosts. Infection is often asymptomatic in endemic areas, but symptomatic cases develop encephalitis with a high mortality and incidence of residual neurological deficit. Precaution against mosquito bites should be taken.

*Disease risk areas.* South-east Asia including China, Thailand, India and low-lying areas of Nepal. Epidemics occur following the rainy season when mosquitoes are most active.

### Vaccine

Japanese B encephalitis vaccine is a formaldehyde-inactivated whole cell virus. Two or three doses are given subcutaneously over a period of 4 weeks for maximum protection. Boosters are required 2- to 3-yearly.

Vaccination is recommended especially for those going to rural areas, staying for long periods (e.g. more than 1 month) or for repeated visits. It is especially recommended for infants and children in whom the illness can be more severe. Vaccine is available on a named patient basis as it is not licensed in Britain.

An urticarial rash sometimes occurs usually 1–2 days after the inoculation. It may be severe enough to warrant a short course of steroids and antihistamines.

## Tick-borne encephalitis

Tick-borne encephalitis is caused by a flavivirus transmitted to humans by a bite from an infected tick. Ticks are most active in the spring and autumn. A meningoencephalitis with paresis may be seen in the acute illness and recovery may be slow. Death is rare.

Passive vaccination with specific hyperimmune globulin is protective if given within 4 days of the tick bite.

*Disease risk areas.* Tick-borne encephalitis is endemic in forested areas of Scandinavia, Austria and Germany, Eastern Europe and countries of the former Soviet Union.

## Vaccine

Tick-borne encephalitis vaccine virus is grown in chick embryo cells and is inactivated with formalin.

Two doses of vaccine are given intramuscularly with an interval time of 2–4 weeks. Initially a booster is required after 1 year, but subsequently only 3-yearly. The vaccine is given in Bavaria as part of the routine childhood vaccination schedule.

Vaccine is recommended for those likely to be exposed to tick bites in forested infected areas, for example campers and rural workers. Efforts should be made to avoid bites, and to carefully and promptly remove ticks if bitten.

Local reactions may occur post-vaccination. Vaccination should be avoided if there is serious egg allergy.

## Hepatitis B

Hepatitis B has a mortality of 0.1% in the acute phase. Five per cent of those infected become long-term carriers (greater than 6 months) and carriers may be at risk of future chronic liver disease and hepatocellular carcinoma. Spread is perinatally (mother to child), by blood to blood contact or by sexual intercourse.

*Disease risk areas.* Worldwide but there is a higher incidence of carriers in West Central Africa, Southeast Asia and South America.

## Vaccine

Hepatitis B vaccine is a recombinant vaccine containing hepatitis B surface antigen (anti-HbS) produced from yeast cells. The prepared vaccine is adsorbed onto aluminium hydroxide as an adjuvant. The vaccine is advised for those at occupational risk and also for long-stay expatriates. A history of recent exposure in the unimmunised is an indication for specific immune globulin while a course of active vaccine is commenced.

Three doses of intramuscular vaccine are given over a period of 6 months (0, 1 and 6 months). An accelerated course can be given with four doses

of vaccine over 6 months (0, 1, 2 and 6 months). Anti-HbS levels are usually checked for those at occupational risk to ensure an adequate level of protection has been achieved (>100 IU/l).

Of those vaccinated 5–10% fail to develop an adequate response even after three or more doses.

Further boosters are usually given at 3- to 5-yearly intervals or depending upon the level of anti-HbS.

Possible adverse reactions include fever, arthralgia, myalgia and mildly deranged liver function tests.

## Meningococcal meningitis

Meningococcal meningitis can be rapidly fatal, and is caused by an invasive Gram-negative diplococcus (*Neisseria meningitidis*), leading to septicaemia and meningitis. In the United Kingdom the most common antigenic groups are B and C, although serotype C prevalence has markedly declined since the introduction of the Meningococcal type C vaccine. Group A and less commonly group W135 and Y may be associated with epidemics in sub-Saharan Africa. Transmission is by respiratory droplet spread and epidemics occur in the dry season.

*Disease risk areas.* Epidemics occur in sub-Saharan Africa and have occurred unpredictably in northern India, Nepal and parts of Brazil.

## Vaccine

A quadrivalent vaccine is now available. This is a polysaccharide vaccine against serogroups A, C, W135 and Y. Vaccination is advised for travellers visiting areas with epidemic meningococcal disease who are going to be in close contact with the local population, especially if they are likely to be away from medical services, e.g. trekking in Nepal, travelling in sub-Saharan Africa or on the Hajj to Mecca. It is not normally advised for package tourists staying in hotels with other expatriates.

One dose of vaccine is required subcutaneously or intramuscularly, which is effective in 7 days.

Boosters are required 5-yearly. Vaccine response is poorer in children under 2 years of age.

## Rabies

Rabies is a neurotropic rhabdovirus with an animal reservoir in canines and bats. Infection is usually by inoculation of infected saliva from a bite of a rabid animal. Once symptomatic, rabies is invariably fatal. It occurs in all continents except Australasia and Antarctica.

### Vaccine

The rabies vaccine licensed in Britain is a whole cell virus cultured on human diploid cells and inactivated by propiolactone. Pre-exposure vaccine is offered to those involved in animal husbandry in infected areas, or to travellers who may be more than 24 h away from a source of post-exposure vaccine. The vaccine gives protection if given immediately after exposure but should ideally be used in conjunction with specific immune globulin.

Three injections over a period of 1 month (0, 7 and 28 days) provide protection, but the traveller should still seek urgent medical advice if put at risk for extra doses to ensure maximum antibody levels. Specific immune globulin is not needed in these circumstances. Boosters are required 3-yearly.

Local reactions rarely occur, with systemic reactions such as fever, headache and rashes being occasionally reported.

Post-exposure management in the unimmunised includes the administration of rabies-specific immunoglobulin (mainly around the wound) and the administration of 1 ml rabies vaccine i.m. at 0, 3, 7, 14 and 28 days. In the immunised patient WHO recommends the administration of two booster doses separated by 2 days.

## Plague

*Yersinia pestis* causes bacteraemic or pneumonic plague. The disease is associated with flea-infested rats and, therefore, travellers are rarely at risk. It occurs in India, Vietnam, Madagascar, rural South America and Central Africa.

### Vaccine

Two doses of killed plague vaccine are given subcutaneously over 1 month. Boosters are required 6-monthly. Vaccine is no longer available in the United Kingdom and has to be imported from the United States. It is usually more practical to give tetracycline to travellers unavoidably exposed to plague, with advice to start treatment promptly if they become ill.

## Malaria prevention and treatment

Forty per cent of the world's population is at risk of malaria and 90% of cases occur in sub-Saharan Africa. It causes an estimated 300 million clinical infections and more than 1 million deaths annually. Children and non-immune adults are at most risk of severe infection and death. In the United Kingdom, non-immune travellers to malarious areas are at great risk unless the appropriate precautions are taken and there are about 2000 cases of imported malaria each year with approximately 10 deaths.

Malaria is caused by the *Plasmodium* genus of protozoans. Four species cause disease in man:
1 *P. falciparum* is the most serious and potentially life-threatening form of malaria.
2 *P. malariae* causes quartan malaria as it may produce fever every third day. Infection is occasionally complicated by a glomerulonephritis. Relapse has been recorded in patients up to 40 years after leaving the tropics.
3 *P. vivax* and *P. ovale* are known as tertian malaria as they may give fever on alternate days after the disease has become established. These species of malaria have a hypnozoite stage, where the parasite has the ability to lie dormant in the liver for months before reactivating.

*P. malariae*, *P. vivax* and *P. ovale* are rarely life-threatening and are referred to as benign malaria. Co-infection with different parasites may occur.

### Life cycle

Parasites are introduced into humans via the bite of the female anophiline mosquito. After an infected bite sporozoites invade hepatocytes where they undergo pre-erythrocytic shizogeny. At this stage *P. vivax* and *P. ovale* may become dormant, producing hypnozoites. Hepatocyte rupture leads to merozoite release into the circulation with subsequent erythrocyte invasion where they undergo further development into schizonts (erythrocytic shizogeny) or gametocytes, which are the sexual form. Gametocytes are taken up by the mosquito during a blood meal and further sexual reproduction of the parasites takes place in the mosquito gut. Clinical signs of malaria occur at the time of red cell invasion and rupture. In the case of *P. falciparum* sequestration in the venules of the deep organs (particularly the CNS, liver, kidneys and lungs) accounts for many of the severe features of the infection. The pathophysiology of severe malaria is complex and is dependent on a number of factors including the parasite, its interaction with endothelium and the host immunological response to the infection.

The cardinal symptom of malaria is fever often with rigors, followed by profuse sweating, headache and myalgia. Falciparum malaria may result in severe anaemia, jaundice and cerebral malaria which is manifested by confusion, coma, seizures and death if untreated. Other complications of severe malaria are renal failure and respiratory failure due to adult respiratory distress syndrome.

*Disease risk areas*. Malaria is endemic in the tropics and subtropics below altitudes of 2000 m (see Fig. 19.1). Optimal conditions for the vector are an ambient temperature of 16–33°C. The most serious risk areas for *P. falciparum* malaria are sub-Saharan Africa, South-east Asia (including rural Thailand, Laos, Cambodia, Burma and Vietnam) and Amazonia in South America.

## Chemoprophylaxis against malaria

Malaria prevention through chemoprophylaxis is not absolute. Avoidance of mosquito bites is fundamental in preventing malaria. Therefore, long sleeves and trousers should be worn, especially after sunset when the female mosquito is most active. The importance of insect repellents and mosquito nets impregnated with an insecticide should be emphasised.

The choice of antimalarial is decided by the likelihood of exposure, the prevalent species and local resistance patterns of the parasite. Chemoprophylaxis is primarily directed against *P. falciparum* in which resistance to chloroquine is now widespread.

Prophylaxis should be commenced 1 week before travel (3 weeks for mefloquine and 1 or 2 days for malarone) to ensure adequate blood levels and to detect those likely to get side effects, during the whole time of exposure and for 4 weeks after visiting a malaria area to cover the 'incubation' phase of malignant malaria.

Despite adequate precautions, malaria infection remains possible; thus any febrile illness should be promptly investigated and treated, sometimes empirically, within 1 year of return from a malarious area. Commonly used prophylactic agents are shown in Table 19.4.

## Drug resistance

Drug resistance in *P. falciparum* occurs directly as a consequence of antimalarial drugs causing resistance in parasites. Resistance leads to delayed response to treatment of clinical infections, early recrudescence and increased transmission. This increases the parasite reservoir and leads to an increase in infections and greater use of antimalarials. Malarial prophylaxis recommendations alter as a result of changing patterns of resistance. Currently, chloroquine resistance in *P. falciparum* is widespread in Africa, Asia and much of South America. Mefloquine resistance is now well established in South-east Asia. Fansidar resistance in Africa and South-east Asia is also well established. The artemsinin derivatives (e.g. artemether) are now widely used in the treatment of severe malaria and in combination in non-severe *P. falciparum* in South-east Asia particularly. They are not advised for use in prophylaxis. Resistance to these compounds has been described. When deciding on suitable prophylaxis for travellers, up-to-date advice should always be sought from specialist

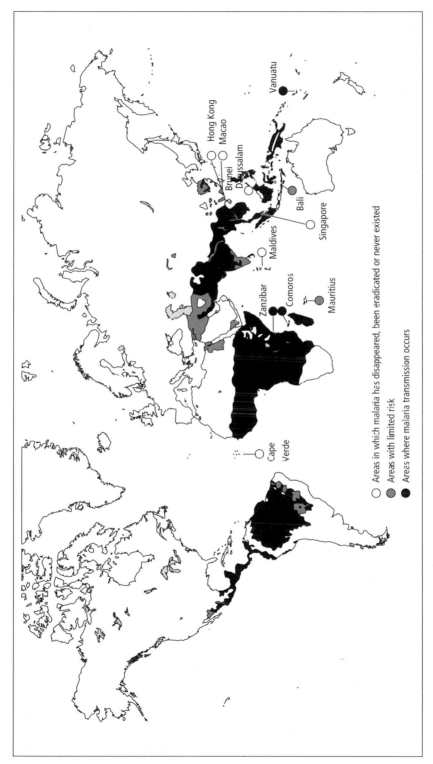

Hong Kong
Macao

Vanuatu

Brunei
Darussalam

Bali

Singapore

Maldives

Zanzibar

Comoros

Mauritius

Cape
Verde

○  Areas in which malaria has disappeared, been eradicated or never existed

●  Areas with limited risk

●  Areas where malaria transmission occurs

**Figure 19.1**  Areas requiring malaria prevention. The map has been kindly provided by *International Travel and Health* (1999, WHO, Geneva).

**Table 19.4** Antimalarial drugs.

| Drug | Mechanism of action | Use | | Adverse effects/cautions |
| --- | --- | --- | --- | --- |
| | | Treatment | Prophylaxis | |
| Chloroquine | Inhibits erythrocytic phase of plasmodial development | Non-falciparum malaria | In combination with proguanil in some areas of the world | GI upset, rash, headaches avoid in epilepsy. Caution in renal/hepatic dysfunction. Arrhythmia, seizure, visual loss in over dose |
| Proguanil | Inhibits dihydrofolate reductase, preventing plasmodial tissue development | Uncomplicated falciparum combined with atovaquone (see malorone) | In combination with chloroquine or atovaqoune (malorone) | GI upset, apthous ulcers Caution in severe renal failure. Folate supplements in pregnancy |
| Mefloquine | Unknown; quinine derivative. Destroys asexual parasites (trophozoites) | Uncomplicated falciparum in combination with artesunate derivative; effective against other species but chloroquine preferred | Yes, but resistance in SE Asia and increasing in Africa | GI upset, dizziness, erythema multiforme, cardiac conduction defects Neuropsychiatric disturbances. Contraindicated in renal and severe hepatic impairment, history of psychiatric illness, epilepsy, cardiac conduction defects, lactation and pregnancy. Avoid co-administration with other agents that may prolong the QT interval |
| Doxycycline | Inhibits protein synthesis | In combination with quinine in *P. falciparum* | Chloroquine/mefloquine resistance or when contra-indicated | GI upset, photosensitivity, interactions with warfarin Contraindicated in pregnancy, lactation and in children under 12 years of age |
| Atovaquone with proguanil (Malarone) | Interferes with pyrimidine biosynthesis. Acts on pre-erythrocytic stage of development | Initial treatment of uncomplicated falciparum malaria | Start 1–2 days prior to travel and can be stopped one week following return. | Nausea, mouth ulceration, hyponatraemia Contraindicated in pregnancy and lactation |

| Drug | Mode of action | Treatment use | Prophylaxis use | Adverse effects |
|---|---|---|---|---|
| Pyrimethamine/dapsone (Maloprim) | Dapsone is sulfone with antifolate activity | No | Used as prophylaxis in patients with epilepsy who cannot take chloroquine or mefloquine | Haemolytic anaemia, bone marrow suppression, haemolysis in those with G6PD deficiency |
| Pyrimethamine/ sulfadoxine (Fansidar) | Pyrimethamine inhibits Plasmodium folate metabolism; sulfadoxine also interferes with microbial folate synthesis | Yes; adjunctive therapy of P. falciparum malaria that has some resistance | No | Severe drug rash including Stevens–Johnson syndrome, but very rare when given as single dose |
| Primaquine | Inhibits Plasmodium mitochondrial transport | Used to eradicate liver forms of P. ovale and P. vivax | No | Nausea, vomiting, methaemoglobinaemia and haemolytic anaemia Contraindicated in G6PD deficiency, pregnancy and lactation |
| Quinine | Cidal vs. all four asexual parasite species. Mode of action not understood | Treatment of P. falciparum in combination with doxycline or with a single dose of Fansidar | No | Ventricular arrhythmias (avoid with other agents that prolong QT interval), hypoglycaemia, blurring of vision, tinnitus, deafness and rarely haemolysis |
| Artemesinin derivatives (artemether, artemesinin, artesunate) | Rapidly cidal vs. young trophozoites | Use oral forms alone or in combination with mefloquine or lumefantrine (Riamet) in uncomplicated falciparum. i.m. or i.v. forms used in severe falciparum | No | Well tolerated; serious adverse effects rare Neurotoxicity in animals not demonstrated in man Lumefantrine may cause arrhythmias |

centres or continually updated on-line databases such as TRAVAX (described above) or recently published guidelines such as those produced by the Health Protection Agency's advisory committee on malaria prevention.

## Treatment of malaria

Malaria treatment should be considered in the context of the infecting species, the severity of the infection and the health-care setting in which the patient is being managed. The emergence of drug resistance impacts on treatment options as well as on

prophylaxis. The benign forms of malaria (*P. vivax, P. ovale* and *P. malariae*) can be treated with short-course chloroquine. *P. vivax* and *P. ovale* require an additional 2-week course of primaquine (assuming G6PD status is normal and patient is not pregnant) to eradicate hypnozoites from the hepatocytes.

Non-severe *P. falciparum* can be treated with either oral quinine plus doxycycline, ratovaquone/proguanil (malarone), mefloquine, or artesunate (an artemesinin derivative). In patients with partial immunity in endemic areas pyrimethamine/sulfadoxine (Fansidar) is still frequently used. There is increasing interest in

**Table 19.5** Selected parasitic infections of medical importance.

| Parasite | Disease | Antimicrobial therapy | Alternative (Alt) or Adjunct (Adj) therapy |
|---|---|---|---|
| Protozoa | | | |
| *Entamoeba histolytica* | Amoebic colitis and liver abscess | Metronidazole | Diloxanide fumarate (Adj) |
| *Giardia lamblia* | Giardiasis | Metronidazole | Tinidazole (Alt) |
| *Leishmania* sp. | Visceral Leishmaniasis and New world cutaneous leishmanisis | Sodium Stibogluconate | Amphotericin B (Alt), Miltefosine (Alt) |
| *Trypanosome* sp. | African Trypanosomiasis | | |
| | Early | Suramin (rhodesiense) | Pentamidine (gambiense) |
| | Late | Melarsoprol | Eflornithine (Alt) |
| | South American T. (Chaga's) | Nifurtimox | Benzidazole (Alt) |
| Helminths | | | |
| i. Nematodes | | | |
| *Strongyloides* | Strongyloidiasis | Albendazole | |
| *Ancylostoma caninum* and *Necator americanis* | Cutaneous larva migrans | Mebendezole | Albendazole (Alt) |
| *Ascaris lumbricoides* | Ascariasis | Mebendazole | |
| *Wuchereria bancrofti, Brugia malayi* | Lymphatic filariasis | Diethylcarbamazine (DEC) | Albendazole (Alt), Ivermectin (Adj) |
| *Onchocerca volvulus* | River blindness, skin nodules | Ivermectin | Doxycycline (Adj) |
| ii. Trematodes | | | |
| *Schistosome* sp. | Schistosomiasis | Praziquantil | Artemesinin (Alt) |
| iii. Cestodes | | | |
| *Taenia solium* (pork tape worm) | Neurocystercicosis | Albendazole | Praziquantel (Alt) Steroids (Adj) |
| *Echinococcus granulosus* (canine tape worm) | Hydatid disease | Albendazole | Surgical excision |

combination therapy with artesunate and mefloquine. This strategy appears to rapidly destroy the parasites and may reduce the risk of resistance emerging. Co-formulated artemether and lumefantrine (Riamet) is available in the United Kingdom for the treatment of uncomplicated falciparum malaria.

Severe *P. falciparum* malaria should be treated with intravenous quinine. A loading dose of 20 mg/kg (maximum 1400 mg) should be given unless the patient has previously received mefloquine. Subsequent dosing is 10 mg/kg 8-hourly. Doxycycline should also be given in case of quinine resistance. An alternative to quinine is intramuscular artemether or intravenous artemisinin. These agents are derived from sweet wormwood, a ubiquitous weed, used for centuries in China in the treatment of fever. The artemsinin derivatives are associated with a more rapid drop in parasitaemia than quinine and have no recognisable serious adverse effects in comparison. Neurotoxicity found in animals following high dosing has not been observed in clinical trials in man. Although not associated with improved survival in severe malaria, the artemisinin derivatives are useful in quinine resistance or intolerance. Drug therapy of *P. falciparum* malaria is usually 7 days. Drugs used in the treatment of malaria are outlined in Table 19.4.

Severe malaria is a multi-system disorder and close attention should be paid to adjunctive measures, including intravenous rehydration, blood transfusion and correction of hypoglycaemia and acidosis. Co-existent bacterial sepsis should also be sought and managed with parenteral antibiotic therapy.

## Treatment of other common imported parasitic infections

There are a great variety of other parasitic infections (protozoal and helminthic) which may affect any organ system. The most common or serious parasitic infections in the returning traveller include (by system) gastrointestinal (giardiasis, amoebiasis, schistosomiasis, strongyloidiasis and ascariasis), genitourinary (schistosomiasis), cutaneous (cutanous larva migrans, onchocerciasis, leishmaniasis), lymphatic (filariasis), multi-system (malaria, leishmaniasis) and neurological (cystercicosis, trypanosomiasis). An overview of treatment of the more common or important infections is given in Table 19.5.

## Further reading

Bradley, D.J. & Bannister, B. (2003) Guidelines for malaria prevention in travelers from the United Kingdom for 2003. Commun Dis Public Health 6(3): 180–199.

Gill, G. & Beeching, N. (2004) *Lecture Notes on Tropical Medicine*, 5th edn. Blackwell Science Ltd, Oxford.

Walker, E., Williams, G. & Raeside, F. (1997) *ABC of Healthy Travel*, 5th edn. BMJ Publishing Group, London.

World Health Organization (2005, updated annually) *International Travel and Health*. WHO, Geneva. http://www.who.int/ith/

# Part 3

# Practical aspects of prescribing

# Chapter 20

# Poisoning and drug overdose

Poisoning results from the effects of excess expo-sure to a drug or chemical. Presentations with acute poisoning are a common cause of hospital admis-sion in the United Kingdom and worldwide. They account for approximately 10% of patients, but the aetiology of the poisoning varies in different countries— being principally due to pharmaceuti-cals in the developed world, and principally due to chemicals, particularly pesticides, or natural toxins such as envenomations in the developing world. There is some overlap in mechanisms involved be-tween adverse reactions and poisoning.

Poisoning is the commonest form of self-harm, and types of poisoning are generally classified into five groups:

1 Intentional (self-harm)
2 Accidental
3 Occupational
4 Environmental
5 Deliberate (by others).

In the hospital setting intentional poisoning is the commonest seen, but a relatively small propor-tion of such patients have organic psychiatric dis-ease. In the majority intentional poisoning forms part of a self-harm profile. Accidental poisoning is particularly common in very young children un-der the age of five. Self-harm now begins at around 10 years old, and increases into the teens. Very rarely poisoning in children may be a feature of the Munchausen's Syndrome by Proxy in the parent.

## General approach to the poisoned patient

Patients with overdose should be treated and man-aged like all medical patients. This would in-clude an appropriate history, appropriate profes-sional care and treatment designed specifically to manage the relevant toxin. Patients who self-harm should also have a formal psychiatric or psychological assessment prior to discharge. Self-harm is a future risk factor for further self-harm episodes.

Many hundreds of different chemicals and drugs are and result in poisoning. The commonest agents in the United Kingdom in recent years are shown in Table 20.1. It is important for doctors to be familiar with these common drugs. In cases of complex overdoses, multiple ingestions or for un-usual or rarer cases advice should be sought. In the United Kingdom accident and emergency de-partments have free on-line access provided to the UK database TOXBASE, the database run by the UK National Poisons Information Service (NPIS), which can be found at http://www.spib.axl.co.uk. This should be used to access information ini-tially. Should further details on management be required a UK 24-h national telephone informa-tion line is available on 0870 600 6266, supported by a 24-h rota of consultant clinical toxicologists (Table 20.2).

**Table 20.1** Twenty Common UK poisons in order of frequency of accesses to TOXBASE in 2004.∗

| |
|---|
| Paracetamol |
| Salicylates |
| Ibuprofen |
| Codeine |
| Hypochlorite (Bleach) |
| Petroleum distillate (White spirit) |
| Ethanol |
| Diazepam |
| Zopiclone |
| Menthol |
| Fluoxetine |
| Venlafaxine |
| Citalopram |
| Dihydrocodeine |
| Amitriptyline |
| Ferrous sulphate |
| Methylenedioxymethamphetamine |
| Dextropropoxyphene |
| Methanol |
| Diphenhydramine |
| Diclofenac sodium |

∗ A total of >800,000 individual agents were accessed in this year.

## Assessment and diagnosis

Airway—ensure airway is clear and protected

Breathing—ensure ventilation is adequate

Circulation—measure pulse, blood pressure and look for signs of shock

Disability—assess level of consciousness

Exposure—look at patient for clues as to drugs taken, e.g. skin colour, needle track marks, blisters

Appropriate resuscitation procedures may be required to be commenced before full details of the ingestion are known. It is important to document

**Table 20.2** Poisons information services.

| |
|---|
| UK National database TOXBASE: |
|   http://www.spib.axl.co.uk |
| UK National telephone number for more complex |
|   enquiries: 0870 600 6266 |

any co-morbidity, particularly cardiovascular or respiratory as this may affect the patients response to both the toxin and any treatment provided.

A history of the event will often provide important clues as to potential substances ingested. Any containers from which material has been consumed should be carefully checked. Co-ingestion of alcohol, and co-ingestion of more than one drug is common in overdose patients. In accidental poisoning usually one agent is involved, and in the majority of cases in children the risk to the patient is low and hospital admission is not encouraged. In self-harm patients' admission is often required both to monitor the course of poisoning in appropriate cases, and also for psychological assessment and management. Patients should be assessed with respect to cardiovascular and respiratory status, and a number of clinical 'toxidromes' are recognised which result from the effects of certain poisons (Table 20.3). Assessment of the central nervous system (CNS) function is often done in emergency departments using the Glasgow Coma Scale (GCS), but this is not designed for assessing poisoning and a similar scale, the AVPU scale (Table 20.4), is quick, easy and useful in practice. The P level (non-responding to pain) equates approximately to GCS 8 and patients below this level are in danger of respiratory obstruction and should be carefully monitored and considered for transfer to a more intensive care setting.

The onset of toxicity and time profile of toxicity varies from compound to compound depending on the mode of action. Metabolic poisons (e.g. paracetamol) may present with symptoms for more than 24 h after ingestion, whereas rapidly acting agents such as opiates or insulin will present within minutes of administration, particularly if given intravenously. Most toxins are ingested but they may be absorbed through the respiratory tract (e.g. glue sniffing) or through the skin (e.g. paraquat, hydrofluoric acid). A careful history and clinical examination may be far more valuable than laboratory analyses, particularly as for many toxins laboratory analyses are not available rapidly, and there is often a poor correlation between single

**Table 20.3** Examples of symptoms associated with specific toxins.

| Agitation | Anticholinergics, amphetamine, cocaine, ethanol, solvents, tricyclic antidepressants |
| --- | --- |
| Coma | Barbiturates, benzodiazepines, ethanol, ethylene glycol, gamma hydroxy butyrate (GBH), methanol, opiates, solvents, tricyclic antidepressants |
| Convulsions | Amphetamine, cocaine, Ecstasy, organophosphates, phenothiazines, theophylline, tricyclic antidepressants |
| Constricted pupils | Organophosphates, opiates, GBH |
| Dilated pupils | Anticholinergics, cocaine, phenothiazines, quinine, sympathomimetics, tricyclic antidepressants |
| Cardiac arrythmias | Anti-arrhythmics, anticholinergics, phenothiazines, quinine, sympathomimetics, tricyclic antidepressants |
| Pulmonary oedema | Aspirin, ethylene glycol, irritant gases, opiates, organophosphates, tricyclic antidepressants |
| Metabolic acidosis | Aspirin; ethanol; ethylene glycol; methanol |
| Hyperthermia | Anticholinergics, cocaine, Ecstasy and monoamine oxidase inhibitors |
| Hepatic failure | Paracetamol, organic sovents, toxic mushrooms |
| Renal failure not related to hypotension or rhabdomyolysis | Ethylene glycol, lithium, methanol, NSAIDs, paracetamol |

plasma concentration measurements and effect, particularly if timing is not accurate and in patients who are habituated to drugs such as addicts.

Examination should include not only the normal physical signs, but also the assessment of airway (for burns, mouth blisters or odour—alcohol and volatile solvents) and the skin for needle marks or burns. In patients who have been found unconscious after taking an overdose some hours before, other complications of importance include pressure areas, and blistering (non-specific) and rhabdomyolysis, particularly of limbs that may have had pressure applied across them during unconsciousness. The latter may result in a com-

partment syndrome, which although uncommon, may need urgent surgical decompression to avoid the need for amputation.

## Toxicological analyses

In a conscious patient who presents a clear history these are only necessary where plasma concentration guides management (e.g. paracetamol, digoxin, methotrexate). Biochemical tests may also be helpful, however, in providing clues to likely ingested compounds, and Fig. 20.1 provides some examples. A 12-lead ECG may also be helpful, in particular in cases of antidepressants (prolonged QRS) or antipsychotics and other drugs such as terfenadine or diphenhydramine that block potassium (Ki) channels (prolonged QT) since these findings are likely to indicate the risk of arrhythmia.

**Table 20.4** The AVPU scale.

| A | **A**wake |
| --- | --- |
| V | Responds to **V**erbal commands |
| P | Responds to **P**ainful stimuli |
| U | **U**nresponse to stimuli |

*Note:* the more detailed Glasgow coma scale may be used in accident departments and intensive care.

## Immediate management

Apart from routine medical supportive therapy, some aspects of the management of poisoning

**Interpretation of investigations in poisoning of unknown cause**

Blood gases
Metabolic acidosis [low pH/high $H^+$ with low $CO_2$]
Carbon monoxide
- Ecstasy
- Iron salts
- Methanol
- Paraldehyde
- Theophylline
- Cyanide
- Ethylene glycol
- Metformin
- Paracetamol
- Salicylates
- Tricyclic antidepressants

Respiratory acidosis [low pH/high $H^+$ with high $CO_2$]
- Barbiturates
- Benzodiazepines
- Opiates
- Tricyclic antidepressants

Respiratory alkalosis [high pH/low $H^+$ with low $CO_2$]
- Ecstasy
- Salicylates
- Theophylline

Hypokalaemia
- $\beta$-Agonists (e.g. salbutamol)
- Diuretics
- Insulin
- Sulphonylureas
- Theophylline

Hyperkalaemia
- Digoxin

Hypoglycaemia
- Ethanol
- Insulin
- Salicylates
- Sulphonylureas
- Agents that cause hepatic failure (paracetamol, iron)

treatments to be effective, as they only work if performed early after overdose. The preferred method of gastric decontamination is now *activated charcoal*, normally given at a dose of 50 g to adults or 1 g/kg in children. Charcoal binds or adsorbs approximately one tenth of its weight of active drug. It requires physical contact with the ingested compound to be effective. Charcoal should be given within 1 h of drug ingestion, although some experts consider that administration up to 2 h may be appropriate in patients who have ingested drugs that delay gastric motility, such as antidepressants or opiates. There is little point giving charcoal to patients who have vomited, and in patients who have respiratory depression the airway must be protected prior to administration.

*Gastric aspiration* (as opposed to lavage) should be considered in patients who have ingested potentially life-threatening high doses of drugs not adsorbed by the normally recommended oral antidote-activated charcoal. These include lithium and iron (Table 20.5).

*Induced emesis* is no longer recommended, as it is ineffective and potentially hazardous. It may mask the features of poisoning, confuse diagnosis and cause unnecessary delay in discharge for children with minor overdose.

*Whole bowel irrigation* may be considered for ingestions involving slow-release formulations or in drug users whole have swallowed drugs in a container or wrapping. Efficacy is uncertain.

For most ingested drugs onset of clinical features is likely to occur within 4–6 h after ingestion, and more intense monitoring is required for drugs affecting the CNS and cardiovascular systems during this time.

have changed over the past 10 years. Routine *gastric decontamination* by lavage or emesis is no longer recommended in poisoning, following international guidelines published in the mid-1990s. Specific hazards of *gastric lavage* include hypoxia, 'wash on' of gastric contents causing increased rate of absorption and increased toxicity, oesophageal perforation and aspiration pneumonia. Most patients present too late for these

**Table 20.5** Agents not adsorbed by charcoal.

| Acids | Iron salts |
|---|---|
| Alcohols, e.g. ethanol, methanol | Glycols, e.g. ethylene glycol |
| Cyanide | Lead, mercury and other heavy metals |
| Lithium salts | Organic solvents |

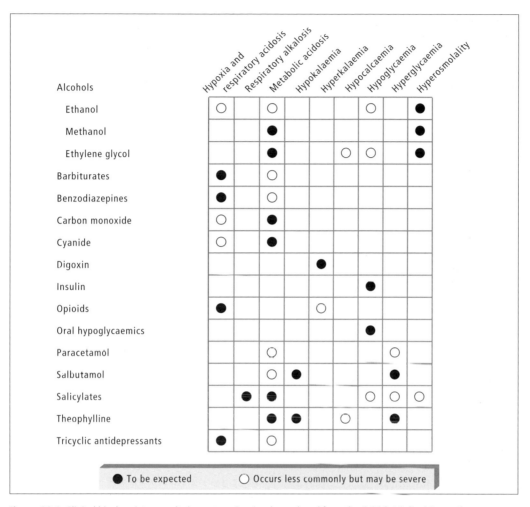

**Figure 20.1** Clinical biochemistry: results in acute poisoning (reproduced from the *British Medical Journal*).

In cases of poisoning simple treatments are preferred, and there are relatively few true antidotes (see later). Most patients will therefore recover with sensible nursing support. Avoid using drugs without specific indications and understanding the implications of their use when managing poisoned patients.

## The management of specific complications

*Convulsions*—diazepam or lorazepam.
*Agitation*—diazepam or lorazepam, if severe consider haloperidol.

*Arrhythmias*—correct acidosis with intravenous sodium bicarbonate, treat torsades de pointes with magnesium. Note: Anti-arrythmic drugs may increase toxic effects, always discuss with a senior colleague or the NPIS before use.
*Temperature abnormalities*—hypothermia may be present in patients who have consumed vasodilators, including alcohol, and have remained outside, particularly in winter. Careful warming and support for complications including rhabdomyolysis is usually all that is required, with specific treatment for any relevant toxin. Hyperthermia is most frequently caused by drugs of abuse, particularly cocaine and amphetamine derivatives such

**Clinical features in poisoning** (these may be complicated if more than one agent is ingested)

Tachycardia
- Anticholinergics
- Amphetamines
- β-Agonists (salbutamol)
- Cocaine
- Ecstasy
- Monoamine oxidase inhibitors
- Phenothiazines
- Theophylline
- Tricyclic antidepressants
- Sympathomimetic drugs

Bradycardia
- Beta-blockers
- Cyanide
- Digoxin
- Organophosphates

Hypertension
- Amphetamines/ecstasy
- Cocaine
- MAOIs

Hypotension
- Is common in severe poisoning from any cause, particularly with CNS depressants

Hypertonia and hyperreflexia
- Amphetamines
- Ecstasy
- Anticholinergics (may have upgoing plantars)
- Carbamazepine
- MAOIs
- Theophylline
- Tricyclic antidepressants (may have upgoing plantars and divergent squint)
- Carbon monoxide (may have upgoing plantars)

Hypotonia and hyporeflexia
- Alcohol
- Barbiturates
- Benzodiazepines
- Haloperidol
- Opiates
- Phenothiazines

Tachypnoea
- Amphetamines/ecstasy
- Cyanide
- Ethylene glycol
- Methanol
- Salicylates
- Theophylline

as methylenedioxymethamphetamine (MDMA). The treatment for these is benzodiazepines and cooling. Malignant neuroleptic syndrome is uncommon in overdose.

*Dystonic reactions* such as oculogyric crisis (with metoclopramide or antipsychotics in young adults) should be treated with either diazepam or an intravenous anticholinergic.

## Specific treatments

The stomach acts as a reservoir for ingested drugs and while drugs (apart from corrosives) are in the stomach they are essentially harmless. Once absorption from the gut occurs then the onset of clinical features will depend on mode of action. The most important principle in managing a poisoned patient is not to conduct an intervention that may increase risk of toxicity or be ineffective. Lack of good clinical trials makes advice on management often empirical, based on a body of expert opinion.

## Enhanced drug elimination

Most drugs are lipid-soluble compounds, which are excreted primarily by drug metabolising enzymes in the liver. In overdose the normal pharmacokinetics seen after therapeutic doses may change, sometimes because of delayed absorption from the gut, and sometimes because of saturation of enzyme metabolising pathways. Patients should always be treated on the basis of their clinical picture, not on the anticipated kinetic predictions from a textbook. For a small number of drugs, for example aspirin, urinary excretion forms a significant part of elimination at therapeutic concentrations. Manipulation of urinary pH may, in this circumstance, increase elimination. For weakly acidic drugs, such as aspirin, alkalinisation of urine increases urinary excretion. This is because aspirin has a pKa close to physiological pH and thus ionisation is altered significantly by small changes in urinary pH, and in an alkaline urine aspirin becomes ionised preventing reabsorption across lipid layers in the kidney. In practice it is often difficult to achieve adequate alkalisation in a metabolically sick patient, and other techniques are used to remove aspirin. Increasing urine flow alone is an inadequate means of increasing drug elimination, and runs the risk of precipitating fluid overload or pulmonary oedema.

## Haemodialysis

For water-soluble compounds such as aspirin, ethanol, methanol, ethylene glycol and lithium, haemodialysis will effectively remove drug from the blood passing across the dialysate membrane. The rate of removal is crucially dependant upon the flow rate across this membrane, and the benefits of the treatment relate directly to the increase in clearance produced by haemodialysis. Thus, although it is possible to show dialysate clearance for many drugs, in practice only for a very few is haemodialysis an effective means of removal. In the case of lithium intoxication prolonged dialysis is necessary because lithium is more widely distributed than the other compounds mentioned. Care should be taken to ensure that the most efficient form of dialysis is adopted, as systems designed for management of chronic haemodialysis patients such as veno–veno systems are less effective than conventional techniques.

## Haemoperfusion

Haemoperfusion is effective in removing compounds with relatively small volumes of distribution, such as theophylline, providing adequate clearances can be achieved across the charcoal column. For the vast majority of drugs, however, the increased clearance achieved by charcoal is inadequate to warrant therapy using this technique. Since patients require to be anticoagulated, there is significant risk in a patient who is suicidal of disconnection of lines and haemorrhage.

## Physiological support systems

Occasionally cardiopulmonary resuscitation may involve direct cardiac pacing, use of aortic balloon pumps or very rarely use of heart–lung machines. Recent experimental studies suggest that albumin dialysis for the management of hepatic failure may have a role in the support of patients with established drug-induced intoxication, but for the present there is little evidence that they have a role in active management of the intoxicated patient prior to the establishment of organ toxicity. They should not be used for this purpose until further clinical trials have been done.

## Features of common drug overdose

In clinical practice almost anything may be taken by a patient in emotional distress. The epidemiology of drug overdose changes with time and, at present in the United Kingdom the most common poisonings seen clinically are paracetamol, benzodiazepine and related sedatives, non-steroidal anti-inflammatories, antidepressants and antipsychotics, opioid and drugs of abuse (Table 20.1). An outline understanding of these drugs is important, and in addition it is useful to understand clinical implications of the mechanisms of effect of a few rare poisons. A list of some antidotes that may be advised in clinical practice is shown in Table 20.6. When managing any case of poisoning it is sensible to consult TOXBASE and print off an appropriate factsheet from that database to act as an *aide-memoire* in the management of the patient during their inhospital stay.

## Antidepressant drugs

### Tricyclic antidepressants

These drugs inhibit the uptake of monoamines into central neurones, but also have anticholinergic (antimuscarinic), sodium channel blocking and $\alpha$-adrenoceptor antagonist effects. Clinical features are due to a combination of these effects. Anticholinergic effects predominate early (dry mouth, dilated pupils, tachycardia, drowsiness and urinary retention). More severe cases are drowsy, develop prolongation of the QRS complex due to sodium

**Table 20.6** List of antidotes and their mechanism of action.

| Poisons | Antidotes | Mechanism of action |
|---|---|---|
| Anticoagulants (Warfarin type) | Vitamin K (phytomenadione) | Cofactor for synthesis of clotting factors |
| β-Adrenergic blockers | Isoprenaline | Competitive agonist at β-receptor |
| | Glucagon | Stimulates myocardial adenyl cyclase |
| Carbon monoxide | Oxygen (normo or hyperbaric) | Competitive displacement of carbon monoxide from haemoglobin molecule |
| Cyanide | Dicobalt edetate | Chelating agent |
| | Sodium nitrate | Forms methaemoglobin that combines with cyanide |
| | Sodium thiosulphate | Accelerates detoxification of cyanide by action with rhodanase |
| | Hydroxocobalamin | Combines with cyanide to form cyanocobalamin |
| Digoxin and digitoxin | Fab antidote fragments | Antidote forms an inert complex with poison |
| Ethylene glycol or methanol | Ethanol | Competitive substrate for alcohol dehydrogenase, slows toxic metabolite production |
| | Fomepizole | Inhibitor of alcohol dehydrogenase |
| Benzodiazepines | Flumazenil | Competitive antagonist at benzodiazepine receptors |
| Heavy metals (lead, mercury, arsenic) | DMSA (2,3-dimercaptosuccinic acid) | Chelating agent |
| | DMPS (2,3-dimercaptopropane-1-sulphonate) | Chelating agent |
| | Sodium calcium edetate | Chelating agent |
| | Dimercaprol | Chelating agent |
| Hydrofluoric acid | Calcium gluconate | Forms an inert complex (calcium fluoride) |
| Iron salts | Desferrioxamine | Chelating agent |
| Narcotics (dextropropoxyphene, heroin, co-proxamol, etc.) | Naloxone | Competitive antagonist at opioid receptors |
| Organophosphates | Atropine | Competitive antagonist at acetylcholine receptor |
| | Pralidoxime | Cholinesterase reactivator |
| Paracetamol | Acetylcysteine | Accelerate detoxification of potentially toxic metabolite (glutathione precursor and SH donor) |
| Thallium | Berlin Blue | Chelating agent |

channel blockade and then develop ventricular arrhythmias and convulsions. Patients who are AVPU 'P' or greater are at significant risk of these complications.

Activated charcoal is indicated in early presentations. Routine 12-lead ECG should be performed to check for QRS duration, and if the patient becomes obtunded, it should be repeated. Prophylactic use of intravenous sodium bicarbonate is advised in the management of arrhythmias, particularly if the QRS duration increases beyond 110 ms. Prolonged cardiac massage is appropriate in patients with tricyclic poisoning, and recovery has been reported after cardiac massage of several hours. In recovery agitation is frequent, and should be managed by benzodiazepines after ensuring that there is no urinary retention.

## Specific serotonin reuptake inhibitors

Specific serotonin reuptake inhibitors (SSRIs) are more specific than tricyclics in that they block the uptake of serotonin only. In overdose they may cause a serotonin syndrome, particularly if co-ingested with other antidepressants or with drugs of abuse such as ecstasy. Features include agitation, myoclonic jerks, hyperreflexia, hyperthermia, rhabdomyolysis and in severe cases renal failure. GI symptoms such as nausea, vomiting and diarrhoea are frequent. Serotonin syndrome can be managed by using serotonin antagonists (e.g. cyproheptadine), but is usually treated with benzodiazepines.

## Other antidepressants

Venlafaxine is more closely aligned to tricyclic antidepressants, acting on reuptake of noradrenaline. Its clinical features in overdose are similar to tricyclic antidepressants, but it may also cause more rhabdomyolysis. It is more toxic in overdose than SSRIs. Mirtazapine, a centrally acting pre-synaptic $\alpha_2$-receptor antagonist, causes drowsiness in overdose, but is otherwise benign.

## MAOIs

Monoamine oxidase inhibitors are particularly toxic in overdose and cause severe cardiovascular instability with hypertension and tachycardia. Features similar to serotonin syndrome may also develop. Patients who have ingested significant quantities of MAOIs require specialist treatment in intensive or high dependency units.

## Sedatives and benzodiazepine related compounds

Benzodiazepines, e.g. diazepam, and related drugs, such as zopiclone and zolpidem, cause drowsiness. If taken alone they are relatively safe, and patients should be treated by good nursing care. Dangers arise when patients vomit and inhale down an unprotected airway, or combine benzodiazepines with other CNS depressants, particularly opioids. Patients with pre-existing chronic obstructive airways disease may be more sensitive to the respiratory depressant effects of this category of drugs.

Clinical features include drowsiness, hyporeflexia, respiratory depression and hypotension in keeping with the level of CNS depression.

Treatment is primarily symptomatic and supportive. Although flumazenil is a specific benzodiazepine antagonist, it should not be used as a diagnostic test or in cases of mixed overdose. In patients who are benzodiazepine-dependent it may cause convulsions, and in mixed overdose it may precipitate fits making management of patients more complex. The half-life of flumazenil is much shorter than any of the marketed benzodiazepines.

## Opioids

A wide range of drugs have opioid agonist properties, including morphine, diamorphine (heroin), pethidine, codeine, dihydrocodeine, dextropropoxyphene, buprenorphine and methadone. Features of opioid poisoning classically include drowsiness, coma and respiratory depression with pinpoint pupils. Nausea and vomiting are common particularly in opioid naïve patients. The time course of opioid poisoning depends primarily on the route of exposure. Intravenous injection and inhalation from smoking ('chasing the dragon') cause rapid clinical effects, whereas absorption from the GI tract is slower. Dextropropoxyphene also has sodium channel blocking properties, causing cardiac arrhythmias and for this reason it is being withdrawn. Dihydrocodeine and codeine are converted to active metabolites (dihydromorphine and morphine) and morphine itself has an active metabolite, morphine 6-glucoronide, which accumulates in renal impairment. Onset of toxicity of methadone is much slower than other agents in this category and is maximal 4–6 h after ingestion. Tramadol is an analgesic with effects on both opioid receptors and 5HT receptors. In addition to causing the classical features of opioid poisoning it also causes convulsions.

### Management

The specific treatment for opioid poisoning is naloxone, a competitive antagonist. In cases with presumed opioid ingestion naloxone is titrated in doses of up to 2.5–5.0 mg in severe cases to match clinical response. The target is to maintain adequate respiration, but in addicts not to fully reverse the opioid effects, otherwise an acute withdrawal syndrome will be precipitated. The duration of action of naloxone is short, 45–90 min, and in patients with severe poisoning, or following ingestion of slow-release or long-acting opioids such as methadone, a naloxone infusion may be required.

## Non-steroidal anti-inflammatory agents

Ibuprofen is widely available over the counter and is now frequently encountered in overdose. Non-steroidals as a class are of relatively low toxicity, with a primary toxicity being on the kidney (acute renal failure) and in patients with co-morbidity cause fluid retention. These effects are due to interaction with prostaglandin mechanisms, in the case of the kidney impairment of vascular tone affecting glomerular filtration. In severe overdose coma, convulsions and hepatic damage has been reported. Mefenamic acid is a non-steroidal anti-inflammatory but is unusual in that it causes fits. Fits are managed conventionally with diazepam or lorazepam.

## Salicylates

Aspirin is now rarely encountered as a serious overdose, and the toxicity is predictable from dose ingested, with doses of 250 mg/kg likely to lead to moderate toxicity and above 500 mg/kg severe toxicity. Clinical features include vomiting, tinnitus, deafness, sweating and hyperventilation due to direct stimulation of the respiratory centre. As aspirin is an acid metabolic disturbance includes a mixed respiratory alkalosis and metabolic acidosis. Subsequent metabolic complications include hyperpyrexia (uncoupling of oxidative phosphorylation and direct CNS effects), hypoglycaemia, thrombocytopaenia, coagulopathy and renal failure. As the distribution of aspirin across lipid membranes depends on its ionisation, patients who develop significant metabolic acidosis are more at risk from CNS penetration of aspirin, causing confusion, impaired consciousness, convulsions and death. Consequences of salicylate poisoning are therefore dependent upon the ability to resist the metabolic acidosis, and this is particularly problematical in young children and the elderly. In severe cases (plasma concentration above 700 mg/l with metabolic complications) or in patients with renal failure, haemodialysis is the treatment of choice.

## Paracetamol

Paracetamol overdose contributes to between 30 and 40% of acute hospital admissions with overdose. Precise mortality figures are uncertain, but are well below 0.1% for inhospital mortality, definitely due to paracetamol. Many deaths previously attributed to paracetamol toxicity were most likely due to the combination product co-proxamol and to the dextropropoxyphene content.

At normal therapeutic doses paracetamol is safe. Paracetamol is metabolised in the liver to inactive conjugates. The intermediate step in the formation of one of these conjugates involves conversion of paracetamol to a reactive N-acetyl benzoquinonimine metabolite by hepatic microsomal enzymes. This metabolite is then conjugated with glutathione in the liver. The conjugate is inactive and non-toxic. In the absence of adequate glutathione stores, particularly when large doses of paracetamol are taken in overdose, the reactive metabolite then binds to sulphydril groups in other protein molecules, specifically enzymes, causing hepatic necrosis.

High-risk groups for paracetamol toxicity are therefore those with inadequate glutathione stores such as the malnourished, patients with eating disorders and malabsorption syndromes, possibly HIV positive patients and alcoholics. A second category is in patients who have hepatic enzyme induction, secondary to drugs such as carbamazepine, phenytoin, barbiturates, rifampicin or St John's wort.

Patients often expect paracetamol to cause symptoms, especially drowsiness early after ingestion, but this is in practice unlikely although nausea may occur. Hepatic necrosis usually presents 36–72 h after overdose with jaundice and right upper quadrant pain. This is often followed by the onset of renal failure, although in rare cases renal failure can occur without major hepatic impairment.

## Management

Management of paracetamol poisoning depends on the time elapsed from overdose to presentation. The risk is determined from the paracetamol treatment nomogram published in the British National Formulary (BNF) and available on TOXBASE (Fig. 20.2). Before 4 h paracetamol concentration is not interpretable, and treatment is unnecessary at this stage. Between 4 and 8 h after presentation it is sensible to do a paracetamol level and determine the need for treatment based on the graph. It is important to make sure paracetamol levels are done speedily, and that the results are accessed. Between 8 and 12 h risk of hepatic damage is increasing, and depending on the time before levels are available treatment should be started based on the history of ingestion. Certainly beyond 12 h this is the appropriate step, with a dose of level for active intervention in patients who have no increased risk of hepatic toxicity of 150 mg/kg.

Beyond 20 h evidence of efficacy in preventing liver damage is absent, and by this stage hepatic necrosis is usually well established. Use of antidotes late in the management of paracetamol poisoning may be indicated if liver function tests are abnormal, but here the treatment is to prevent hepatic encephalopathy, not liver damage itself.

## Treatment

The recommended treatment of paracetamol poisoning in the United Kingdom is intravenous N-acetylcysteine. The dose is given in an initial loading dose, followed by two subsequent lower infusions over a period in total of 20 h. Methionine is no longer generally recommended, and in patients where intravenous access is impossible N-acetylcysteine can be given orally. N-acetylcysteine replaces the glutathione that is lacking, and in this way prevents hepatic damage. N-acetylcysteine causes a pseudo allergic reaction in up to 10% of patients. Treatment should be *temporarily* discontinued, an antihistamine or bronchodilator given and treatment recommenced.

## Assessing severity of hepatic damage

At presentation risk of hepatic damage can be predicted from the paracetamol level, although the degree of metabolic acidosis also correlates with severity of overdose. It is important to check the response to treatment, and three blood tests are necessary. Firstly, a measure of the transaminase in order to assess if liver damage has occurred. A normal transaminase indicates normal hepatic function with no further action required. If the transaminase is abnormal a prothrombin time is needed, and this is the best predictor of outcome in hepatic function. In addition it is important to check renal function. Changes in renal function are slower than in hepatic function, and an increase in serum creatinine during the period of N-acetylcysteine infusion should be rechecked to exclude insipient renal failure. A prothrombin time that is longer in seconds (measured using the Manchester reagent) than the number of hours since the overdose indicates a poor prognosis. Such cases should be discussed with the NPIS or a liver unit. Clotting disturbance in paracetamol poisoning should never be corrected with vitamin K, or clotting factors before such discussion has occurred, as this is the most sensitive outcome

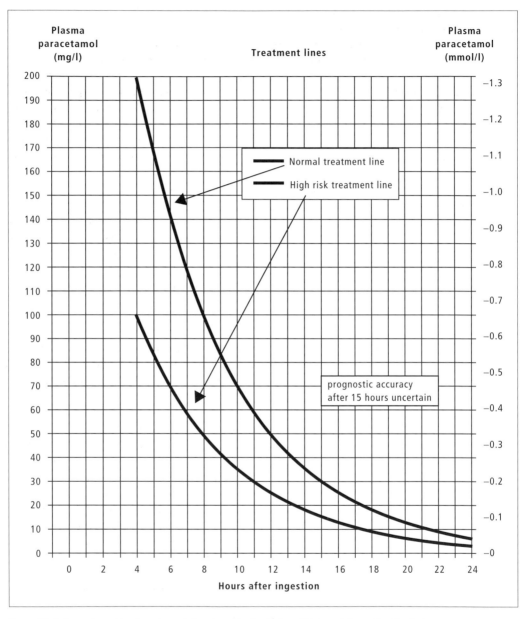

**Figure 20.2** Paracetamol treatment graph (produced by the National Poisons Information Service).

measure. In severe hepatic failure liver support systems, or transplantation may be indicated. Patients being considered for such treatment should be seen by a psychiatrist before they develop a hepatic coma in order that an assessment can be made.

## Drugs of abuse

Common drugs of abuse include opioids (see above) and stimulants including in particular MDMA, cocaine and amphetamines. All these drugs act on central amine receptor systems to cause excitation, with the risk of tachycardia, blood pressure change and convulsions. MDMA causes a syndrome similar to the serotonin syndrome (see section on SSRIs) but also stimulates antidiuretic hormone release, causing water retention. In patients who drink excess water (e.g. at raves) significant hyponatraemia may occur resulting in fits and brain damage. Treatment is supportive with control of hyperthermia using benzodiazepines. Specific 5HT antagonists such as cyproheptadine may be considered.

Amphetamines cause convulsions and cardiac arrhythmias. Management is supportive using benzodiazepines to 'turn off' central stimulation.

Cocaine has local anaesthetic (sodium channel blocking) activities, as well as direct and indirect amine effects. It is absorbed rapidly across the buccal and nasal mucosa causing a rapid 'high'. It causes surges in blood pressure with vasoconstriction and may result in stroke, acute myocardial infarction and gut infarcts. It also causes hyperpyrexia and convulsions. Management is by use of large doses of benzodiazepines to sedate, combined in hyperpyrexia with ice baths. Myocardial infarction should be managed conventionally.

## Other substances

### Digoxin

Digoxin poisoning is uncommon, the features are vomiting and cardiac conduction abnormalities. Severe arrhythmias may require active treatment with a specific Fab antibody. As digoxin blocks sodium–potassium channels hyperkalaemia is a normal feature of severe digoxin intoxication. When taken in acute overdose the onset of digoxin poisoning may be delayed up to 12 h. The typical features of severe poisoning include complete heart block.

### Lithium

Lithium is used in the management of bipolar depression. It is excreted by the kidney and there are well-recognised interactions with NSAID's, diuretics and ACE inhibitors causing lithium retention. Presentation in chronic poisoning, in patients who develop renal impairment secondary to lithium, a recognised adverse effect of this therapy, present insidiously with confusion, nausea, vomiting, tremor, nystagmus and ataxia. As coma progresses irreversible damage to the brain occurs. In patients on lithium therapy it is therefore mandatory to monitor lithium levels regularly and avoid interacting drugs. In this situation plasma concentrations of lithium correlate well with clinical features. In contrast, in acute overdose, plasma concentrations rise and then fall quite quickly as lithium distributes quickly to tissues. Here management is based on clinical features as much as plasma concentration. Lithium is excreted via the kidney, and in patients with CNS features the treatment of choice is dialysis, which may be prolonged.

### Iron

Iron produces toxicity as a metabolic poison, but also causes acute gastritis. It is also present with vomiting and haematemesis. Clinical features of iron poisoning reflect the onset of metabolic poisoning, particularly on mitochondrial systems, which result in metabolic acidosis, coma and death. Iron poisoning tends to come on in phases, initially presenting with vomiting, haematemesis, GI upset, drowsiness, metabolic acidosis, acute hypotension, coma and convulsions. This phase lasts between 30 min and 6 h. This is often followed by a short interval in which symptoms may appear to improve, but as the onset of the metabolic complications develop over 12–24 h the patient becomes more unwell and hepatic failure with metabolic acidosis, hypoglycaemia and cardiovascular collapse, renal failure and pulmonary oedema. If patients survive this, small bowel and upper GI strictures may form in phase IV.

Assessment of iron poisoning is difficult and is based on a mixture of the clinical features seen, specifically degree of acidosis and hepatic and renal function, and the iron levels. These will often rise rapidly and then fall in the early phases of poisoning, and on their own may be only a partial index of the wider clinical prognosis.

X-ray of patients who have ingested iron has been recommended, but is of doubtful benefit. The specific chelating agent desferrioxamine will bind iron, and will increase urinary excretion. In the context of severe iron poisoning large doses of desferrioxamine may be administered, outwith normal guidelines after discussion with poisoning specialists.

## Lead

Lead toxicity occurs from occupational exposure in industry, and occasionally environmentally, particularly in houses with lead paints. Some children develop the syndrome of pica in which they eat material containing lead. Lead causes multisystem toxicity and interacts with cations such as calcium, zinc and iron. Clinical features are only partially related to plasma concentrations following acute exposure, since lead distributes well into tissues, and assessment will therefore depend both on lead concentration and on clinical features. In young children there is some evidence that high lead levels are associated with impaired intellectual development, and in some countries screening programmes for lead concentrations are undertaken in the community. Features of chronic lead poisoning include GI disturbance, peripheral neuropathy, anaemia and wrist and ankle drop. Encephalopathy may be seen. Investigations include blood lead levels, x-rays if there is a suspicion of lead ingestion may be important. Blood films show a classical basophilic stippling and iron and calcium studies may be relevant. Chelating agents are available including DMSA, but prevention of exposure is the primary treatment of lead poisoning.

## Mushrooms

A number of toxic mushrooms are present in the environment; mushrooms in the amanita family cause hepatic necrosis. There are no specific treatments for these. 'Magic mushrooms' (psylocybe) cause acute psychosis and agitation, but no long-lasting effects.

Many other compounds are ingested, and specific details of toxicity should be sought from TOXBASE.

# Chapter 21

# Drugs you may need in a hurry

Most drugs are not given in a hurry. There is time to check facts or seek further advice. However, sometimes events move very quickly and there are some drugs, used under these circumstances, for which it is very useful to have facts and figures at your fingertips.

The purpose of this brief chapter is to provide that information for drugs used in circumstances that a newly qualified doctor might expect to encounter.

## Adrenaline (epinephrine) for anaphylaxis

### Why give it?

Most deaths from anaphylaxis occur in the first hour and most of these are a consequence of severe bronchospasm, increased capillary permeability or circulatory failure caused by vasodilatation. Adrenaline is given to prevent death from these causes, particularly by raising blood pressure and reversing bronchospasm.

### Mechanism

Adrenaline is a potent agonist at both $\alpha$- and $\beta$-adrenoceptors. It reduces bronchospasm by $\beta_2$-mediated airway smooth muscle relaxation, raises blood pressure by $\alpha_1$-mediated vasoconstriction and may also reduce the release of inflammatory mediators by a $\beta_2$-mediated increase in mast cell cyclic AMP.

### How to give it

Intramuscular injection—adrenaline acts quickly by this route, provided the circulation is adequate.

The adult dose is 500 µg to 0.5 ml of the 1:1000 preparation.

If there is severe shock and a serious question over absorption from muscle, adrenaline can be given intravenously slowly, at the rate of 100 µg/min for 5 min or until a response is obtained, using ECG monitoring if possible. Five millilitres of the 1:10,000 preparation is used.

### Pitfalls

- Confusing the 1:1000 and 1:10,000 preparations
- Ventricular arrhythmias (particularly in people taking tricyclic antidepressants)
- Adrenaline may not be effective in relieving bronchospasm in people taking non-selective beta-blockers (intravenous salbutamol will be needed under these circumstances)
- Blood pressure may rise quite dramatically—and even cause cerebral haemorrhage—in people on non-selective beta-blockers because of unopposed $\alpha_1$-mediated vasoconstriction.

## Chlorphenamine for anaphylaxis

### Why give it?

To counteract the histamine-mediated components of anaphylaxis and to help prevent a relapse.

### Mechanism

Many substances are released during an anaphylactic reaction, but histamine is probably the main cause of increased capillary permeability, where histamine $H_1$-receptors play a significant role. Chlorphenamine is a potent $H_1$-receptor antagonist and is very effective at limiting the increased capillary permeability. Interestingly, it has little influence on the vascular and respiratory aspects of anaphylaxis, for which adrenaline (epinephrine) must be given.

### How to give it

After adrenaline has been given and begun to work, chlorphenamine is given by intravenous injection of 10–20 mg over a minute. This drug is continued for 24–48 h.

### Pitfalls

Usually none under these circumstances, but hypotension or cerebral stimulation can occur.

Steroids also have a role in the management of anyphylactoid reactions (Chapter 10); however, their effects take hours rather than minutes to manifest themselves, and hence in emergency situations the delivery of adrenaline and chlorpheniramine should be prioritised.

## Adrenaline (epinephrine) for cardiac arrest

### Why give it?

To start the heart.

### Mechanism

Adrenaline is a potent agonist at the $\beta_1$-receptor and is therefore a powerful cardiac stimulant, with effects on myocardial contractility and rate.

### How to give it

Hundred microgrammes intravenously—as 10 ml of 1:10,000 preparation. Preferably through a central line, or if through a peripheral line flushed with 20 ml of 0.9% sodium chloride to ensure entry to the circulation.

### Pitfalls

As above.

## Amiodarone for cardiac arrest

### Why give it?

Amiodarone is used in cardio-pulmonary resuscitation when ventricular fibrillation or pulseless ventricular tachycardia persists despite defibrillation.

### Mechanism

Amiodarone is effective against most tachyarrhythmias (Chapter 6). It has a wide spectrum of pharmacological activity and the precise mechanism(s) of its action are not known.

### How to give it

Intravenous—300 mg from a pre-filled syringe or in a glucose solution.

### Pitfalls

Usually none in this context, although anaphylaxis can occur.

## Atropine for cardiac arrest

### Why give it?

To block vagal activity in patients with asystole or severe bradycardia.

### Mechanism

Atropine is a competitive antagonist of the action of acetylcholine at muscarinic $M_2$-receptors on the sinoatrial and atrioventricular (AV) nodes. It therefore increases heart rate and speeds AV conduction.

## How to give it

A single intravenous dose of 3 mg (the drug is quite long-acting, so repeat doses are not needed).

## Pitfalls

Although many of the well-described effects of atropine can occur, there are usually no serious side effects in this context.

## Adenosine for supraventricular tachycardia

### Why give it?

To revert supraventricular tachycardias to sinus rhythm.

### Mechanism

Stimulation of adenosine $A_1$-receptors in the sinoatrial and atrioventricular nodes leads to a transient slowing of sinus rate, reduced AV node conduction and increased AV node refractoriness (Chapter 6).

### How to give it

Rapid intravenous injection of 3 mg, followed at intervals of 1–2 min by 6 mg and 12 mg if necessary, with cardiac monitoring. Adenosine has a very short half-life of a few seconds. Patients usually feel some chest tightness and breathlessness.

### Pitfalls

- Heart block
- Avoid in asthmatics because adenosine can cause severe bronchospasm
- Patients with heart transplants are very sensitive to adenosine because of denervation sensitivity
- Patients taking dipyridamole (an adenosine reuptake inhibitor) are very sensitive to adenosine and should be give a starting dose of 0.5–1 mg

## Loop diuretic for acute left ventricular failure

### Why give it?

Acute left ventricular failure (LVF) is terrifying for the patient—who is dying by drowning in their own fluid—and dramatic for the doctor. The purpose of giving a loop diuretic—usually furosemide or bumetanide—is to relieve symptoms of severe breathlessness and prevent death.

### Mechanism

Loop diuretics act more quickly in acute LVF than would be expected from their diuretic actions alone (Chapter 6). There are probably two mechanisms at work.

Reduction of left ventricular filling pressure by increasing systemic venous capacitance. This vascular effect has been recognised for many years but is not fully understood.

Powerful diuresis by inhibition of the $Na^+$-$K^+$-$2Cl^-$ symporter in the ascending limb of the loop of Henle.

### How to give it

Intravenously—for example, furosemide 40 mg followed if necessary by 40 mg every 15 min up to a maximum of 160 mg.

### Pitfalls

Usually none at this dose. Tinnitus can occur following rapid injections of high doses, but rarely seen in this context.

## Morphine for acute left ventricular failure

### Why give it?

Morphine is given in acute LVF for two reasons. One is to relieve distress, but the other is because it has rapid and dramatically beneficial cardiovascular effects.

## Mechanism

The cardiovascular actions of morphine have been recognised for many years but are still not fully understood. Morphine causes both arteriolar and venous dilatation, which is partially reversed by histamine $H_1$-receptor antagonists, but fully reversed by naloxone, an opioid μ-receptor antagonist (Chapter 15).

## How to give it

Intravenously—2 mg/min up to a maximum of 10 mg.

## Pitfalls

- Nausea—give an antiemetic such as metoclopramide
- Respiratory depression—reverse with naloxone

## Lorazepam for status epilepticus

### Why give it?

Lorazepam has two advantages over diazepam in this condition. One is that it has a longer duration of action (diazepam enters the brain quickly, but leaves quite quickly too because of redistribution to adipose tissue). The other is that diazepam is more likely to cause thrombophlebitis.

## Mechanism

All benzodiazepines limit seizure activity by GABA-mediated inhibitory effects (Chapter 17).

## How to give it

Intravenous—absorption from intramuscular injection is too slow. Adult dose is 4 mg into a large vein; if resuscitation equipment is not readily available, give initial dose of 2 mg.

## Pitfalls

Respiratory arrest.

## Rectal diazepam for status epilepticus

### Why give it?

The rectal formulation of diazepam is useful when intravenous access is not possible.

## Mechanism

As for lorazepam.

## How to give it

Normal adult dose is 500 μg/kg up to a maximum of 30 mg given as diazepam rectal solution (elderly, 250 μg/kg up to a maximum of 15 mg).

## Pitfalls

Rectal absorption can sometimes be unpredictable.

## Naloxone for opioid poisoning

### Why give it?

Opioid poisoning leads to respiratory depression, hypotension and can be fatal. Naloxone is given to reverse these effects.

## Mechanism

Drugs such as heroin (diamorphine) cause respiratory depression by acting on the μ-opioid receptor and a significant part of their cardiovascular effects are also mediated through this receptor. Naloxone is an antagonist at this receptor and has no agonist activity (Chapter 15).

## How to give it

Intravenous—the adult dose is 0.4–2 mg, repeated at intervals of 2 min until a maximum of 10 mg has been reached. Naloxone is very fast-acting and a reversal of respiratory depression and dilation of the pupils is normally seen in about a minute.

## Pitfalls

• Naloxone acts for 1–4 h so repeated doses may be necessary following large opioid overdoses.
• Opioid addicts may experience withdrawal reactions.
• Naloxone only partially antagonises the respiratory depression caused by pentazocine (which acts mainly at the κ-opioid receptor) and buprenorphine (which appears to bind particularly avidly to the μ-receptor).

## Glucagon for hypoglycaemic coma

### Why give it?

Hypoglycaemic coma can be treated either by intravenous glucose or by intravenous or intramuscular glucagon. The latter approach can be very useful if venous access is difficult.

### Mechanism

Glucagon increases plasma glucose by stimulating glycogenolysis and reducing glycogen synthesis.

### How to give it

One milligram by intramuscular or intravenous injection.

### Pitfalls

Glucagon causes the release of catecholamines from a phaeochromocytoma.

# Chapter 22

# Prescribing and its pitfalls

Most doctors will prescribe drugs on a daily basis. Approximately 640 million prescriptions are written in the United Kingdom annually, equivalent to 10 prescriptions per year for each member of the UK population. Although perceived as a routine and mundane component of the work of most clinicians, the process of good prescribing requires significant skill and care and should not be undertaken without due thought and consideration. Good prescribing involves the recommendation of the correct dose and formulation of an appropriate drug, accompanied by clear instruction regarding when, how and for how long it should be taken. A prescription should be written only when in possession of adequate clinical information about the patient and thesymptoms, and ideally following solicitation of the patient's preferences and discussion of alternative treatment strategies. The need for thorough training in the skill of prescribing is highlighted by the high frequency with which drugs are prescribed at the wrong dose, through the wrong route or for the wrong condition. The likelihood of patient injury occurring as a result of a drug error has been estimated at approximately 3% per inpatient stay, an error rate that would not be tolerated by major airlines handling passengers' baggage, and surely not acceptable in modern hospitals given the potential severity of the consequences. This chapter reviews the components of good prescribing practice and discusses the pitfalls inherent in the process.

## Good prescribing: questions to ask yourself before picking up the pen

### (a) Is drug treatment really necessary?

It is obvious that while appropriate drug therapy can be of great benefit, inappropriate therapy is not harmless. On all occasions, there should be a positive reason for prescribing a drug. Drug treatment should never become a routine. In hospital it is still not uncommon to find 'routine' prescriptions for hypnotics, analgesics and purgatives without any consideration of individual need. Many patients may expect a consultation to result automatically in the prescription of a medicine, the provision of unnecessary antibiotic therapy for a viral illness being a common example. These situations are clearly undesirable and represent bad prescribing practice.

### (b) Which drug should I choose?

When drug treatment is indicated, it is mandatory that the most appropriate agent is given in the correct dose and in a regimen that results in optimum treatment with minimum adverse effects. Selection of the best drug requires consideration of factors that relate not only to the range of drugs available, but also to both the patient and the condition being treated. Age and disease may influence kinetics and dynamics to a significant degree (see Chapter 3) and should be reflected in the choice of agent. Choosing the wrong drug (such as diclofenac over paracetamol for mild headache in a patient with renal impairment) may aggravate existing medical conditions. As discussed later in this chapter, concomitant therapy for co-morbid conditions may interact with any new prescription, with occasionally catastrophic results (see p. 291).

## (c) By what route should it be administered?

Certain drugs (for example, the third-generation cephalosporin antibiotic cefotaxime) can only be administered intravenously. A choice of routes of administration is available for most drugs, however, and this should be considered when writing a prescription. In the context of emergencies (e.g. antibiotic treatment of severe sepsis), drug administration through the intravenous route is preferred due to the rapid, predictable delivery of treatment. Alternative routes may also be preferred in those patients unable to swallow (e.g. rectal administration of aspirin to dysphagic stroke patients).

## (d) What dose and how often?

Recommended doses and dosing intervals are given in the *British National Formulary* (BNF; see below), which should be consulted when prescribing any drug with which you are not intimately familiar. Particular care should be taken when the patient's ability to metabolise or excrete a drug may be compromised, for example patients with hepatic or renal impairment. These considerations are discussed in more detail in Chapter 3.

## Writing the prescription: practical aspects

Once the choice of drug, route of administration, dose and dosing interval has been made, it must be communicated with clarity to the dispensing pharmacist. All prescriptions for medicine should be printed or handwritten clearly and in ink. Whenever a prescription is written, the following guidelines should be adhered to:

1 Specify the patient's full name, address and age, although the legal requirement is 'age if under 12'.

2 Indicate clearly the drug or medicine. As discussed below, in most cases use of the approved or generic name rather than the proprietary (brand) name is preferred.

3 Specify precisely the strength of tablets, capsules or mixtures. It is good prescribing practice to indicate these in words and figures and mandatory for prescriptions of controlled drugs.

4 Indicate the dose frequency and total quantity to be supplied or the duration of treatment. Once again it is good practice to include these in words and figures as this is a legal requirement for controlled drugs.

5 Do not leave large blank spaces on the prescription, which may be filled in by unscrupulous individuals to obtain unauthorised supplies of drugs of abuse.

6 Sign the prescription, date it and indicate your name and address. Addition of a telephone number assists the pharmacist in contacting the prescriber in the case of a prescription for an unusual drug or dose regimen.

## Should generic or brand name prescribing be used?

Drugs available on prescription have approved or generic names. Individual manufacturers give their own preparations proprietary (brand or trade) names. Brand names are usually distinctive, often easier to remember than the generic name (for example, that GP2b IIIa receptor antagonist abciximab is generally referred to as 'Reopro', for obvious reasons). When a proprietary name is used on a prescription, the pharmacist is obliged to dispense that product rather than a generic equivalent which may be cheaper and more readily available. Unlike generic names, proprietary names give no clear indication of the active constituents of the medicine. This may lead to inadvertent oversupply of a drug common to two prescribed medicines, such as Solpadeine and Panadol both of which contain paracetamol. For these reasons, in most instances, prescription by generic name is recommended. An exception to this recommendation occurs when drugs with a narrow therapeutic index (such as theophylline and lithium) are prescribed in a sustained release preparation. Clinically significant differences in absorption profiles of these drugs may exist between proprietary brands, hence brand name should be specified when these drugs are used.

The generic and proprietary names of all drugs in clinical use can be found in the BNF, a useful reference which is published every 6 months and provided free to doctors and medical students in the United Kingdom. Details of recommended doses together with brief notes on adverse effects, contraindications and interactions are provided. It is widely used as a reference by doctors and pharmacists, and is particularly practical when used in conjunction with formularies compiled and published at a local hospital or general practice level. These formularies are now very common and essentially serve to indicate which drugs will be readily available to prescribers in a particular locality or hospital.

## General pointers on good prescribing

The ability to prescribe drugs in a safe, effective and thoughtful manner is one of the defining characteristics of a good clinician. It can be a deceptively difficult skill to acquire, and requires constant maintenance as the range of drugs available expands. The following advice is distilled from many years of experience of prescribing and is offered to provide some general principles applicable to most situations.

1 Wherever possible, minimise the number of drugs and total number of doses to be given. Always satisfy yourself that a prescription is necessary before considering a pharmacological solution to the problem. Compound preparations are helpful in achieving this goal when there is an established therapeutic need for all the constituents, and where the combination of two or more drugs aids compliance.

2 Make an effort to ensure that the patient understands the reason for the prescription, and is aware of how it should be taken.

3 Familiarise yourself with a limited number of well-established drugs with known effects and side effects. Do not chop and change amongst equivalent preparations on whim or fancy. Avoid trying out new preparations simply because of novelty or extensive commercial promotion.

4 Check the dose carefully each time you prescribe. Do not trust to memory and be particularly careful when doses are in the microgram range or when prescribing for children and the elderly.

5 Finally, always review drug prescriptions regularly: every day in hospital patients or weekly or monthly as appropriate in outpatients or general practice. When reviewing prescriptions ask the following questions:

(a) Is the drug treatment still necessary?

(b) Is the optimum dose regimen being followed?

(c) Is the desired effect being achieved?

(d) Are there any symptoms or adverse effects that could be secondary to drug treatment?

(e) In general practice, has a maximum of one month's supply been prescribed?

Do not continue treatment by repeating prescriptions over long periods of time without assessing the response in the patient, or worse still, without seeing the patient.

*Comment.* The basis of good prescribing is a sound training in clinical methods and pathophysiology, which, together with an understanding of pharmacodynamic and pharmacokinetic properties of the drugs being used, permits maximum benefit to be achieved with the minimum risk of adverse effects. Prescriptions are legal documents. They should consist of clear, legible instructions to the pharmacist. Illegible, incomplete or ambiguous prescriptions are not only bad medicine, but they are also illegal.

## When prescribing goes wrong

Any drug can be harmful if used improperly. The mechanisms through which drugs may injure patients are many and varied: problems may arise solely as a result of one drug (adverse drug reactions) or as a consequence of prescription of combinations of agents (drug interactions). This section reviews the more commonly encountered problems in this area and discusses methods of reducing the burden of adverse events related to drug prescribing.

## Adverse drug reactions

Adverse drug reactions comprise any unwanted effect of a drug. They are best considered in two broad groups: *predictable* (and usually dose-related) effects and *unpredictable* (or idiosyncratic) effects. Predictable effects are relatively common and usually seen shortly after the drug is initiated, increased or in some cases discontinued. Conversely, unpredictable effects occur less frequently and need not necessarily be dose-dependent.

## Predictable effects

Predictable adverse drug effects are due to excessive pharmacological activity of the drug in question. This arises particularly with central nervous system depressants, cardioactive, hypotensive and hypoglycaemic agents. Specific examples of this type of reaction are:

1 Respiratory depression in patients given morphine or benzodiazepine hypnotics
2 Hypotension resulting in stroke, myocardial infarction or renal failure in patients receiving excessive doses of antihypertensive drugs
3 Bradyarrhythmias in patients receiving excessive digoxin doses

Less obvious but equally important are predictable adverse effects where the particular pharmacological effect involved is not the one for which the drug was initially administered. For example, a patient receiving an antihistamine for the prevention of motion sickness may become drowsy.

All patients are at risk of developing this type of reaction if high enough doses are given. However, certain subgroups are particularly susceptible and include those with renal disease, liver disease, the very young and the elderly. Specific considerations relating to these more vulnerable groups are discussed in Chapter 3.

## Withdrawal symptoms or rebound responses after discontinuation of treatment

This type of reaction is unusual in that it occurs in the absence of the causative agent. The abrupt interruption of therapy is followed by a characteristic withdrawal syndrome:

1 Extreme agitation, tachycardia, confusion, delirium and convulsions may occur following the discontinuation of long-term central nervous system depressants such as barbiturates, benzodiazepines and alcohol.
2 Acute Addisonian crisis may be precipitated by the abrupt cessation of corticosteroid therapy.
3 Withdrawal symptoms may be characterised by agitation and autonomic overactivity after discontinuation of narcotic analgesics.

## Unpredictable effects

The most frequently encountered unpredictable effects relate to drug allergy and hypersensitivity. They occur only in a small proportion of the population exposed to the drug, and it is usually impossible to determine in advance which patients may experience this response. The reactions may vary from a mild erythematous skin rash to a major anaphylactoid reaction which carries significant risk of death. An allergic adverse effect of a drug is characterised by the fact that:

1 The reaction does not resemble the expected pharmacological drug effect.
2 There is delay between first exposure to the drug and the development of a reaction.
3 The reaction recurs upon repeated exposure even to traces of the drug.

The drugs most frequently associated with allergic skin reactions are the penicillins, the sulphonamides and the blood products.

## Genetic factors

Adverse drug reactions may arise in certain individuals with a particular genotype or genetic make-up. Hereditary disorders such as pseudocholinesterase deficiency prevent affected individuals from metabolising the muscle relaxant succinylcholine, causing a potentially fatal syndrome of prolonged paralysis and apnoea following its use (Chapter 15). A further example is glucose-6-phosphate dehydrogenase deficiency, a disorder particularly prevalent in Sephardic Jews and Black populations, which predisposes to acute haemolysis after exposure to a wide variety of drugs, including the antimalarial drug primaquine and antibiotics such as the sulphonamides and nitrofurantion.

Genetically, variability in activity of the enzyme *N*-acetyl transferase causes clinically significant differences in response to a number of drugs metabolised by this enzyme. In contrast to the genetic factors described above, this polymorphism causes delayed adverse effects that may not be immediately apparent to the patient or treating physician. Drugs such as isoniazid, hydralazine and procainamide are metabolised in the liver by the enzyme. There is a bimodal distribution of acetylator capacity in the population, with some individuals being slow and others fast acetylators (Chapter 1). Slow acetylators of isoniazid given standard doses are much more likely than fast acetylators to suffer from peripheral neuropathy. The drug-induced lupus syndrome is much more common in slow acetylators receiving hydralazine or procainamide. In the future, tissue typing may help to predict susceptibility to these genetically determined adverse effect of drugs.

## Idiosyncratic drug reactions

The term idiosyncrasy is used primarily to cover unusual, unexpected or bizarre drug effects that cannot readily be explained or predicted in individual recipients.

Also included in this type of reaction are drug-induced fetal abnormalities such as phocomelia (limb deformity), which develop in the offspring of mothers receiving thalidomide in early pregnancy.

Drug-induced malignant disease is fortunately rare and may be considered an idiosyncratic drug effect:

1 Analgesic abuse may rarely cause cancer of the renal pelvis.

2 Long-term oestrogens without coincidental progestogens may induce uterine cancer.

3 Immunosuppressive drugs may induce lymphoid tumours.

4 Intramuscular iron preparations may cause sarcomata at the site of injection.

5 Thyroid cancer may develop in patients who have received $^{131}$I-therapy in the past.

## Drug interactions

When administration of one drug influences the effect of another, the term 'drug interaction' is used. Interactions account for approximately one quarter of all adverse drug reactions, and are most commonly seen in elderly people taking a variety of drugs for multiple problems. Many hundreds of interactions have been described, and this section focusses upon the general principles involved, using more commonly encountered interactions as illustrative examples. Drug interactions commonly involve interference with any of the pharmacokinetic or pharmacodynamic processes described in Chapters 1 and 2. More rarely they may arise as a consequence of a direct chemical reaction between two agents, for example precipitation of chalk following administration of sodium bicarbonate and calcium salts through the same intravenous catheter. A further, more recent concern is the potential for "herbal remedies" purchased over the center to interact with prescribed drugs. St. John's Wort, a substance sometime taken without prescription for depressive symptoms, may cause failure of the oral contraceptive pill.

The most commonly encountered drug interaction causing the need for hospital admission involves warfarin and antibiotic treatment. Antibiotics may influence warfarin's effects through a number of mechanisms, including disturbance of intestinal flora with subsquent reduction in vitamin K production, induction of malabsorbtion of vitamin K or direct inhibition or potentiation of warfarin metabolism. Caution should always be used when prescribing antibiotic treatment for a patient already on warfarin, and careful monitoring of INR in this circumstance is mandatory.

**Table 22.1** Examples of pharmacokinetic interactions.

---

**Absorption interactions**

Tetracyclines chelate calcium and magnesium salts leading to reduced antibiotic absorption.

Cholestyramine reduces warfarin absorption by binding to it.

**Distribution interactions**

Aspirin displaces warfarin from plasma proteins, potentiating the anti-coagulant effect.

Valproate displaces phenytoin from plasma proteins, increasing plasma-free phenytoin.

**Metabolism interactions**

*Induction*

Carbamazepine induces enzymes which metabolise phenytoin, necessitating larger doses of phenytoin.

Phenytoin induces enzymes responsible for metabolism of estrogens and progestogens in the oral contraceptive pill, so increasing the risk of unplanned pregnancy.

*Inhibition*

Warfarin may be potentiated by metronidazole, which inhibits metabolism of the warfarin molecule.

Allopurinol potentates the cytotoxic effect of azathioprine by inhibiting xanthine oxidase, the enzyme responsible for its enzymatic degradation.

---

## Pharmacodynamic interactions

These tend to involve the administration of two drugs with similar effects. Such interactions may involve two agents acting at one receptor (attenuation of salbutamol's bronchodilatory effect by non-specific beta-blockers) or through a less specific effect upon particular tissues (potentiation of the sedative effect of benzodiazepines by alcohol). Pharmacodynamic interactions at one receptor may have therapeutic use, such as the reversal of opiate toxicity by naloxone. The clinical effects are largely predictable and can be prevented by thoughtful prescribing.

## Pharmacokinetic interactions

These interactions involve interference with absorption, distribution or metabolism of one drug as a consequence of the administration of another. They tend to be less easy to predict than pharmacodynamic interactions, although the consequences may be no less severe. Some commonly encountered pharmacokinetic interactions are summarised in Table 22.1.

An exhaustive list of all potential interactions lies outwith the scope of this text. Appendix 1 of the BNF provides a useful reference, and should be consulted whenever the question of a potential interaction arises.

## What can we do to minimise drug-related harm to patients?

Although the age of the patient is often cited as a determinant of the frequency of adverse drug reactions, the total number of drugs taken by the patient is a more important factor. Many studies have demonstrated a rise in frequency of adverse drug reactions as the number of drugs increases, and significantly the frequency of these interactions falls following rationalisation of drug therapy. As a ballpark figure, long-term treatment with two drugs will lead to drug-related adverse effects in 10–15% of patients: this figure rises to more than 50% in patients taking five drugs on a regular basis. Careful prescribing and the application of the principles described above will minimise the problems caused by predictable adverse reactions; however, other idiosyncratic, unpredictable or rare adverse effects may be encountered even following the most assiduous prescribing. These effects are particularly prevalent in new drugs, as despite the extensive evaluation which occurs before a drug is marketed, some adverse drug effects only become apparent when the drug is used in clinical practice.

A framework for the detection, analysis and reporting of these less common effects is necessary.

In the United Kingdom, the 'yellow card' scheme fulfils this role. Medical professionals and more recently patients and carers are invited to report any suspected adverse reaction or drug interaction they encounter by filling in a 'yellow card', which requests details of the drug, the reaction and the characteristics of the patient concerned. The information collected on yellow cards is then evaluated by the regulatory authorities who assess the causal relationship between drug and reaction, and may recommend changes in the use of the drug to minimise the risk of future problems arising. Similar schemes exist in all European countries: they play a vital role in the continuing surveillance of all medicines and the minimisation of drug-related harm.

# Index

Page numbers in *italic* refer to Figures and those in **bold** refer to tables.